Innovative Technologies and Translational Therapies for Deafness

Innovative Technologies and Translational Therapies for Deafness

Editors

Olivier Sterkers
Ghizlène Lahlou
Huan Jia

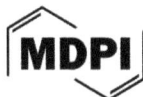

Basel • Beijing • Wuhan • Barcelona • Belgrade • Novi Sad • Cluj • Manchester

Editors

Olivier Sterkers
Service ORL
Paris
France

Ghizlène Lahlou
Hopital Pitié Salpêtrière
Paris
France

Huan Jia
Shanghai Ninth People's Hospital
Shanghai
China

Editorial Office
MDPI AG
Grosspeteranlage 5
4052 Basel, Switzerland

This is a reprint of articles from the Special Issue published online in the open access journal *Journal of Clinical Medicine* (ISSN 2077-0383) (available at: https://www.mdpi.com/journal/jcm/special_issues/Innovative_Deafness).

For citation purposes, cite each article independently as indicated on the article page online and as indicated below:

Lastname, A.A.; Lastname, B.B. Article Title. *Journal Name* **Year**, *Volume Number*, Page Range.

ISBN 978-3-7258-1901-0 (Hbk)
ISBN 978-3-7258-1902-7 (PDF)
doi.org/10.3390/books978-3-7258-1902-7

© 2024 by the authors. Articles in this book are Open Access and distributed under the Creative Commons Attribution (CC BY) license. The book as a whole is distributed by MDPI under the terms and conditions of the Creative Commons Attribution-NonCommercial-NoDerivs (CC BY-NC-ND) license.

Contents

Mariam Alzaher, Chiara Valzolgher, Grégoire Verdelet, Francesco Pavani, Alessandro Farnè, Pascal Barone and Mathieu Marx
Audiovisual Training in Virtual Reality Improves Auditory Spatial Adaptation in Unilateral Hearing Loss Patients
Reprinted from: *J. Clin. Med.* **2023**, *12*, 2357, doi:10.3390/jcm12062357 1

Lore Kerkhofs, Anastasiya Starovoyt, Jan Wouters, Tristan Putzeys and Nicolas Verhaert
Optical Coherence Tomography-Based Atlas of the Human Cochlear Hook Region
Reprinted from: *J. Clin. Med.* **2023**, *12*, 238, doi:10.3390/jcm12010238 15

Thierry Mom, Mathilde Puechmaille, Mohamed El Yagoubi, Alexane Lère, Jens-Erik Petersen, Justine Bécaud, et al.
Robotized Cochlear Implantation under Fluoroscopy: A Preliminary Series
Reprinted from: *J. Clin. Med.* **2023**, *12*, 211, doi:10.3390/jcm12010211 32

Luc Boullaud, Hélène Blasco, Eliott Caillaud, Patrick Emond and David Bakhos
Immediate-Early Modifications to the Metabolomic Profile of the Perilymph Following an Acoustic Trauma in a Sheep Model
Reprinted from: *J. Clin. Med.* **2022**, *11*, 4668, doi:10.3390/jcm11164668 42

Renato Torres, Jean-Yves Tinevez, Hannah Daoudi, Ghizlene Lahlou, Neil Grislain, Eugénie Breil, et al.
Best Fit 3D Basilar Membrane Reconstruction to Routinely Assess the Scalar Position of the Electrode Array after Cochlear Implantation
Reprinted from: *J. Clin. Med.* **2022**, *11*, 2075, doi:10.3390/jcm11082075 54

Ki Wan Park, Peter Kullar, Charvi Malhotra and Konstantina M. Stankovic
Current and Emerging Therapies for Chronic Subjective Tinnitus
Reprinted from: *J. Clin. Med.* **2023**, *12*, 6555, doi:10.3390/jcm12206555 66

Anissa Rym Saidia, Jérôme Ruel, Amel Bahloul, Benjamin Chaix, Frédéric Venail and Jing Wang
Current Advances in Gene Therapies of Genetic Auditory Neuropathy Spectrum Disorder
Reprinted from: *J. Clin. Med.* **2023**, *12*, 738, doi:10.3390/jcm12030738 85

Athanasia Warnecke, Hinrich Staecker, Eva Rohde, Mario Gimona, Anja Giesemann, Agnieszka J. Szczepek, et al.
Extracellular Vesicles in Inner Ear Therapies—Pathophysiological, Manufacturing, and Clinical Considerations
Reprinted from: *J. Clin. Med.* **2022**, *11*, 7455, doi:10.3390/jcm11247455 104

Stephen Leong, Aykut Aksit, Sharon J. Feng, Jeffrey W. Kysar and Anil K. Lalwani
Inner Ear Diagnostics and Drug Delivery via Microneedles
Reprinted from: *J. Clin. Med.* **2022**, *11*, 5474, doi:10.3390/jcm11185474 122

Madeleine St. Peter, Athanasia Warnecke and Hinrich Staecker
A Window of Opportunity: Perilymph Sampling from the Round Window Membrane Can Advance Inner Ear Diagnostics and Therapeutics
Reprinted from: *J. Clin. Med.* **2022**, *11*, 316, doi:10.3390/jcm11020316 133

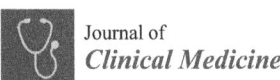

Article

Audiovisual Training in Virtual Reality Improves Auditory Spatial Adaptation in Unilateral Hearing Loss Patients

Mariam Alzaher [1,2,*], Chiara Valzolgher [3,4], Grégoire Verdelet [4,5], Francesco Pavani [3,4,6], Alessandro Farnè [3,4,5], Pascal Barone [1] and Mathieu Marx [1,2]

1. Research Center of Brain and Cognition, CerCo, CNRS, 31000 Toulouse, France
2. ENT Department, University Hospital of Purpan, 31000 Toulouse, France
3. Center for Mind/Brain Sciences—CIMeC, University of Trento, 38100 Trento, Italy
4. Impact Team of the Lyon Neuroscience Research Centre INSERM U1028 CNRS UMR5292, University Claude Bernard Lyon I, 69000 Lyon, France
5. Neuroimmersion, Lyon Neuroscience Research Center, 69000 Lyon, France
6. Centro Interuniversitario di Ricerca "Cognizione, Linguaggio e Sordità"—CIRCLeS, University of Trento, 38100 Trento, Italy
* Correspondence: mariam.alzaher@cnrs.fr

Abstract: Unilateral hearing loss (UHL) leads to an alteration of binaural cues resulting in a significant increment of spatial errors in the horizontal plane. In this study, nineteen patients with UHL were recruited and randomized in a cross-over design into two groups; a first group ($n = 9$) that received spatial audiovisual training in the first session and a non-spatial audiovisual training in the second session (2 to 4 weeks after the first session). A second group ($n = 10$) received the same training in the opposite order (non-spatial and then spatial). A sound localization test using head-pointing (LOCATEST) was completed prior to and following each training session. The results showed a significant decrease in head-pointing localization errors after spatial training for group 1 ($24.85° \pm 15.8°$ vs. $16.17° \pm 11.28°$; $p < 0.001$). The number of head movements during the spatial training for the 19 participants did not change ($p = 0.79$); nonetheless, the hand-pointing errors and reaction times significantly decreased at the end of the spatial training ($p < 0.001$). This study suggests that audiovisual spatial training can improve and induce spatial adaptation to a monaural deficit through the optimization of effective head movements. Virtual reality systems are relevant tools that can be used in clinics to develop training programs for patients with hearing impairments.

Keywords: spatial adaptation; audiovisual training; virtual reality; unilateral hearing loss; head movements

1. Introduction

One of the fundamental functions of binaural integration is sound source localization and the perception of targets in the presence of competing noise [1]. In the case of acquired unilateral hearing loss (UHL), the symmetrical integration of interaural time and intensity differences is severely altered, leading to a significant disruption in spatial hearing. Despite the spatial deficit, there is growing evidence that compensation after UHL takes place due to the plasticity of central auditory processing and an adaptation and recovery in spatial auditory performance [2,3]. Animal studies that examined the effect of UHL on cortical activation suggest a possible weakening of the neural representation of the deaf ear accompanied by a strengthening of the neural representation of the opposite intact ear in monaural listening situations. This pronounced reorganization in favor of the better ear in the case of asymmetrical hearing can also be observed in unilateral cochlear implantation after profound symmetrical deafness in cats [4] and in children [5]. Parallel to neural adaptation, different studies tried to understand the behavioral changes that accompany monaural hearing conditions [6]. They suggest that listeners with UHL learned to make use of the spectral shape cues due to the direction-dependent filtering of the pinna in the intact ear to better judge sound direction. The important role of monaural cues was shown, for example, in experiments with pinna shape modification that led to an increase in localization errors [7]. Experiments on monaural plugging in ferrets showed that spatial adaptation took place, and that is presumably related to the use of the spectral cues of the better ear [8]. In humans, Slattery and Middlebrooks (1994) propose that the use of these spectral cues can be learned and enhanced in some patients with UHL [6]. In addition to spectral pinna cues, the subsequent work of Hendrikse et al. and Friedman et al. [9,10] noted an important implication of the head shadow effect (HSE) in sound localization. The HSE interferes with the perception of sound intensity; in a free field, a stimulation is filtered and attenuated, especially in the azimuth, due to the acoustic properties of the head; therefore, extracting horizontal spatial information from intensity analyses is possible. However, it is unknown to what extent the HSE can play a role in detecting accurate azimuth sound sources [9].

It has also been shown that the reliance on both the HSE and monaural cues can be enhanced in active listening, i.e., localization using head movements [11]. The first to document the importance of head rotation in reducing spatial ambiguities and front–back confusions was Wallach in 1940. Recent studies using virtual reality and motion tracking confirmed that sound localization accuracy could be improved with the use of head movements [12–15]. These studies suggested that modifying interaural cues using head movements produces a change in the angle specified initially by these cues, and the dynamic change of this angle during active listening can disambiguate spatial information and enable spatial discrimination and localization of a single sound source [9]. All these factors can be helpful for patients with UHL to adapt to their monaural hearing conditions. Middlebrooks, in 1994, showed that despite the binaural deficit, some patients manage to surpass the spatial deficit and present near-normal spatial accuracy in the horizontal plane [6]. Although the experimental procedure of Middlebrooks, 1994, did not provide additional information on the potential mechanisms involved in monaural adaptation, it seems that the factors cited above could have variable interindividual contributions.

Visual integration was found to have a significant impact on spatial auditory functions. In the animal model, for example, studies on owls reared with binocular prisms placed over their eyes to displace the visual field from the first day of eye-opening, without any change in their acoustic cues, revealed a spatial auditory shift towards the direction of the altered visual representation field [12]. In the case of altered binaural cues, studies on ferrets showed rapid spatial recovery due to audiovisual training [13]. In humans, the introduction of minimal visual cues in a virtual reality task changes spatial auditory performance in normal-hearing participants [14]. In the case of monaural listening, audiovisual spatial training improved sound localization even in an auditory-only condition [15]. These findings indicate that the possible adaptation to monaural hearing outside the training programs can be enhanced and accelerated if a rigorous and regular audiovisual training program are applied.

Although it remains unclear how UHL patients adapt to monaural hearing, the growing evidence mentioned above shows that these compensatory mechanisms must be studied in a testing procedure able to control all the features that can interfere with spatial auditory behavior. To date, the majority of experimental designs used to evaluate spatial functions do not have full control over the possible factors involved in spatial auditory perception. Classical methods usually evaluate spatial hearing in one dimension, with a limited number of speakers and thus limited angular positions. In addition to weak control of the possible effects of the visual environment and visual references during the experiment, the control of the implication of head movements (the number and reaction times) remains rare. A recent study by Valzolgher et al. [14] was able to validate the utility of a virtual reality (VR) tool using a head-mounted display (HMD_VIVE) in assessing spatial behavior. Notably, the VR system was able to track head movement behavior, including the angle of movements, reaction times, and the number of movements. Additionally, the VR system can provide the participant with an immersive experience where different conditions can be easily manipulated and tested (visual and non-visual).

In the present study, we aimed to explore the behavioral mechanisms adopted by adults with UHL to compensate for their binaural deficit. Our main objective was to assess the efficacy of the spatial training program on the localization abilities of participants with unilateral moderate to profound hearing loss, as has already been performed in previous studies on normal-hearing participants with monaural plugs [16] and bilateral cochlear implants [17]. We also aimed to decipher the adaptive behavioral mechanisms used to improve spatial skills by UHL participants. The present study can be an open door for future clinical implications of the VR approach in training programs that provide extensive and rapid adaptation to UHL.

2. Materials and Methods

2.1. Population

Twenty patients with unilateral moderate to profound hearing loss (Age = Mean ± SD, 51.4 ± 11.8, 10 right deafness, and 12 women) were recruited from the Ear, Nose, and Throat Department of Toulouse University Hospital. One patient did not complete the protocol and was eliminated from the study. The experiments took place in the Brain and Cognition Research Center in Toulouse (CerCo), France. All participants underwent an audiometric test to verify their hearing levels at the following frequencies, 250, 500, 1000, 2000, and 4000 Hz for both ears separately. The average of pure tone audiometry for each patient at each ear is presented in Figure 1, and the age, gender, and side and etiology of deafness of the 19 participants are presented in Table 1.

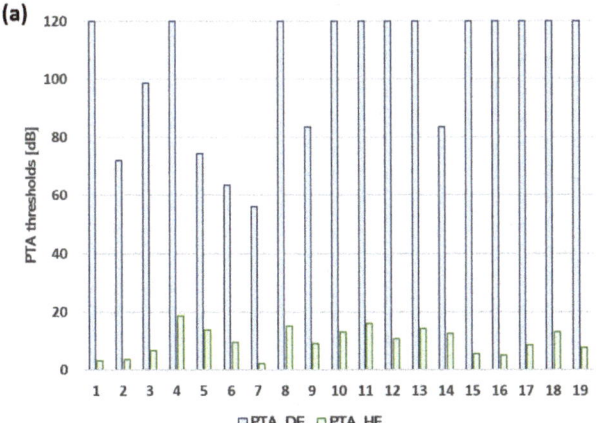
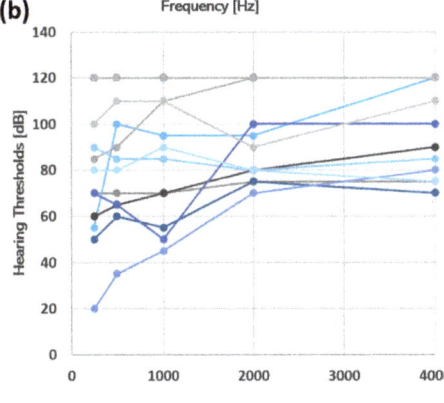

Figure 1. (**a**) Levels of hearing loss for the 19 unilateral hearing loss patients. The green histogram bars represent the hearing level in the healthy ears of the patients. The blue histogram bars represent the hearing level in the deaf ears of the patients. Abbreviations: PTA_HE = 'Pure Tone Audiometry in the Healthy Ear'; PTA_DE = 'Pure Tone Audiometry in the Deaf Ear'. (**b**) Individual hearing thresholds. The hearing thresholds are presented for the deaf ear of each patient at the tested frequencies (250, 500, 1000, 2000, and 4000 Hz).

Table 1. Demographic information about the 19 unilateral hearing loss patients.

ID	Gender	Age	D. Onset	Side of Deafness	Etiology of Deafness
UHL 01	M	37	5	R	Sudden
UHL 02	M	20	16	R	Congenital
UHL 03	F	43	12	R	Granulome
UHL 04	F	56	7	L	Facial paralysia
UHL 05	F	55	21	L	Unknown
UHL 06	M	44	2	R	Unknown
UHL 07	F	47	8	R	Sudden
UHL 08	F	70	64	L	Tympanic lesion
UHL 09	M	60	13	L	Unknown
UHL 10	F	65	5	L	Vestibular schwanoma
UHL 11	M	69	3	L	Vestibular schwanoma
UHL 12	F	56	3	L	Vestibular schwanoma
UHL 13	F	59	4	L	Congenital
UHL 14	M	48	10	L	Neurinoma
UHL 15	M	55	5	R	Vestibular schwanoma
UHL 16	M	55	11	R	Intracochlear schwanoma
UHL 17	F	47	8	R	Unknown
UHL 18	F	59	59	L	Congenital
UHL 19	F	43	1	R	Cholestéatome

D. Onset for Deafness Onset, F for Female, M for Male, L for Left, and R for Right. White lines correspond to participants belonging to group 1, and gray lines correspond to participants belonging to group 2.

2.2. Experimental Sessions

The protocol comprised two sessions separated by a washout phase that lasted two to four weeks. In each session, patients underwent a pre- and post-test that we will call the LOCATEST and one training type (spatial training or non-spatial training). The order of the training types was counterbalanced between the 19 participants in a within-subject cross-over design. Nine participants underwent spatial training in the first session and non-spatial training in the second session (group 1). Ten participants performed the opposite order of the sessions, with non-spatial training in the first session and spatial training in the second session (group 2). There was no significant difference between group 1 and group 2 in terms of hearing loss thresholds in the deaf ear (104.33 ± 24.03 vs. 103.25 ± 23.21; $p = 0.92$) and in terms of age (52.56 ± 14.51 vs. 51.50 ± 8.32; $p = 0.86$).

2.3. Description of the VR material

Virtual reality and kinematic tracking were implemented using the HTC Vive (Vive Enterprise). The VR system used for this experiment was validated for experimental use in research [14]. The system comprises a head-mounted display (HMD, 1800 × 1200 px) with two base stations positioned at two opposite angles of the room with a distance of 4 m to detect position and motion of HTC Vive objects. The base stations continuously scanned and tracked the moving objects inside a play surface defined by the experimenter before the beginning of the experiment. The moving objects tracked by the base station in real-time were the HMD, the controller held by the patients in their hands during the training, and the tracker positioned above the speaker used to deliver the sound.

2.4. Experimental Procedure of Head-Pointing Localization Test (LOCATEST)

The first test was a sound localization task using the head-pointing method. The participants sat in the center of the room on a rotating armless chair with the HMD mounted on their heads. The participants were immersed in a room with green walls with the same dimensions as the real experimental room of the lab (2.65 m × 2.85 m, width = 4.90 m). The sound stimulation was delivered in a free field at four different azimuth positions ($-67.5°$, $-22.5°$, $22.5°$, and $67.5°$) and two elevation positions ($+5°$ and $-15°$) at a constant distance of 55 cm from the center of the patient's head. The experimenter positioned the speaker in each location by following instructions visible on a monitor. The sound consisted of a

3 s white noise burst and amplitude modulated at 2.5 Hz with an intensity of 65 dB at the participant's head (for more details about the procedure, check [15,18]) (Figure 2).

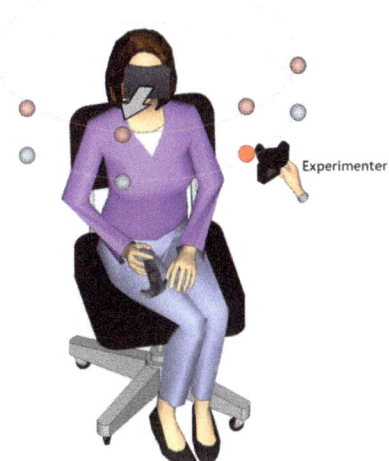

Figure 2. Experimental setup of head-pointing localization task (LOCATEST). The illustration shows the participant wearing the head-mounted display (HMD) during the LOCATEST. The eight spheres indicate predetermined speaker positions, which were not visible in the HMD. The hand holding the speaker near the red sphere was the experimenter's hand, who moved the speaker to reach the target position.

Patients were asked to localize the emitted sound by pointing, with their heads, towards the sound direction. They were also informed that they were free to move their head in any direction and that the sound could come from any position in the 3D plane. At the beginning of each trial, a central fixation cross appeared in the HMD; the fixation cross helped the participants to easily point their heads towards the sound source using the cross as a visual reference of their movements. There were no additional visual cues added to the visual scene. After sound emission, patients were asked to direct their heads toward the sound source direction and to validate their head position (their answer) by clicking on a controller that was held in their right hand. The experimenter explained that the response should be carried out using the head-pointing only, with no hand-pointing using the hand controller, which would only be used for head position validation. The LOCATEST was completed after 40 trials and was applied twice in every session, before and after the spatial and the non-spatial training.

2.5. Experimental Procedure of Spatial Training

The spatial training took place in the same experimental room with the same experimental condition as the LOCATEST. When the participants wore the HMD, they could see a virtual array of 13 loudspeakers arranged in a semicircle spanning from −72° at the left to +72° at the right, with the circular array falling into the visual field of the participant to maximize the efficiency of the use of visual cues with a 12° angular separation between each speaker at a distance of 55 cm from the participants' heads. Small angle separation was important to evaluate the efficiency of the audiovisual spatial training. The sound was randomly delivered through the 13 positions using two different types of sound stimulation. Half of the stimuli were amplitude modulated at 2 Hz, and the remaining half was modulated at 3 Hz, with a total of 156 stimuli at the end of the training.

The participants were holding a controller in their hands. They were asked to judge the spatial location of the emitted sound by touching the virtual speaker using the hand-held controller; participants were free to move their heads. The sound stimulation was continuous, and it only stopped when the participant touched the correct speaker. In the case where the participant touched the wrong speaker, the correct speaker would light up in red, and the participant was invited to correct their answers by touching the speaker lit up in red. Figure 3.

2.6. Experimental Procedure of Non-Spatial Training

The stimulation procedure of spatial and non-spatial trainings was the same. The only difference was that in the non-spatial training, patients were not asked to judge the spatial location of the sound; instead, they were asked to judge the sound quality (or amplitude modulation) by pointing their hand-held controller upwards (above the central speaker) if the stimulation sounded fast (amplitude modulation at 3 Hz) and downwards (below the central speaker) if the stimulation sounded slow (amplitude modulation at 2 Hz). If the participant reported an incorrect answer, for example, pointing upwards when the sound was amplitude modulated at 2 Hz, the central speaker would light up in red with an indication of the correct direction. Similarly to the spatial training, the stimulation only ended when the participant reported a correct answer (Figure 3).

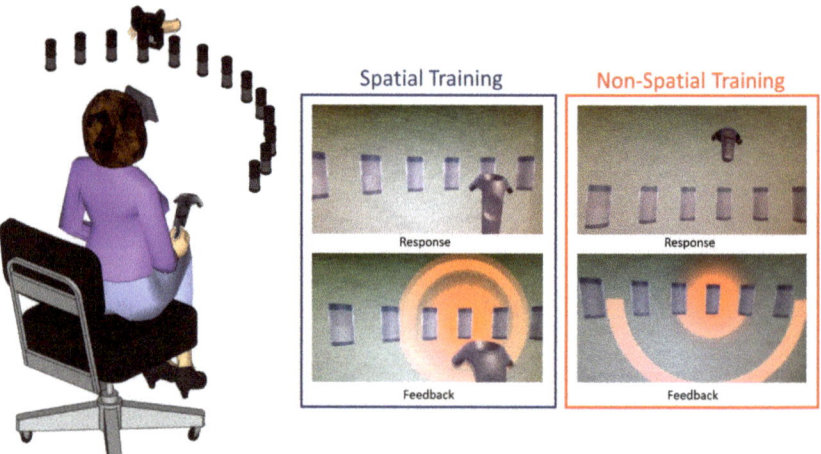

Figure 3. Experimental setup of both spatial and non-spatial trainings. In the spatial training, the participant was asked to judge the spatial location of the sound by touching the corresponding speaker with the controller held in their right hand. In the non-spatial training, the patient was asked to judge the quality of the sound by positioning the controller up if the sound was amplitude modulated at 3 Hz and down if the sound was amplitude modulated at 2 Hz. In both trainings, visual feedback was provided in the case of a wrong response.

2.7. Data Analysis

2.7.1. Head-Pointing Localization Performances (LOCATEST)

In the LOCATEST, two types of variables were analyzed. (1) The azimuth head-pointing localization error (absolute error), designated by the angular distance between the speaker position and the patient's head-pointing projection in the azimuth at the moment of the response validation. (2) The number of head movements during and after the sound emission. The head movements were manually selected by visualizing the velocity and the spatial rotation using a custom-made toolbox in MATLAB 2020. We fitted the absolute head-pointing localization error in the azimuth and the number of head movements in linear mixed-effect (LMER) models using the following statistical packages in R software (emmeans, lme4, and lmerTest).

2.7.2. Performances during Audiovisual Training

For the spatial training, we decided to study the variation of the hand-pointing errors, the number of head movements, and the head reaction times across the 156 trials to check if there was an effect of the audiovisual spatial training on auditory spatial behavior within the training session. We averaged the hand-pointing localization errors committed at each trial by the 19 participants (the average of 19 responses by trials), and we evaluated the linear regression of the errors across the 156 trials. We performed the same procedure for the reaction times (sec) and the number of head movements.

All the data visualizations were plotted using the function ggplot in R studio 3 February 2022.

3. Results

3.1. Performances in Head-Pointing Localization (LOCATEST)

Before analyzing the data on the group level ($n = 19$), we decided to test the variation between each group separately according to the order of the session. We fitted the absolute horizontal errors collected during the LOCATEST in a linear mixed-effect model with the group (group 1 and group 2), session (day 1 or day 2), and phase (pre- and post-) as the fixed factors and the participants as the random factor (the intercept and slope). We found an effect of the phase ($X^2(1,N = 19) = 40.3, p < 0.001$) and session ($X^2(1,N = 19) = 40.3, p < 0.001$) but no effect of the group ($p > 0.05$). However, importantly, we found an interaction between the groups, session, and phase ($X^2(1,N = 19) = 4.46, p < 0.05$). This interaction was induced by a significant reduction of errors in session 1 for group 1 but not for group 2 and a slight reduction in session 2 for group 2 but not for group 1, as illustrated in Figure 4. Group 1 (the spatial training first) showed a significant reduction of absolute azimuth errors in session 1 after the spatial training (24.85 ± 15.8 vs. 16.17 ± 11.28; $p < 0.001$). This spatial gain was maintained after the washout (pre-sessions 2: 16.05 ± 15.37) and was not influenced by the non-spatial training (post-session 2: 16.75 ± 13.46; $p = 0.977$), where the azimuth error remained low. For group 2 (the non-spatial training first), no significant change was noted after the non-spatial training during session 1 (27.37 ± 30.52 vs. 25.83 ± 26.42; $p = 0.846$). The horizontal errors were significantly reduced after the washout phase in session 2 (day 1, post-, 25.83 ± 26.42 vs. day 2, pre-, 19.75 ± 19.15; $p < 0.05$). The significant drop in the errors during the washout phase was driven by the performance of two patients who presented atypical performance compared to the 17 participants: patient number 19, who drastically reduced her errors from 74° (post-session 1) to 33° (pre-session 2), and patient number 15, who reduced his errors from 65° (post-session 1) to 56° (pre-session 2). The eight patients left in group 2 maintained a regular reduction of errors of 2.3° ± 5.6°, which is comparable to the reduction in group 1 (1.8° ± 3°); thus, after the spatial training was applied on the second day, the errors seemed to slightly reduce within the session for the whole of group 2 ($n = 10$); however, this reduction was not statistically significant (day 2, pre-, 19.75 ± 19.15 vs. day 2, post-, 17.78 ± 18.49; $p = 0.772$) (Figure 4).

To study the impact of the spatial training on our 19 participants, we used a linear mixed-effect model with the training (spatial and non-spatial) and phase (pre- and post-) as the fixed factors and the participants and session as the random factors. The analysis showed an effect of the phase ($X^2(1,N = 19) = 5.37; p < 0.05$) and an interaction between the phase and training ($X^2(1,N = 19) = 4.28; p < 0.05$) on head-pointing precision in the horizontal plane. The horizontal errors in the LOCATEST significantly decreased after the spatial training (pre-, 22.17 ± 17.8, vs. post-, 16.51 ± 15.54; $p < 0.05$), while no significant change was noted after the non-spatial training (pre-, 22.21 ± 24.6, vs. post-, 21.53 ± 21.7; $p > 0.05$), as shown in Figure 5.

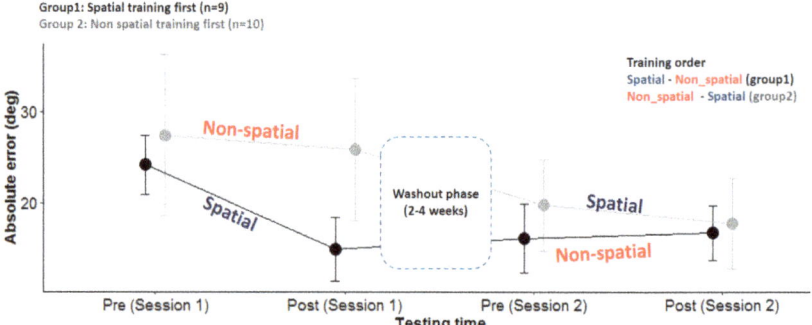

Figure 4. Head-pointing localization errors (LOCATEST) for each group pre- and post-spatial and non-spatial trainings. Session 1 designates the session on the first day. Session 2 designates the session on the second day, 2 to 4 weeks after the first session.

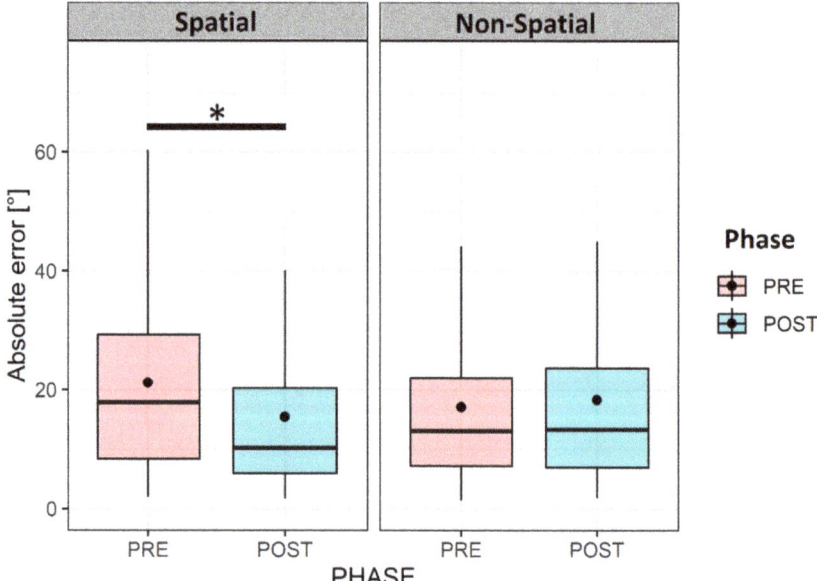

Figure 5. Horizontal errors' variation according to training type and phase. Illustration of the variation of the absolute horizontal head-pointing errors in the LOCATEST, regardless of the order of the session in the 19 UHL patients. The asterisk (*) symbol in the legend denotes statistical significance at the alpha level of 0.05.

We wanted to step further into the details of the spatial improvement after the audiovisual spatial training, and we decided to test the variation of the absolute horizontal error as a function of the stimulation side (the deaf and healthy ears); we noticed that the decrease in the horizontal errors after the spatial training was mainly on the side of the deaf ear. The errors significantly decreased from (24.99 ± 20.52) to (16.33 ± 16.30) ($p < 0.05$) on the side of the deaf ear, while no significant change was noted on the side of the healthy ear pre- (19.34 ± 14.18) and post- (16.7 ± 14.85) training ($p > 0.05$), as shown in Figure 6.

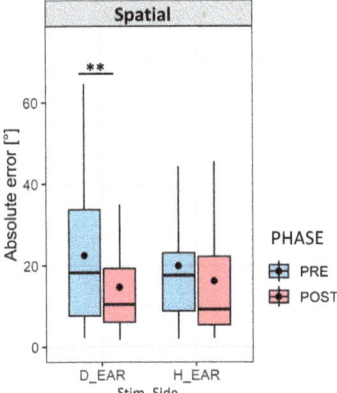

Figure 6. Variation of localization errors according to stimulation side. The box plots represent the variation of the horizontal absolute head-pointing error on the side of the deaf ear (D_EAR) and on the side of the healthy ear (H_ear) before (PRE) and after (POST). Abbreviations: Stim_Side: 'stimulation side'; H error: 'horizontal error'. The asterisk (**) symbol in the legend denotes statistical significance at the alpha level of 0.01.

In addition to the effect of the stimulation side, we assumed that head movements could also play an important role in guiding and orienting the participants. Therefore, we wanted to investigate the influence of the two training types on the number of head movements. Using the LME model, we analyzed the variation in the number of head movements as a function of the training and phase. We noticed that after the spatial training, the number of head movements increased during the task (pre-: 1.77 ± 0.52 vs. post-: 2.01 ± 0.83; $p < 0.01$), while this number decreased when the non-spatial training was applied (pre-: 1.9 ± 0.57 vs. post-: 1.78 ± 0.45; $p < 0.01$) (Figure 7).

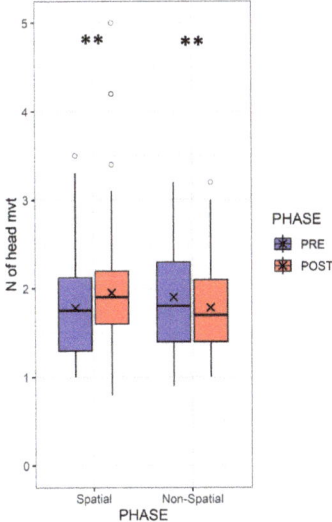

Figure 7. Variation of the number of head movements according to the training type. Box plots representing the variation of the number of head movements in the head-pointing task (LOCATEST) before and after the spatial and the non-spatial training for the 19 patients with UHL. The asterisk (**) symbol in the legend denotes statistical significance at the alpha level of 0.01.

3.2. Performance during Audiovisual Training

In the previous section, we showed that spatial training had an impact on both the spatial errors and the number of head movements (Figure 8). We wanted to step further into the strategies used during the spatial training. Therefore, we decided to study the behavioral changes across 156 trials during the spatial training. We studied the ability of the trial number to predict the hand-pointing errors, number of head movements, and head reaction time using a simple linear regression model. We found a significant relationship ($p < 0.001$) between the trial number and hand response errors ($R^2 = 0.1053$), and we also found a significant relationship ($p < 0.001$) between the trial number and head reaction time ($R^2 = 0.0038$); however, this relationship was not significant ($p = 0.82$) for the number of head movements, which did not change across 156 trials. The hand response errors were significantly reduced from ($18.94° \pm 32.81°$) in the first trial to ($6.94° \pm 9.22°$) in the 156th trial. Similarly, the head reaction time, designated by the first head movement during the stimulation, was significantly reduced (trial 1: 1.17 sec $\pm$ 0.41 and trial 156: 1.05 sec $\pm$ 0.58), while the number of head movements did not change (trial 1: 2.36 $\pm$ 1.11 and trial 156: 3 $\pm$ 1.76).

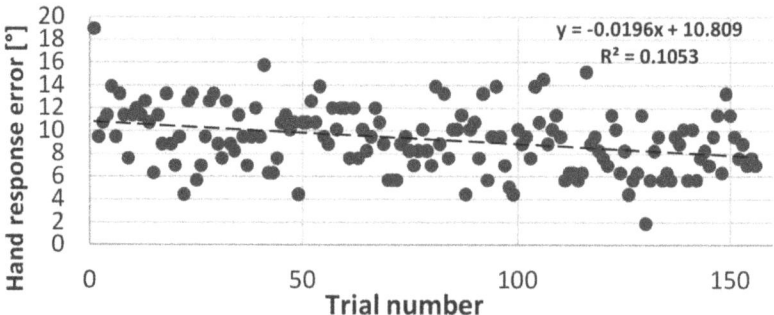

Figure 8. Variation of hand-pointing errors across trials. Scatter plot representing the horizontal errors of hand-pointing during the spatial training with 156 trials.

4. Discussion

4.1. Effect of Audiovisual Training on Spatial Hearing Abilities in UHL

The aim of this study was to evaluate the effectiveness of audiovisual spatial training on auditory spatial behavior displayed by UHL patients to compensate for their binaural deficit. The cross-modal approach in treating auditory deficits has indeed shown effectiveness in improving spatial perception [14,15]. Anatomical and electrophysiological studies in animal models showed the involvement of multisensory processing in the early stages of sensory perception, with this multisensory processing helping to re-calibrate unisensory modalities independently [19]. Anatomically, this can be explained by the presence of direct projections originating from the representation of the peripheral visual fields in the pre-striate cortex [20] towards the caudal areas of the auditory cortex, which are involved in spatial processing [21]. A large body of studies proved that multisensory stimulation that includes visual feedback is more effective than unisensory stimulation in normal-hearing participants with monaural plugs [15,16,18,22] and in patients with cochlear implants [17,23]. The study of [15] suggests that unisensory auditory training, applied to normal-hearing participants with ear plugs, showed no improvement in spatial behavior. However, when a visual cue was added, the horizontal errors decreased significantly on the side of the plugged ear. In the animal model, the seminal work of [24] proved the existence of a strong relationship between the width of the field of best vision and auditory spatial acuity, suggesting that the common behavior between mammals when hearing a sound is the motor reflex of eye orientation, followed by a head orientation to explore space.

In the present study, multisensory training played a crucial role in guiding vision towards the auditory stimulus, but it led to an improvement of spatial behavior even in the unisensory task of head-pointing without visual cues (LOCATEST). In the LOCATEST, where no visual cue can indicate the location of the sound, patients had to point with their heads toward the sound source. Despite their hearing loss level (the average hearing loss = 103 dB), these patients were able to improve their spatial localization after the audio-visual spatial training. This result is consistent with the findings of [16] on normal-hearing participants fitted with monaural plugs, where the same audiovisual spatial training improved spatial performance in the unisensory auditory spatial task by decreasing the degree of head-pointing localization errors from 19.3° before the spatial training to 11.5° after the training [16].

This effect of multisensory training on unisensory experience was also found in adult patients with bilateral cochlear implants (BCIs); a study by [22] showed faster improvement after multisensory spatial training compared to training in the auditory modality only. Although both populations (UHL and BCIs) have different adaptation strategies, they both rely on visual sensory inputs to optimize environmental spatial mapping [25]. Adding a new informative cue about sound location, such as vision in this case, is a helpful experience that minimizes listening effort and improves rapid learning [26].

4.2. Re-Learning to Move the Head Effectively

Spontaneous head movements are used in daily life to direct vision and localize visual and auditory objects [24]. Thus, the use of head movements by the listeners helps them to optimize the advantage of binaural cues by continuously changing the ITD (interaural time difference) and ILD (interaural intensity difference) [9]. The spontaneous reaction of turning the head and body towards a sound source has been found to be an important factor in weighing auditory cues [27,28]. Studies comparing static and active listening conditions showed better spatial performance when head movements were allowed [18,22,29].

In the case of UHL, binaural symmetry is disrupted, leading to a disruption in the auditory spatial acuity [28,30]. In this case, head rotations can play a strategic role in compensating and guiding spatial behavior by enhancing the head shadow effect and by guiding the head towards a sound position [31–33].

Most of the studies examining spatial auditory behavior in hearing-impaired participants tested spatial localization in conditions where the head was immobilized [28,34]. Nonetheless, this condition does not reflect the ecological situation, where listeners are continuously exploring their environment through the motor orientation of the eyes, head, and body.

Thus, studies that tended to assess spatial behavior in monaural listening with the head immobilized showed a significant increase in errors in the side of the plugged ear [6,31,32]. Head shadow effects can be more effective when moving the head by masking unnecessary noise and concentrating on the target sound [11]. This benefit is due to the spatial advantage extracted from the HSE, which is able to attenuate and filter sound due to the head's properties, especially in azimuth. Varying sound intensity in the unplugged ear during head movements to optimize the head shadow advantage is an efficient provider of spatial information [33]. This improvement is noted in both horizontal and vertical planes [11]. This advantage explains the common behavior adopted by UHL patients to project their localization answers towards the side of the hearing ear [6]. The UHL patients displace their better ear towards the source location by rotating their head in order to increase the level of sound in the hearing ear and to reduce spatial ambiguities [35,36].

This "better ear preference" is also present in our UHL population, as shown in Figure 6. The advantage of our task in the LOCATEST is that we included head movements not only by allowing mobilization but also by using head-pointing as a localization task. In the head-pointing localization task, before the spatial training, localization errors were higher on the side of the deaf ear compared to the non-deaf ear (24.9° vs. 19.3°). Interestingly, the decrease in localization errors after the spatial training was on the side of the deaf ear only (from 24.9°(pre-) to 16.3° (post-)). In our study, the specific improvement of spatial accuracy on the side of the deaf ear can be explained by a "re-learning" to move the head effectively in order to optimize the advantage from the head shadow effect. Thus, when we analyzed head movement behavior during the audiovisual spatial training, we found no change in the number of head movements; however, the head reaction times and hand-pointing errors decreased at the end of the training. Even though the number of head movements did not change during the spatial training, patients used their head movements in a more effective manner.

The advantage of the task in the LOCATEST, as mentioned earlier, is that it forced the patient to use head movements in a unisensory task where no visual feedback was used as an orienting cue for the eyes and the head. We also used a stimulus duration of 3 s to make sure that dynamic tracking of the sound, which usually starts after 300 ms, was taking place [27,28]. Although the localization modality in the spatial training was different (hand-pointing vs. head-pointing in the LOCATEST), patients rapidly learned how to use their heads effectively. Valzolgher et al. [16] noted the same rapid adaptation in simulated monaural hearing, suggesting that participants learn to explore wider angles of the space after spatial training. The study of Valzolgher [16] also noted the importance of hand reaching to sound as a guiding tool that provides additional motor interaction with the sound; this could explain the significant decrease in the head reaction times at the end of the spatial training. The reaching-to-sound procedure can also maximize head movement accuracy and, therefore, accelerates spatial learning in this population [16,18].

4.3. Clinical Relevance of Motion-Tracked Virtual Reality in Treating Auditory Deficit

This novel technique permits continuous tracking of the head and body interaction with sound and allows us to control different factors involved in auditory behavior that are difficult to evaluate in classical methods [14].

Using this approach, we can deliver a wide variety of stimulus types at different spatial positions in the free field. A free field sound emission allows us to target different types of hearing impairments, including patients with hearing aids and cochlear implants. In addition to the ability of the device to control multiple factors involved in auditory behavior, the device is user-friendly and accessible to different age ranges, including children, which makes its utility in clinics more relevant.

In the present design, we aimed to verify the feasibility of audiovisual training in the spatial rehabilitation of UHL. Auditory spatial behavior improved after one session of spatial training; however, the present protocol can be optimized in order to maintain a long-term benefit and improve spatial perception in daily life. In future studies, we could increase the number of training sessions; although one session showed an effect on spatial behavior that lasted even after the non-spatial training (group 1), the frequency of the training can be an important factor in consolidating spatial gain. Studies on monaural-plugged ferrets showed quick and extensive improvement in spatial performance when spatial training was provided regularly in daily sessions. In the study of [15] on monaurally plugged normal hearing controls the number of sessions of spatial audiovisual training was five training sessions during one week (one session per day). A recent study by Coudert et al. [22] on bilateral cochlear implants showed that intensive spatial training of eight sessions over 10 weeks significantly improved spatial performance and also performance in the speech in noise, which was evaluated by a matrix test, while four sessions spread over 2 weeks seemed to be insufficient. Such results indicate that the number of sessions and the duration between each session are important factors for the efficiency of a training program. All of the mentioned studies that used VR showed its clinical relevance in developing training programs for patients with hearing deficits. Thus, to eliminate the possibility of device habituation that might have an effect on behavior, an evaluation of spatial performance outside of the VR before and after training can be useful. This could help explain, for example, the significant reduction of head-pointing errors for participants number 15 and number 19 during the washout phase. To eliminate such a possibility in the future, and in order to control the VR habituation effect, a control condition of a sound localization task outside of VR is useful. In addition, spatial testing in VR can be ameliorated by adding natural audiovisual presentations, such as the use of realistic, immersive scenes with more realistic sounds.

5. Conclusions

Unilateral hearing loss disrupts binaural integration and alters spatial function. However, adaptation to monaural listening conditions can be enhanced and accelerated by a regular audiovisual training program, allowing for active listening in motion-tracked virtual reality devices, which can become clinically useful tools that control all possible factors involved in spatial auditory behavior.

Author Contributions: Conceptualization: F.P. and A.F.; Data curation: M.A.; Formal analysis: M.A.; Funding acquisition: F.P., A.F., P.B. and M.M.; Investigation: M.A. and C.V.; Methodology, M.A., C.V. and F.P.; Project administration, M.A., F.P. and A.F.; Resources, C.V. and G.V.; Software, G.V.; Supervision: F.P., A.F., P.B. and M.M.; Validation: F.P., A.F., P.B. and M.M.; Visualization, M.A.; Writing—original draft, M.A.; Writing—review & editing, M.A., C.V., F.P., A.F., P.B. and M.M. All authors have read and agreed to the published version of the manuscript.

Funding: This work was supported by the ANR (Agence Nationale de la Recherche), AgeHear (ANR-20-CE28-0016), and ANR Hearing 3D (ANR 16-CE17-0016). MA is an employee at the university hospital of Purpan, Toulouse.

Institutional Review Board Statement: The study was conducted in accordance with the Declaration of Helsinki, and approved by the national ethics committee in France (Ile de France X, N° ID RCB 2019-A02293-54), and recorded in clinicaltrials.gov (NCT04183348).

Informed Consent Statement: All participants signed an informed consent before starting the experiment.

Data Availability Statement: The data are not publicly available due to the quality of personal health data containing information that could compromise the privacy of research participants. Given the nature of the data and in order to comply with the Sponsor's data protection policy, a data-sharing agreement must be established with the Toulouse University Hospital before the access.

Acknowledgments: We would like to thank Julie Gatel, Soumia Taoui, and Iholy Rajosoa for their administrative support; we would also like to thank the participants for taking the time to participate in the study. Lastly, we would like to thank Jessica Foxton for providing a critical review of the article.

Conflicts of Interest: The authors declare no conflict of interest.

References

1. Bronkhorst, A.W.; Plomp, R. Binaural speech intelligibility in noise for hearing-impaired listeners. *J. Acoust. Soc. Am.* **1989**, *86*, 1374–1383. [CrossRef] [PubMed]
2. Keating, P.; King, A.J. Developmental plasticity of spatial hearing following asymmetric hearing loss: Context-dependent cue integration and its clinical implications. *Front. Syst. Neurosci.* **2013**, *7*, 123. [CrossRef] [PubMed]
3. Keating, P.; Rosenior-Patten, O.; Dahmen, J.C.; Bell, O.; King, A.J. Behavioral training promotes multiple adaptive processes following acute hearing loss. *Elife* **2016**, *5*, e12264. [CrossRef] [PubMed]
4. Barone, P.; Lacassagne, L.; Kral, A. Reorganization of the Connectivity of Cortical Field DZ in Congenitally Deaf Cat. *PLoS ONE* **2013**, *8*, e60093. [CrossRef] [PubMed]
5. Gordon, K.; Kral, A. Animal and human studies on developmental monaural hearing loss. *Heart Res.* **2019**, *380*, 60–74. [CrossRef]
6. Slattery, W.H.; Middlebrooks, J.C. Monaural sound localization: Acute versus chronic unilateral impairment. *Heart Res.* **1994**, *75*, 38–46. [CrossRef]
7. Hofman, P.M.; van Riswick, J.G.; van Opstal, J. Relearning sound localization with new ears. *Nat. Neurosci.* **1998**, *1*, 417–421. [CrossRef]
8. King, A.J.; Parsons, C.H.; Moore, D.R. Plasticity in the neural coding of auditory space in the mammalian brain. *Proc. Natl. Acad. Sci. USA* **2000**, *97*, 11821–11828. [CrossRef]
9. Hendrikse, M.M.E.; Grimm, G.; Hohmann, V. Evaluation of the Influence of Head Movement on Hearing Aid Algorithm Performance Using Acoustic Simulations. *Trends Heart* **2020**, *24*. [CrossRef]

10. Ausili, S.A.; Agterberg, M.J.H.; Engel, A.; Voelter, C.; Thomas, J.P.; Brill, S.; Snik, A.F.M.; Dazert, S.; Van Opstal, A.J.; Mylanus, E.A.M. Spatial Hearing by Bilateral Cochlear Implant Users with Temporal Fine-Structure Processing. *Front. Neurol.* **2020**, *11*, 915. [CrossRef]
11. Perrett, S.; Noble, W. The contribution of head motion cues to localization of low-pass noise. *Percept. Psychophys.* **1997**, *59*, 1018–1026. [CrossRef]
12. Knudsen, E.; Knudsen, P. Vision calibrates sound localization in developing barn owls. *J. Neurosci.* **1989**, *9*, 3306–3313. [CrossRef]
13. Kacelnik, O.; Nodal, F.R.; Parsons, C.H.; King, A.J. Training-Induced Plasticity of Auditory Localization in Adult Mammals. *PLoS Biol.* **2006**, *4*, e71. [CrossRef]
14. Valzolgher, C.; Alzhaler, M.; Gessa, E.; Todeschini, M.; Nieto, P.; Verdelet, G.; Salemme, R.; Gaveau, V.; Marx, M.; Truy, E.; et al. The impact of a visual spatial frame on real sound-source localization in virtual reality. *Curr. Res. Behav. Sci.* **2020**, *1*, 100003. [CrossRef]
15. Strelnikov, K.; Rosito, M.; Barone, P. Effect of Audiovisual Training on Monaural Spatial Hearing in Horizontal Plane. *PLoS ONE* **2011**, *6*, e18244. [CrossRef]
16. Valzolgher, C.; Todeschini, M.; Verdelet, G.; Gatel, J.; Salemme, R.; Gaveau, V.; Truy, E.; Farnè, A.; Pavani, F. Adapting to altered auditory cues: Generalization from manual reaching to head pointing. *PLoS ONE* **2022**, *17*, e0263509. [CrossRef]
17. Valzolgher, C.; Gatel, J.; Bouzaid, S.; Grenouillet, S.; Todeschini, M.; Verdelet, G.; Salemme, R.; Gaveau, V.; Truy, E.; Farnè, A.; et al. Reaching to Sounds Improves Spatial Hearing in Bilateral Cochlear Implant Users. *Ear Heart* **2022**, *44*, 189–198. [CrossRef]
18. Valzolgher, C.; Verdelet, G.; Salemme, R.; Lombardi, L.; Gaveau, V.; Farné, A.; Pavani, F. Reaching to sounds in virtual reality: A multisensory-motor approach to promote adaptation to altered auditory cues. *Neuropsychologia* **2020**, *149*, 107665. [CrossRef]
19. Nodal, F.R.; Kacelnik, O.; Bajo, V.M.; Bizley, J.K.; Moore, D.R.; King, A.J. Lesions of the Auditory Cortex Impair Azimuthal Sound Localization and Its Recalibration in Ferrets. *J. Neurophysiol.* **2010**, *103*, 1209–1225. [CrossRef]
20. Falchier, A.; Schroeder, C.E.; Hackett, T.A.; Lakatos, P.; Nascimento-Silva, S.; Ulbert, I.; Karmos, G.; Smiley, J.F. Projection from Visual Areas V2 and Prostriata to Caudal Auditory Cortex in the Monkey. *Cereb. Cortex* **2009**, *20*, 1529–1538. [CrossRef]
21. Rauschecker, J.P.; Tian, B. Mechanisms and streams for processing of "what" and "where" in auditory cortex. *Proc. Natl. Acad. Sci. USA* **2000**, *97*, 11800–11806. [CrossRef] [PubMed]
22. Coudert, A.; Verdelet, G.; Reilly, K.T.; Truy, E.; Gaveau, V. Intensive Training of Spatial Hearing Promotes Auditory Abilities of Bilateral Cochlear Implant Adults: A Pilot Study. *Ear Heart* **2022**, *44*, 61–76. [CrossRef] [PubMed]
23. Coudert, A.; Gaveau, V.; Gatel, J.; Verdelet, G.; Salemme, R.; Farne, A.; Pavani, F.; Truy, E. Spatial Hearing Difficulties in Reaching Space in Bilateral Cochlear Implant Children Improve with Head Movements. *Ear Heart* **2021**, *43*, 192–205. [CrossRef] [PubMed]
24. Heffner, R.S.; Heffner, H.E. Visual Factors in Sound Localization in Mammals. *J. Comp. Neurol.* **1992**, *317*, 219–232. [CrossRef]
25. Bulkin, D.A.; Groh, J.M. Seeing sounds: Visual and auditory interactions in the brain. *Curr. Opin. Neurobiol.* **2006**, *16*, 415–419. [CrossRef]
26. Isaiah, A.; Hartley, D.E. Can training extend current guidelines for cochlear implant candidacy? *Neural Regen. Res.* **2015**, *10*, 718–720. [CrossRef]
27. Blauert, J. *Spatial Hearing: The Psychophysics of Human Sound Localization*; MIT Press: Cambridge, MA, USA, 2001.
28. Middlebrooks, J.C.; Green, D.M. Sound Localization by Human Listeners. *Annu. Rev. Psychol.* **1991**, *42*, 135–159. [CrossRef]
29. Gessa, E.; Giovanelli, E.; Spinella, D.; Verdelet, G.; Farnè, A.; Frau, G.N.; Pavani, F.; Valzolgher, C. Spontaneous head-movements improve sound localization in aging adults with hearing loss. *Front. Hum. Neurosci.* **2022**, *16*. [CrossRef]
30. Kumpik, D.P.; King, A.J. A review of the effects of unilateral hearing loss on spatial hearing. *Heart Res.* **2018**, *372*, 17–28. [CrossRef]
31. Makous, J.C.; Middlebrooks, J.C. Two-dimensional sound localization by human listeners. *J. Acoust. Soc. Am.* **1990**, *87*, 2188–2200. [CrossRef]
32. Alzaher, M.; Vannson, N.; Deguine, O.; Marx, M.; Barone, P.; Strelnikov, K. Brain plasticity and hearing disorders. *Rev. Neurol.* **2021**, *177*, 1121–1132. [CrossRef]
33. Van Wanrooij, M.M.; Van Opstal, A.J. Contribution of Head Shadow and Pinna Cues to Chronic Monaural Sound Localization. *J. Neurosci.* **2004**, *24*, 4163–4171. [CrossRef]
34. Freigang, C.; Schmiedchen, K.; Nitsche, I.; Rübsamen, R. Free-field study on auditory localization and discrimination performance in older adults. *Exp. Brain Res.* **2014**, *232*, 1157–1172. [CrossRef]
35. Brimijoin, W.O.; Akeroyd, M. The moving minimum audible angle is smaller during self motion than during source motion. *Front. Neurosci.* **2014**, *8*, 273. [CrossRef]
36. Brimijoin, W.O.; McShefferty, D.; Akeroyd, M.A. Undirected head movements of listeners with asymmetrical hearing impairment during a speech-in-noise task. *Heart Res.* **2012**, *283*, 162–168. [CrossRef]

Disclaimer/Publisher's Note: The statements, opinions and data contained in all publications are solely those of the individual author(s) and contributor(s) and not of MDPI and/or the editor(s). MDPI and/or the editor(s) disclaim responsibility for any injury to people or property resulting from any ideas, methods, instructions or products referred to in the content.

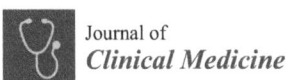

Article

Optical Coherence Tomography-Based Atlas of the Human Cochlear Hook Region

Lore Kerkhofs [1,2,*,†], Anastasiya Starovoyt [1,2,†], Jan Wouters [1,2], Tristan Putzeys [1,2,3] and Nicolas Verhaert [1,2,4]

1. Research Group Experimental Oto-Rhino-Laryngology, Department of Neurosciences, KU Leuven, 3000 Leuven, Belgium
2. Department of Neurosciences, Leuven Brain Institute, KU Leuven, 3000 Leuven, Belgium
3. Laboratory for Soft Matter and Biophysics, Department of Physics and Astronomy, KU Leuven, 3000 Leuven, Belgium
4. Department of Otorhinolaryngology, Head and Neck Surgery, University Hospitals of Leuven, 3000 Leuven, Belgium
* Correspondence: lore.kerkhofs@kuleuven.be; Tel.: +32-16-32-69-04
† These authors contributed equally to this work.

Abstract: Advancements in intracochlear diagnostics, as well as prosthetic and regenerative inner ear therapies, rely on a good understanding of cochlear microanatomy. The human cochlea is very small and deeply embedded within the densest skull bone, making nondestructive visualization of its internal microstructures extremely challenging. Current imaging techniques used in clinical practice, such as MRI and CT, fall short in their resolution to visualize important intracochlear landmarks, and histological analysis of the cochlea cannot be performed on living patients without compromising their hearing. Recently, optical coherence tomography (OCT) has been shown to be a promising tool for nondestructive micrometer resolution imaging of the mammalian inner ear. Various studies performed on human cadaveric tissue and living animals demonstrated the ability of OCT to visualize important cochlear microstructures (scalae, organ of Corti, spiral ligament, and osseous spiral lamina) at micrometer resolution. However, the interpretation of human intracochlear OCT images is non-trivial for researchers and clinicians who are not yet familiar with this novel technology. In this study, we present an atlas of intracochlear OCT images, which were acquired in a series of 7 fresh and 10 fresh-frozen human cadaveric cochleae through the round window membrane and describe the qualitative characteristics of visualized intracochlear structures. Likewise, we describe several intracochlear abnormalities, which could be detected with OCT and are relevant for clinical practice.

Keywords: optical coherence tomography; human organ of Corti; intracochlear anatomy; cochlear implantation

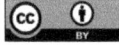

1. Introduction

Sensorineural hearing loss is one of the most common sensory deficits in the world and will affect up to 10% of the world population by 2050, according to the estimates of the World Health Organization [1]. Hearing disability has a large impact on the daily quality of life; it can lead to social isolation and even give rise to dementia, yet possibilities for effective treatment remain limited [2,3]. In the majority of cases, sensorineural hearing loss is due to structural damage of the cochlea, which is often treated with a cochlear implant in patients with severe hearing loss. Unfortunately, the surgical insertion of the stimulating electrode array often traumatizes the delicate intracochlear microstructures, which cannot be visualized intraoperatively. Targeted regenerative inner ear therapies are being researched, but their translation into clinical practice relies on the ability to diagnose the underlying pathology and administer the treatments to specific regions of the cochlea without collateral damage [4,5]. As such, the efficacy of current and future treatments largely depends on the ability to visualize the intracochlear anatomy.

The human cochlea is a very small (4 mm × 7 mm × 10 mm) and complex organ, deeply embedded inside the human skull bone, prohibiting direct visualization of its internal structure [6]. In current clinical practice, magnetic resonance imaging (MRI) or computed tomography (CT) is used for intracochlear diagnostics and preoperative planning. Unfortunately, these techniques fall short in imaging most intracochlear microstructures due to their limited resolution (0.5 mm) [6]. MicroCT and histology can provide high-resolution visualization of the internal cochlear anatomy, but these destructive methods are not viable for future (in vivo) clinical use [7,8].

Recently, the use of optical coherence tomography (OCT) in hearing research has been rising in both morphological and functional studies [9–17]. OCT is a nondestructive high-resolution imaging technique with similar working principles to ultrasonography. It uses low-coherence infrared light instead of sound waves, resulting in a higher micrometer-scale resolution. It was first applied in the field of ophthalmology, and due to its success, the use of OCT rapidly increased in other medical fields, such as oncology, cardiology, and dermatology [18–20].

A main advantage of OCT is the possibility to perform transmembrane OCT imaging, which happens through the round window membrane (RWM), providing the ability to image the first 1–3 mm of the most basal portion of the inner ear, namely the proximal hook region [14]. This eliminates the need to disrupt the cochlear homeostasis by opening it, which makes it a promising tool for atraumatic cochlear implantation, inner ear therapy, and diagnostics. In our previous work, we demonstrated that relevant structures such as the basilar membrane (BM), Osseous Spiral Lamina (OSL), Secondary Spiral Lamina (SSL), and spiral ligament (SL) can be identified in the proximal hook region [14]. However, the interpretation of human intracochlear OCT images is non-trivial for researchers and clinicians who are not yet familiar with this novel technology.

This study aims to extensively augment the knowledge of intracochlear structures by nondestructive transmembrane OCT imaging and to provide otological clinicians and researchers with an atlas of the human cochlear microanatomy. Likewise, we investigated whether abnormalities of the intracochlear structures can be visualized using OCT in fresh and fresh-frozen human temporal bones.

2. Materials and Methods

2.1. Sample Preparation

Seventeen temporal bones were dissected and imaged with OCT in this study. All samples were harvested within 72 h post-mortem: 3 specimens were obtained from an anonymous donor at the Vesalius Institute of the University of Leuven; 14 specimens were retrieved from individuals who underwent a clinical brain autopsy at the University Hospitals of Leuven. Informed consent was obtained from all subjects, their next of kin, or legal guardian(s). No medical history or background information was known from the anonymous donors; only the age and the gender were known from the clinical brain autopsy donors. Harvesting and use of the temporal bones were conducted in accordance with the Helsinki declaration and approved by the Medical Ethics Committee of the University Hospitals of Leuven (S65502). To achieve maximal access to the RWM for transmembrane OCT imaging, the inner ears (approx. 10 mm × 10 mm × 20 mm) were dissected out of the temporal bones according to the previously described method by Starovoyt et al. 2019 [14]. The stapes was preserved to avoid leakage of the intracochlear fluid and entry of air bubbles into the cochlea. No drilling or blue-lining on the cochlea or labyrinthine complex was performed to maximize the structural preservation of the structures. After the surgical dissection, the isolated inner ears were thoroughly evaluated under a surgical microscope to exclude obvious anatomical malformations and trauma to the stapes, the RWM, the cochlear capsule, and the semicircular canals of the vestibular system. In addition, the stapes mobility and the integrity of the RWM were visually evaluated under the surgical microscope by confirming the movement of the RWM, without leakage of the intracochlear fluid, when gentle pressure is applied to the stapes. No pathological findings were detected during the inspection and dissection of the temporal bones. The cochleae were not fixed, dehydrated, or decalcified to avoid damaging the delicate intracochlear structures, such as the vulnerable sensory epithelium on the basilar membrane.

2.2. OCT Imaging

Extracted cochleae were imaged using a commercially available stationary spectral-domain OCT system (Telesto TEL220C1; Thorlabs, Lübeck, Germany), with an optical source having a broadband center wavelength of 1310 nm. The axial resolution of the system was either 4.1 or 5.5 µm for water and air, respectively. An objective lens was used with a working distance of 42.3 mm and an effective focal length of 54 mm (LSM04, Thorlabs), resulting in a lateral resolution of 20 µm. The number of A-lines was 1024, as well as the number of b-scans. Three-dimensional C-scans of the intracochlear structures were acquired through the RWM, whereby the scanning was performed at the rate of 10, 28, and 76 kHz without averaging. With a dimension of $512 \times 512 \times 1024$ pixels for c-scans, the acquisition time was between 7 s (for 10 kHz) and 2 s (for 76 kHz). During imaging, the extracted cochleae were held in place using dental wax. They were viewed and analyzed in ThorImage software, version 5.1.3, whereby the signal range was adjusted to the dynamic range of each dataset. Highly reflective structures will appear as bright (in the grey scale) or red to red-white (in the false color scale) on the OCT images. The refractive index was set to 1.45, the average refractive index of the RWM, measured in two human cochleae according to the method of Tearney et al. [21].

For segmentation, a c-scan was saved as a stack of JPG files, which were then imported into Avizo (FEI Visualization Sciences Group and Thermo Fisher Scientific Inc., Bordeaux, France). In Avizo, the JPG files were manually segmented by experts in cochlear anatomy, who carefully evaluated the results. The voxel size for each dimension was also specified in Avizo.

2.3. Microcomputed Tomography (microCT)

The extracted cochleae were imaged after staining them in contrast for 72 h using a Phoenix Nanotom M MicroCT device (GE Measurement and Control Solutions, Germany) [22–24]. The device was equipped with a tungsten target and had a voxel size of 6.3 µm; it was operating at a voltage of 50 kV and a current of 531 µA, with an exposure time of 500 ms, without using a filter. Over 360°, 2400 frames were taken. The data were processed in Datos | x using scan optimization and exported as 16-bit .tiff slices, which were converted to .jpeg images.

2.4. Histological Preparations

One cochlea was sent for histological analysis. This sample was fixed in a 4% formaldehyde solution for 5 days, dehydrated in ethanol 50% and 70%, and imaged using standard microCT to guide the position of the 2D histological sections. LLS Rowiak (LaserLabSolutions, Hanover, Germany) performed polymethylmethacrylate embedding, OCT-guided sectioning with a laser microtome TissueSurgeon and staining of the slices with eosin-hematoxylin.

3. Results

Seven fresh and ten fresh-frozen were visually inspected by OCT in the three-dimensional plane. The fresh samples were analyzed and imaged within 24 h after the death of the donor, while the fresh-frozen samples were preserved by freezing them at $-18°$ for a longer period of time and were thawed at $4°$ 24 h before OCT imaging was carried out. After visual inspection, fifteen samples were included for further analysis. Two samples were excluded because of the presence of air bubbles in the ST and SV. The sample characteristics are summarized in Appendix A. An overview of transmembrane OCT images of all cochleae is provided in Appendix B. When it comes to scanning rates, our results show that a lower scanning time (e.g., 76 kHz) results in a shorter acquisition time but a lower overall quality due to a decreased signal-to-noise ratio (SNR). On the other hand, a longer scanning time (e.g., 10 kHz) leads to higher overall quality because of an increased SNR, which enabled us to align structures within the sensory epithelium more clearly.

3.1. Intracochlear Microanatomy

First, we investigated intracochlear microanatomy by means of nondestructive transmembrane OCT imaging and studied their appearance on the OCT images. We were able to clearly distinguish previously described intracochlear structures. The RWM separates the inner ear from the middle ear and is the first structure to backscatter the infrared light; it has the brightest intensity in the OCT image. The segmentation of a 3D image in Figure 1A illustrates the relation of the intracochlear structures with respect to the RWM.

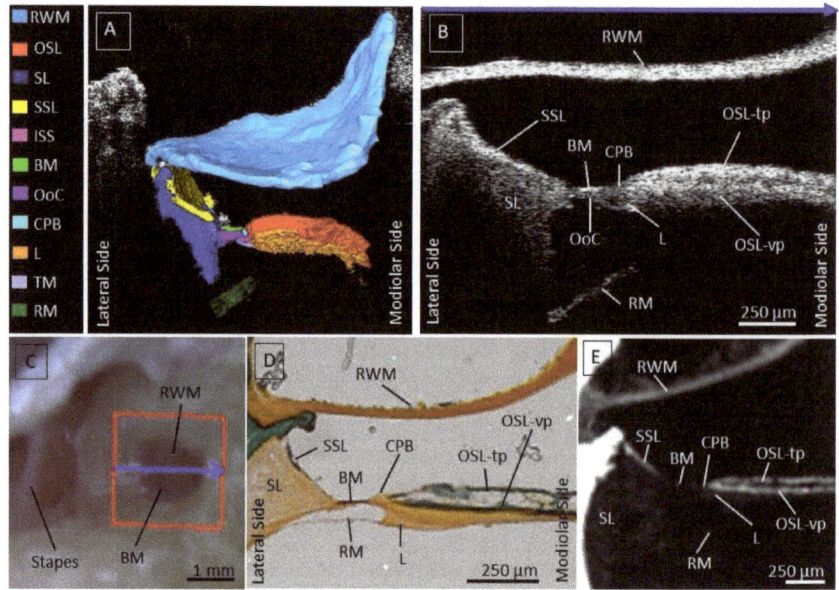

Figure 1. (**A**): Segmentation of a 3D OCT image; each structure is illustrated in a different color indicated in the legend. (**B**): OCT cross-section, with an a-scan rate of 10 kHz. Highly scattering structures result in whiter color, nicely indicating the border between the SSL and SL and CPB and OSL. (**C**): Corresponding microscopic view of the RWM, with the blue arrow indicating the location of the cross-section in (**B**). The location of the BM is visible through the transparent RWM as a dark line beneath the RWM. The stapes is located superior to the RWM. (**D**): Histology with Masson-Goldner staining as a reference to the structures on the OCT images. (**E**): Microcomputed topographical image, providing an extra comparison for the visualized structures on the OCT image in (**B**). Abbreviations: Round window membrane (RWM), Osseous spiral lamina—tympanic plate (OSL-tp), vestibular plate (OSL-vp), cochlear partition bridge (CPB), Basilar Membrane (BM), Organ of Corti (OoC), Secondary spiral lamina (SSL), Spiral ligament (SL), Spiral Limbus (L) and Reissner's Membrane (RM).

Underneath the RWM, the osseous spiral lamina (OSL) separates the scala tympani (ST) from the scala vestibuli (SV). This structure is recognizable on the one hand due to the gap between the vestibular (OSL-vp) and tympanic plate (OSL-tp), indicating the location of the auditory nerve fibers running in between, and on the other hand, due to the high reflectance and intensity of the bony structure, indicated in Figure 1B. The OSL-vp is located underneath the gap, where the nerves run through. The less reflective part underneath the OSL-vp is the tympanic lip of the limbus.

Laterally from OSL, the CPB can be recognized based on lower reflectivity than the OSL. Laterally from the CPB, the BM forms the base for the epithelial cells of the organ of Corti, appearing as a thin, mostly high-scattering layer.

Next to the BM towards the later wall, a triangle-shaped soft tissue structure is visible, the spiral ligament (SL). Besides its typical shape, the soft-tissue SL can be recognized based on its less reflective appearance on the OCT images. The most lateral part of the SL is often shadowed by the bony secondary spiral lamina (SSL) resting on top of the SL at the ST side. The SSL can usually be discerned well from the SL based on its higher reflectivity.

The Scala Media and Scala Vestibuli are separated by the Reissner's membrane, visible on OCT images as a tilted thin layer running underneath the OSL, BM, and SL. The attachment of the Reissner's membrane onto the OSL is often not clearly visible because it is covered by the shadow of the bony OSL. The visualized structures within the OCT image illustrated in Figure 1B, we compared using Masson-Goldner histological staining (Figure 1D, and on the other hand, using microCT (Figure 1E). In the figure, the microscopic view of the RWM was also added, where the blue arrow over the RWM corresponds to the visualized OCT cross-section, indicated by the blue arrow at the top of Figure 1B.

3.2. The Human Organ of Corti

Since the organ of Corti (OoC) is the most crucial part of the human hearing system and the target for various inner ear therapies, we studied its anatomy on OCT more in detail and added a close-up OCT image and additional schematic representation of the visualized structures in a fresh sample (Figure 2). The OCT images have the required resolution to delineate different parts within the OoC, where the tunnel of Corti (TC) and inner spiral sulcus (ISS) are operating as crucial landmarks. The ISS is covered by the tectorial membrane (TM), which separates it from the SM. Besides its typical shape, the TM can be recognized as a structure covering the medial part of the OoC. The TC, the ISS, and the TM form an important indication to estimate the location of the outer and inner groups of cells and can be followed through different cross-sections in a 3D image. The most lateral part of the TM covers the three OHC rows, which rest on top of the Deiter cells (DC) and are neighbored at the medial side by the outer pillar cells (OPC), all of which are located laterally from the TC. At the current resolution (4.73 µm × 4.62 µm × 2.39 µm), the individual cells cannot be distinguished from each other, and we indicated them on the OCT image as a group of 'outer cells'. Likewise, we indicated the 'inner cells' (inner hair cells, inner phalangeal cells, and inner pillar cells) between the TC and the ISS based on the histological slice in Figure 2C.

At the modiolar side, the (thinner) TM is attached to the (thicker) spiral limbus, which can be distinguished from the OSL based on its lower reflectivity. In the proximal hook region, the spiral limbus sits on top of both the CPB and the OSL.

3.3. The Cochlear Partition Bridge and Spiral Limbus

Raufer et al. recently reported that in human cochleae, the OSL connects to the BM through an intermediary structure called the CPB, such that the OoC sits on top of the BM and the CPB [25]. OCT enabled us to study the microanatomy of the most proximal CPB in more detail (Figure 3). This structure could be clearly discerned on OCT images: the reflectivity of the soft-tissue CPB is lower than the bony OSL, and the CPB is thicker than the BM. Since the CPB is the shortest in the base, we were able to only image a small part of it in the proximate hook region. The spiral limbus is neighbored by both OSL and CPB and is visible as a less reflective structure, a soft tissue structure underneath the vestibular plate (Figure 3).

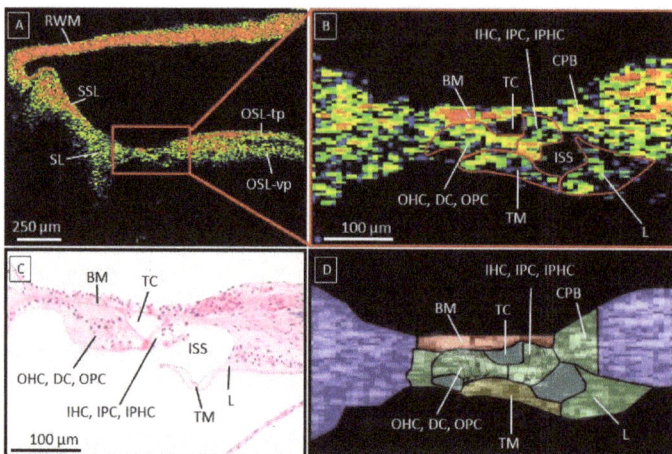

Figure 2. (**A**): illustrates an OCT cross-section (a-scan rate 10 kHz) of a fresh human temporal bone in color scale, with high scattering tissue in red. (**B**): is a zoomed-in cross-section of the OoC, with the cell groups indicated based on important landmarks such as the ISS, TM, and TC. (**C**): Histological section as validation for the OoC anatomy. (**D**): Schematic overview of the recognizable structures within the OoC. Abbreviations; Basilar membrane (BM), tunnel of Corti (TC), inner hair cells (IHC), outer hair cells (OHC), inner spiral sulcus (ISS), Tectorial membrane (TM), Spiral Limbus (L), Reticular Lamina (RL), Osseous Spiral Lamina tympanic plate (OSL-tp), OSL vestibular plate (OSL-vp), Reissner's membrane (RM), Spiral Ligament (SL), Secondary Spiral Lamina (SSL), Round window membrane (RWM). Figure 2C was used with the written permission of the Massachusetts Eye and Ear otopathology temporal bone atlas.

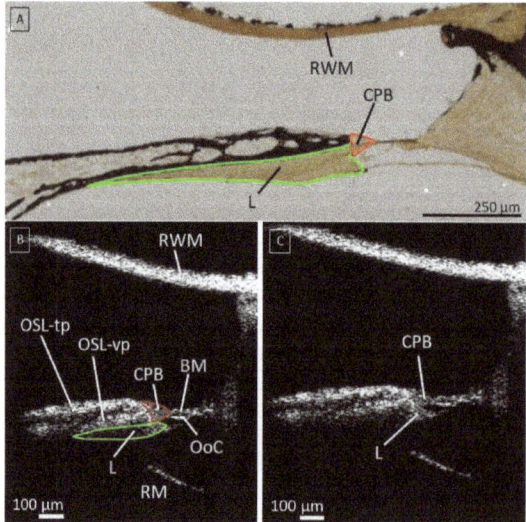

Figure 3. (**A**): Histological slice using von Kossa/von Gieson staining to illustrate the location of the CPB and L. (**B**); The cochlear partition bridge (CPB), aligned in red, is visible as a less reflective structure compared to the osseous spiral lamina illustrated in image (**C**). It is narrow at the base of the cochlea, indicated in the red circle in (**B**). The spiral limbus is aligned in green. (**C**) Same picture without labels and markings. A-scan rate of 10 kHz; Abbreviations: Round window membrane (RWM), Osseous spiral lamina—tympanic plate (OSL-tp), vestibular plate (OSL-vp), cochlear partition bridge (CPB), Basilar Membrane (BM), Organ of Corti (OoC), Spiral Limbus (L) and Reissner's Membrane (RM).

3.4. Deviating Appearance of Intracochlear Structures

Apart from the natural intracochlear anatomy, we investigated if transmembrane OCT also enables the detection of deviating appearance of the structures within the SM, relevant for intracochlear diagnostics. The most common deviation was the disappearance of the Organ of Corti OoC epithelium, leaving only the BM as a straight thin line between the CPB, OSL, and the SL, visible in Figure 4 (after freezing, false color and greyscale OCT), and Appendix B. In one case, transmembrane OCT imaging was performed in a fresh sample received a few hours after the death of the donor, thus before freezing and after freezing for six months at −18°. Before freezing, the sensory epithelium was present on top of the BM so that the combined central thickness amounted to 57 μm. After freezing, the epithelium could no longer be discerned, leaving the BM at a central thickness of 32 μm (Figure 4). The microscopic view on the RWM and Stapes in Figure 4 showed no clear differences before and after freezing. Overall, we saw more remnants of the sensory epithelium in fresh OCT-imaged samples compared to the samples, which were fresh-frozen and needed to be thawed before they were imaged for the first time. This may indicate freezing-induced damage.

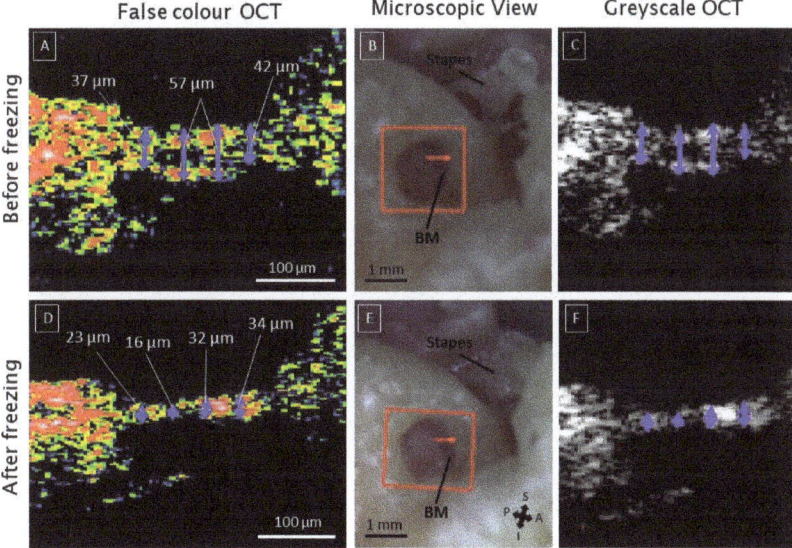

Figure 4. The disappearance of the hearing epithelium in the organ of Corti after freezing. This example is from the same sample at different scanning times. (**A**): the sample was first scanned after the release from the mortuary, and important landmarks within the OoC are visible, such as the ISS and TC. (**B,C**) are the corresponding microscopic and greyscale images, respectively. The red arrow indicates the location of the cross-section of the OCT images. (**D**): shows the same sample but at a later scanning date, where it was frozen and thawed again before the scanning. (**E,F**) are the corresponding microscopic and greyscale images, respectively. The blue arrows and corresponding thickness measures show how the freezing process altered the condition of the sensory epithelium. The a-scan rate of the OCT images was set to 76 kHz. Abbreviations; basilar membrane (BM), superior (S), inferior (I), anterior (A), and posterior (P).

Another non-natural appearance concerns the varying orientation and shape of the TM, visualized in Figure 5. Figure 5A illustrates the original position of the TM, covering the medial part of the sensory epithelium. In some samples, the TM was detached from the OoC, no longer forming a barrier between the ISS and SM and no longer covering the medial part of the sensory epithelium. This detachment was also often accompanied by deformation of the TM shape and closer proximity to the RM (Figure 5B,D). In Figure 5C, only the spiral limbus remains, and the TM appears to have disappeared.

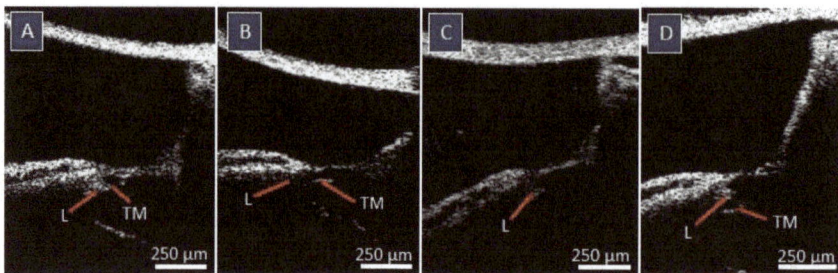

Figure 5. Different shapes, sizes, and orientations of the tectorial membrane (TM). (**A**): the TM in the original position, covering the medial part of the sensory epithelium. (**B**); clear distortions in the shape of the TM. (**C**): the TM disappeared. (**D**): the TM altered towards the SM; however, it must not be confused with the spiral limbus, which got loosened in these images. A-scan rate: 76 kHz Abbreviations: Tympanic membrane (TM) and spiral limbus (L).

Finally, the appearance of the RM varied between samples: in some cochleae, it formed a straight line, as shown in Figure 6A, whereas in the others, the contour of the RM was rather loose and irregular and oftentimes concave towards the SM (Figure 6B).

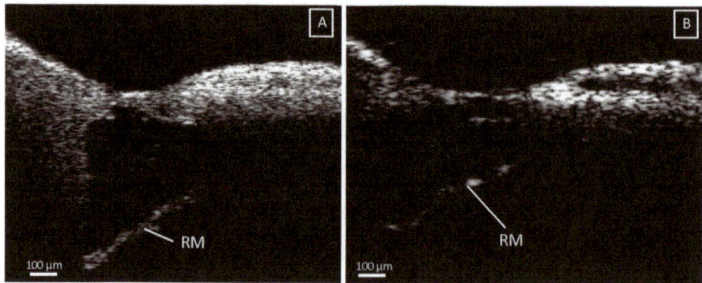

Figure 6. (**A**): Illustration of a straight Reissner's membrane (RM), compared to an irregular, slightly concave towards the scala media (**B**). OCT images were taken with an a-scan rate of 76 kHz. Abbreviations: Reissner's membrane (RM).

3.5. Factors Limiting Imaging through the RWM

In Figure 7, three samples were found to contain a pseudomembrane: one located at the superior rim, one at the anterior rim, and one covering the entire RWM. In Figure 7A,B, the pseudomembrane could be clearly discerned from the RWM as it was never fully attached to the RWM over its entire surface. In Figure 7C, the pseudomembrane covers the entire RWM, making it difficult to differentiate it from the RWM itself. However, it can be distinguished by the thin black line between the membranes, as shown in Appendix B. To clearly align the pseudomembrane covering the entire RWM, multiple cross-sections must be analyzed. On microscopic examination, the pseudomembrane covering the entire RWM appears as a white membrane, while the RWM is typically more transparent (Figure 7(1C)). In some samples, The presence of the pseudomembrane limited the penetration depth of the OCT into the cochlea, making the intracochlear structures less clear (Figure 7B).

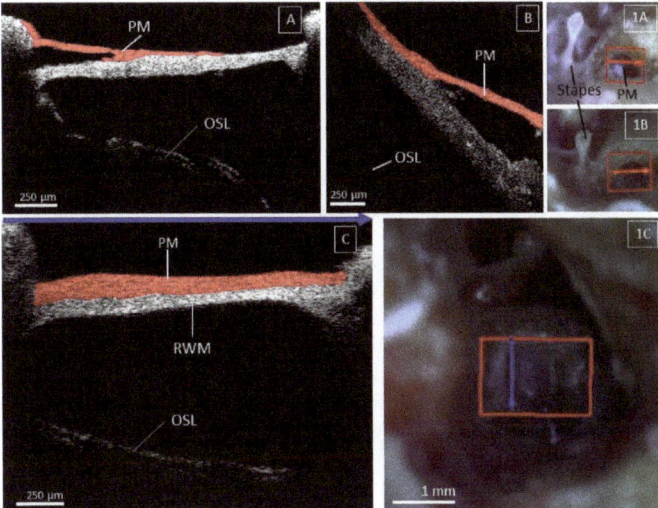

Figure 7. Visualization of pseudomembrane (PM) on top of the round window membrane (RWM). Figure (**1A,1B,1C**) are the corresponding microscopic images, with the blue and red arrows corresponding to the cross-section of the OCT images, indicated by the blue arrow at the top of figure (**C**). The shape, orientation, and extent of the PM were different across all samples and are illustrated in the Figure. (**A,1A**) show a PM covering the RWM at the superior rim. (**B,1B**) show a PM at the anterior rim of the RW niche, limiting the view onto the underlying OSL. (**C,1C**) show a PM covering the entire RWM; due to the perpendicular axis of the internal structures towards the OCT beam, the OSL is still visible; however, it is less reflective. (**A–C**) have an a-scan rate of 10, 76, and 28 kHz, respectively. Abbreviations: Round window membrane (RWM), Pseudomembrane (PM), Osseous spiral lamina (OSL).

4. Discussion

The objective of this study was to provide an OCT-based atlas of the human proximal hook region to aid future clinicians and researchers with the interpretation of transmembrane OCT images of the human cochlea. We performed transmembrane OCT imaging in a series of seventeen human cadaveric cochleae and analyzed the characteristics of the visualized intracochlear structures, which are relevant for inner ear diagnostics and therapies. Our results demonstrate that transmembrane OCT imaging enables nondestructive, high-resolution, 3D visualization of the intracochlear microstructures, which are crucial for hearing function, as well as the detection of abnormalities in these structures. To the best of our knowledge, this was also the first OCT imaging study performed on a large sample size of human cochleae.

We were able to consistently visualize important intracochlear structures in the proximal hook region through the RWM. The RWM is a crucial entry point to the cochlea for inner ear therapies, functional studies, and, most likely intracochlear diagnostics. The proximal hook region is characterized by complex anatomy and is critical for the implementation of inner ear therapies. In particular, the OSL, BM, SSL, and SL, which are structures of interest during cochlear implantation [26,27], could be visualized using transmembrane OCT imaging. Damage occurring at these structures during an electrode insertion can harm residual hearing, causing mechanical-induced hearing loss, inflammation, fibrosis, or ossification of the cochlea [27,28].

Pathologies of the inner ear inducing hearing loss mostly affect the OoC, making it a target structure for the development of gene and inner ear therapies and accurate diagnostics. Based on OCT-based visualization of important landmarks such as the TM, ISS, and TC, we could determine the position of the inner and outer hair cells together with the supporting epithelium surrounding them. At the current resolution, it was not possible to visualize the cells of the sensory epithelium individually; however, in the future, this can be tackled by using functional OCT [11,29–31]. On the other hand, improving the resolution could be achieved by increasing the spectral bandwidth of the light source and enhancing the resolution of the optical spectrometer that records the reflected light's interference spectrum. However, spreading the signal over a larger detection array requires a higher optical output to maintain a similar signal-to-noise ratio (SNR). Some of these challenges have been addressed in a recent study, but these solutions have not yet been implemented in commercially available OCT systems [32].

Recently, the CPB, a soft tissue structure between the OSL and BM, has been identified in humans, differentiating it from the cochlear partition composition of rodents [25]. In this study, we were able to visualize the CPB in the proximal hook region using OCT imaging. Here, the CPB was a remarkably short structure, supporting the most lateral attachment of the spiral limbus. These observations are in line with the description of Raufer et al. [25], stating that the CPB becomes wider from base to apex in the human cochlea. The ability of transmembrane OCT to visualize CPB nondestructively in the proximal hook region of the human cochlea is highly promising for the functional study of inner ear mechanics [25].

In addition, we were able to detect intracochlear abnormalities with unprecedented detail using OCT in an intact human cochlea, which is highly relevant for intracochlear diagnostics and therapy. Out of seventeen specimens, the sensory epithelium was apparent in four fresh samples. In contrast to the other samples, these were not frozen before being imaged with OCT. In one sample, we observed normal sensory epithelium within a few hours post-mortem, but it disappeared after being frozen for six months, suggesting that freezing may have a destructive effect on the sensory epithelium. as it is remarkable that the sensory epithelium was mostly left in fresh samples, compared to fresh frozen samples. This is a significant finding, and on top of that, the sensory epithelium was most likely to be preserved in fresh samples compared to fresh-frozen samples. These findings highlight the importance of using fresh samples for reliable morphological and functional studies of the human cochlea and suggest that further research is needed on the effects of freezing and prolonged frozen storage on the quality of human temporal bones. Additionally, we also observed degenerated sensory epithelium in two fresh cochlear samples. We do not have any otologic background information for these samples, but these results might demonstrate the ability of transmembrane OCT to detect pathological changes in the human organ of Corti, which in clinical practice could be related to ototoxic drugs, noise exposure, aging, genetic factors, or other factors. Furthermore, OCT imaging could be a promising tool to monitor in vivo the efficacy of future regenerating therapies [33].

Other abnormalities were detected at the TM, which is believed to play a key role in hair cell activation in response to acoustical stimulation and undergo significant structural changes and degeneration with aging [34–36]. We were able to visualize detachment of the TM from the limbus, a structural indication that is potentially linked to (the onset of) age-related hearing loss and hence relevant for future studies regarding future inner ear (gene) therapies and nondestructive (preventive) diagnostics [35,36]. While no otologic background information about the donors is known, the median age of the donors was 77 (range between 55 and 90 years) and thus might show signs of age-related hearing loss. However, why hypothesize that aging will not significantly affect the location of the visualized intracochlear structures using OCT but further clinical application in hearing-impaired subjects would be necessary to investigate the effect of aging on the integrity of intracochlear structures.

Additionally, we were also able to evaluate the RM through the RWM. The RM separates the SM from the SV and normally is tense between its attachment at the OSL and the lateral wall. Included in our intracochlear OCT atlas are both a straight tensed RM and a flaccid RM. The cause of the latter appearance is not known, yet in certain pathologies such as Meniere's disease, endolymphatic hydrops in the SM can cause distension of the RM [37]. In OCT images of the isolated cochlea, it is possible that the tension caused by the fluid in the scalae is altered, causing bulging of the RM.

Since OCT imaging was performed through the RWM, any overlying pseudomembrane was also imaged when present [38–41]. A pseudomembrane was noted in 18% of all samples, comparable to the findings of Sahin et al. [41]. Since the RWM is the main access point for transmembrane OCT imaging, the presence of a pseudomembrane could negatively affect the visualization of intracochlear structures. It is not yet clear what the cause of pseudomembranes might be and hence unpredictable whether it is present in a patient who qualifies for inner ear surgery and diagnostics [39]. Regarding inner ear therapy, a pseudomembrane could also negatively affect the diffusion of drugs administered by transtympanic injection into the cochlea [42].

Our results illustrate that transmembrane OCT imaging is a promising tool for clinical practice to nondestructively investigate the intracochlear anatomy in high resolution and in real time. The anatomy of the hook region is individually highly variable, and OCT can be crucial as a tool to anticipate the patient-specific anatomy, decreasing the risk for traumatic CI insertions [43–45]. With the rising interest in residual hearing preservation and atraumatic electrode insertion during CI surgery, understanding the round window area and the anatomy of the proximal hook region is of utmost importance [46]. Additionally, the hook region is also highly relevant regarding safe intratympanic injections, precise diagnostics, gene therapy, and in vivo studies of human intracochlear mechanics [47–49]. OCT meets the needed requirements for in vivo high-resolution imaging, with the advantage of in-depth transmembrane imaging, facilitating the anatomical investigation of the cochlear base without the need for opening the cochlea and disrupting its integrity [14,32,50,51].

OCT imaging does have certain limitations. First, we used extracted cochleae, providing the advantage of determining the optimal imaging angle, which might be unachievable in clinical settings. One solution might be using an endoscopic-based OCT through a transcanal approach, which might account for the limited degree of freedom one experiences within an entire skull [32,51]. To achieve comparable imaging results to a rigid OCT system, an endoscopic OCT system would need to be specially designed and optimized for imaging the cochlea. This might involve using a smaller, more flexible endoscope and a light source with a broader spectrum to improve the resolution and contrast of the images. It would also require advanced imaging algorithms and specialized image processing techniques to improve the overall quality of the images produced [32].

Furthermore, due to the limited imaging depth of the OCT, we were only able to image the approximate hook region. Because of this, the apex of the cochlea remains unreachable with OCT. In the future, fiberoptic tools might provide a solution for this, such as imaging of the intracochlear space during the insertion of a cochlear implant or during the injection of intracochlear therapies [50]. Finally, certain factors may negatively affect the quality of transmembrane OCT imaging: a thickened RWM, pseudomembrane, and remaining debris or fluid on top of the RWM. Lowering the scanning frequency, removing the debris, and aspiration of the fluid can overcome these limiting factors. In many cases, the pseudomembrane also can be carefully removed by the surgeon. The origin of a pseudomembrane is not yet known, but it might be related to middle ear infections. However, clinical evidence for this correlation is still lacking, and further research is needed to investigate this. A mucosal pseudomembrane found adjacent to the surface of the RWM may impact its permeability. They may either inhibit diffusion by acting as an additional barrier, protecting the RWM [41,52]. On the other hand, several pathologies, such as Menière's disease or chronic otitis media, can cause the thickening of the RWM itself, which might negatively affect transmembrane OCT imaging and its future applications [53,54]. Additionally, the presence of blood in a clinical setting on top of the RWM could form an additional challenge, as blood is highly scattered. This could be helped with the aspiration of the blood drops and better control of the blood pressure, as it is currently conducted during cochlear implant surgery.

In summary, various studies investigated intracochlear anatomy using transmembrane OCT imaging; most of these were based on animal research [14,29,30,55–57]. Here, we provide an extensive imaging atlas of the human intracochlear anatomy in the proximal hook region, which would help future otologic researchers and clinicians to familiarize themselves with the features of intracochlear structures on OCT images. We were able to consistently visualize relevant intracochlear microstructures at a very high resolution and illustrated both normal and abnormal anatomical appearances using transmembrane OCT imaging. Being able to disentangle normal and abnormal composition of intracochlear structures, together with the fact that OCT is nondestructive and can be used in real-time in vivo, makes it a highly promising tool for clinical practice. OCT is a step forward towards aiding hearing-impaired patients in getting a safe insertion of inner ear therapies and enabling microstructural inner ear diagnostics, which is currently not possible.

Author Contributions: Conceptualization, L.K., A.S., T.P., J.W. and N.V.; methodology, L.K., A.S., T.P., J.W. and N.V.; validation, L.K., A.S., T.P. and N.V.; formal analysis, L.K. and A.S.; investigation, A.S.; resources, L.K. and A.S.; data curation, L.K. and A.S.; writing—original draft preparation, L.K., A.S., J.W., T.P. and N.V.; writing—review and editing, L.K., A.S., T.P., J.W. and N.V.; visualization, L.K.; supervision, J.W. and N.V.; project administration, L.K., A.S., T.P., J.W. and N.V. All authors have read and agreed to the published version of the manuscript.

Funding: This research was funded by Flemish Research Foundation (FWO), project grant G088619N, senior clinical investigator fund 1804816N, postdoctoral fellowship grant 12Y6919N, and predoctoral fellowship grants 1S78519N, 1S78521N, and 11D5723N.

Institutional Review Board Statement: The study was conducted in accordance with the Declaration of Helsinki and approved by the Institutional Review Board (or Ethics Committee) of the Medical Ethics Committee of the University Hospitals of Leuven (approval No. NH019 2016-06-04).

Informed Consent Statement: Not applicable.

Data Availability Statement: Data available upon reasonable request.

Acknowledgments: The authors thank Alicia Quesnel and her colleagues at the otopathology laboratory of Massachusetts eye and ear institution at Harvard University for the histological image. The authors thank the donors of the temporal bones and the colleagues of the Vesalius Institute and UZ Leuven Mortuary for the harvesting of the temporal bones.

Conflicts of Interest: The authors declare no conflict of interest.

Appendix A

Sample	age	gender	L/R	Fresh/fresh-frozen
1	86	F	L	Fresh-frozen
2	86	M	L	Fresh
3	86	M	L	Fresh-frozen
4	90	F	L	Fresh-frozen
5	72	F	R	Fresh
6	72	F	L	Fresh
7	71	M	R	Fresh-frozen
8	78	F	R	Fresh-frozen
9	88	M	R	Fresh-frozen
10	64	M	R	Fresh-frozen
11	73	M	R	Fresh-frozen
12	55	M	R	Fresh-frozen
13	72	M	R	Fresh
14	77	M	R	Fresh
15	Unknown	Unknown	R	Fresh
16	Unknown	Unknown	R	Fresh-frozen
17	Unknown	Unknown	R	Fresh-frozen

Figure A1. Figure A1 presents information about the characteristics of the samples used in the study. The figure includes information about the age and gender of the donors, as well as which side of the body the sample was taken from. The figure also indicates whether the sample was fresh or fresh-frozen. A fresh sample was imaged within 24 h after the donor's death, while a fresh-frozen sample was first frozen and then thawed before being imaged.

Appendix B

Abbreviations: Round window membrane (RWM), Osseous spiral lamina—tympanic plate (OSL-tp), vestibular plate (OSL-vp), cochlear partition bridge (CPB), Basilar Membrane (BM), Organ of Corti (OoC), Secondary spiral lamina (SSL), Spiral ligament (SL), Spiral Limbus (L), and Reissner's Membrane (RM).

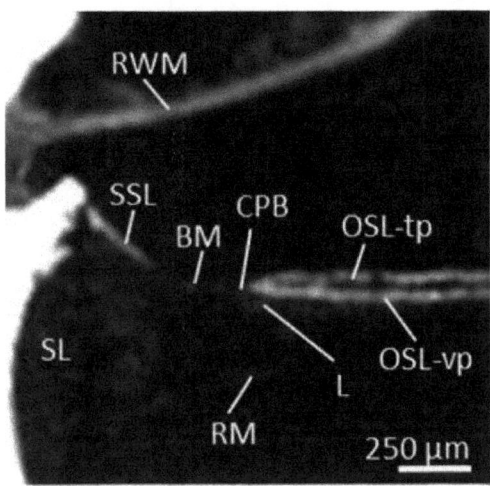

Figure A2. An enlargement of the microCT image in Figure 1E, which corresponds to the OCT image in Figure 1B.

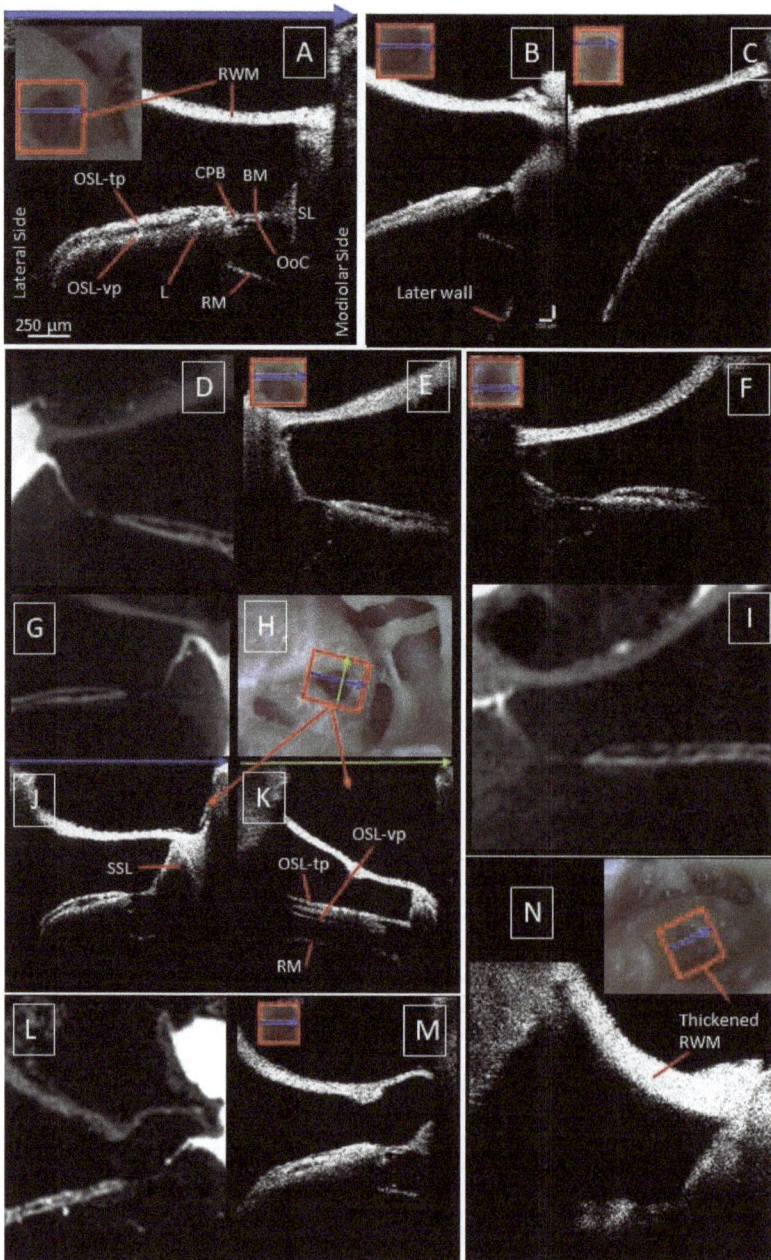

Figure A3. (**A**), the blue arrow on top of the OCT cross-section corresponds to the blue or green arrow at the RWM. In Figure (**B**), a small part of the lateral wall is visible. In (**C**), the BM and RM are shadowed towards the lateral wall. Figure (**D**) is the corresponding microCT image of Figure (**E**). Figure (**F**) corresponds to Figure (**I**), while Figure (**G**) corresponds to Figure (**J**), with the microscopic view and cross-section in the x-direction (green arrow) indicated in Figures (**H**,**K**), respectively. Figure (**L**) corresponds to the OCT cross-section in (**M**). Figure (**N**) includes both the microscopic view and corresponding OCT image. A-scan rates for OCT images from A to N: 76 kHz, 10 kHz, 76 kHz, 10 kHz, 10 kHz, 76 kHz, 76 kHz, 10 kHz, and 10 kHz.

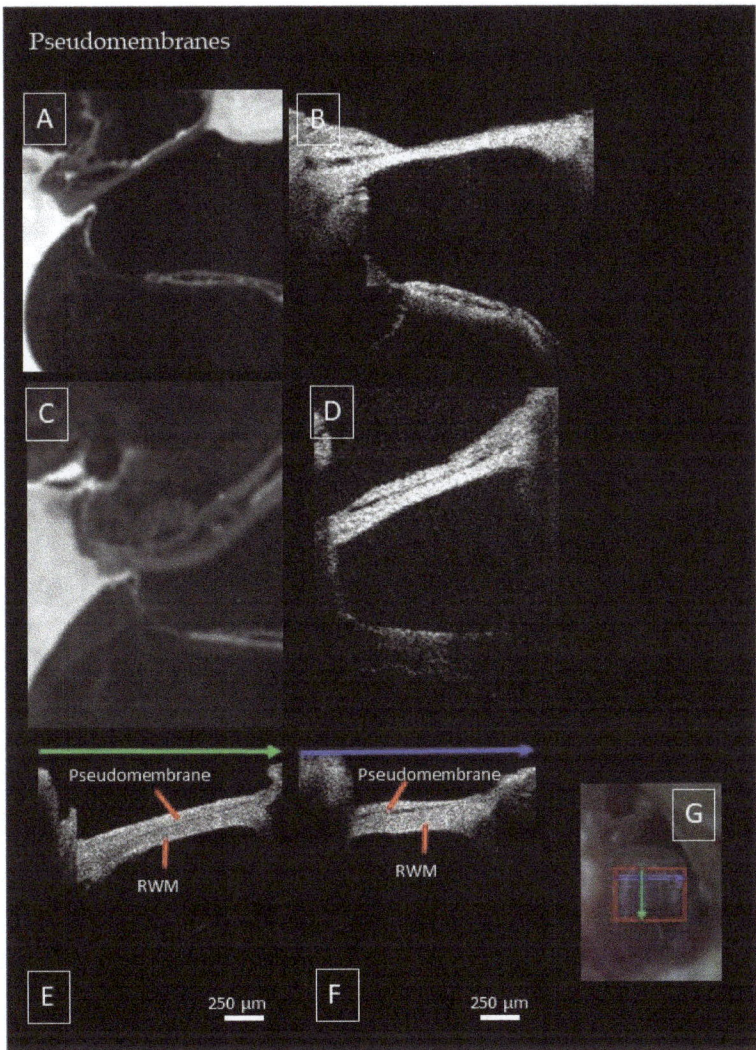

Figure A4. This supplementary Figure illustrates the presence of a pseudomembrane. Figure (**A**) is a microCT image of the same sample as in Figure (**B**), and Figure (**C**) corresponds to Figure (**D**). Figure (**E**) shows a cross-section in the x-direction, indicated by the green arrow on top of the figure and in the microscopic image in Figure (**G**). Figure (**F**) is a cross-section in the y-direction, indicated by the blue arrow on top of the image and in the corresponding microscopic image (**G**). The pseudomembrane is visible as a thin black gap between the pseudomembrane and the RWM. A-scan rates for OCT images (**B**–**F**) are respectively 10 kHz, 76 kHz, 28 kHz, and 28 kHz.

References

1. World Health Organization (WHO). Deafness and Hearing Impairment. Available online: http://www.who.int/news-room/fact-sheets/detail/deafness-and-hearing-loss (accessed on 1 August 2021).
2. Ford, A.H.; Hankey, G.J.; Yeap, B.B.; Golledge, J.; Flicker, L.; Almeida, O.P. Hearing loss and the risk of dementia in later life. *Maturitas* **2018**, *112*, 1–11. [CrossRef] [PubMed]
3. Ciorba, A.; Bianchini, C.; Pelucchi, S.; Pastore, A. The impact of hearing loss on the quality of life of elderly adults. *Clin. Interv. Aging* **2012**, *7*, 159–163. [CrossRef] [PubMed]
4. Devare, J.; Gubbels, S.; Raphael, Y. Outlook and future of inner ear therapy. *Hear. Res.* **2018**, *368*, 127–135. [CrossRef] [PubMed]

5. Minoda, R.; Miwa, T.; Ise, M.; Takeda, H. Potential treatments for genetic hearing loss in humans: Current conundrums. *Gene Ther.* **2015**, *22*, 603–609. [CrossRef]
6. Zanzonico, P. *Basic Sciences of Nuclear Medicine*, 2nd ed.; Khalil, M.M., Ed.; Springer: Berlin/Heidelberg, Germany, 2011.
7. Montgomery, S.C.; Cox, B.C. Whole Mount Dissection and Immunofluorescence of the Adult Mouse Cochlea. *J. Vis. Exp.* **2016**, *2016*, e53561. [CrossRef]
8. Brody, K.M.; Hampson, A.J.; Cho, H.-J.; Johnson, P.; O'Leary, S.J. A new method for three-dimensional immunofluorescence study of the cochlea. *Hear. Res.* **2020**, *392*, 107956. [CrossRef]
9. Matthews, T.J.; Adamson, R. Optical coherence tomography: Current and future clinical applications in otology. *Curr. Opin. Otolaryngol. Head Neck Surg.* **2020**, *28*, 296–301. [CrossRef]
10. Wong, B.J.F.; de Boer, J.F.; Park, B.H.; Chen, Z.; Nelson, J.S. Optical coherence tomography of the rat cochlea. *J. Biomed. Opt.* **2000**, *5*, 367–370. [CrossRef]
11. Iyer, J.S.; Batts, S.A.; Chu, K.K.; Sahin, M.I.; Leung, H.M.; Tearney, G.J.; Stankovic, K.M. Micro-optical coherence tomography of the mammalian cochlea. *Sci. Rep.* **2016**, *6*, 33288. [CrossRef]
12. Mchugh, C.I.; Raufer, S.; Cho, N.H.; Zosuls, A.; Tubelli, A.A.; Ravicz, M.E.; O'connor, K.N.; Guinan, J.J.; Puria, S.; Nakajima, H.H. Human Cochlear Partition Anatomy and Motion Using Optical Coherence Tomography. In Proceedings of the Mechanics of Hearing (MOH) Workshop, Helsingor, Denmark, 24–29 July 2022.
13. Subhash, H.M.; Davila, V.; Sun, H.; Nguyen-Huynh, A.T.; Nuttall, A.L.; Wang, R.K. Volumetric in vivo imaging of intracochlear microstructures in mice by high-speed spectral domain optical coherence tomography. *J. Biomed. Opt.* **2010**, *15*, 036024. [CrossRef]
14. Starovoyt, A.; Putzeys, T.; Wouters, J.; Verhaert, N. High-resolution Imaging of the Human Cochlea through the Round Window by means of Optical Coherence Tomography. *Sci. Rep.* **2019**, *9*, 14271. [CrossRef] [PubMed]
15. Reif, R.; Zhi, Z.; Dziennis, S.; Nuttall, A.L.; Wang, R.K. Changes in cochlear blood flow in mice due to loud sound exposure measured with Doppler optical microangiography and laser Doppler flowmetry. *Quant. Imaging Med. Surg.* **2013**, *3*, 235–242. [CrossRef] [PubMed]
16. Dziennis, S.; Reif, R.; Zhi, Z.; Nuttall, A.L.; Wang, R.K. Effects of hypoxia on cochlear blood flow in mice evaluated using Doppler optical microangiography. *J. Biomed. Opt.* **2012**, *17*, 1060031. [CrossRef] [PubMed]
17. Burwood, G.W.S.; Dziennis, S.; Wilson, T.; Foster, S.; Zhang, Y.; Liu, G.; Yang, J.; Elkins, S.; Nuttall, A.L. The mechanoelectrical transducer channel is not required for regulation of cochlear blood flow during loud sound exposure in mice. *Sci. Rep.* **2020**, *10*, 9229. [CrossRef]
18. Sun, J.G.; Adie, S.G.; Chaney, E.J.; Boppart, S.A. Segmentation and correlation of optical coherence tomography and X-ray images for breast cancer diagnostics. *J. Innov. Opt. Heal. Sci.* **2013**, *06*, 1350015. [CrossRef]
19. Pierce, M.C.; Strasswimmer, J.; Park, B.H.; Cense, B.; de Boer, J.F. Advances in Optical Coherence Tomography Imaging for Dermatology. *J. Investig. Dermatol.* **2004**, *123*, 458–463. [CrossRef]
20. Vignali, L.; Solinas, E.; Emanuele, E. Research and Clinical Applications of Optical Coherence Tomography in Invasive Cardiology: A Review. *Curr. Cardiol. Rev.* **2014**, *10*, 369–376. [CrossRef]
21. Tearney, G.J.; Brezinski, M.E.; Southern, J.F.; Bouma, B.E.; Hee, M.R.; Fujimoto, J.G. Determination of the Refractive Index of Highly Scattering Human Tissue by Optical Coherence Tomography. *Opt. Lett.* **1995**, *20*, 2258–2260. [CrossRef]
22. Kerckhofs, G.; Stegen, S.; van Gastel, N.; Sap, A.; Falgayrac, G.; Penel, G.; Durand, M.; Luyten, F.P.; Geris, L.; Vandamme, K.; et al. Simultaneous three-dimensional visualization of mineralized and soft skeletal tissues by a novel microCT contrast agent with polyoxometalate structure. *Biomaterials* **2018**, *159*, 1–12. [CrossRef]
23. De Bournonville, S.; Vangrunderbeeck, S.; Ly, H.G.T.; Geeroms, C.; De Borggraeve, W.M.; Parac-Vogt, T.N.; Kerckhofs, G. Exploring polyoxometalates as non-destructive staining agents for contrast-enhanced microfocus computed tomography of biological tissues. *Acta Biomater.* **2020**, *105*, 253–262. [CrossRef]
24. De Clercq, K.; Persoons, E.; Napso, T.; Luyten, C.; Parac-Vogt, T.N.; Sferruzzi-Perri, A.N.; Kerckhofs, G.; Vriens, J. High-resolution contrast-enhanced microCT reveals the true three-dimensional morphology of the murine placenta. *Proc. Natl. Acad. Sci. USA* **2019**, *116*, 13927–13936. [CrossRef] [PubMed]
25. Raufer, S.; Guinan, J.J.; Nakajima, H.H. Cochlear partition anatomy and motion in humans differ from the classic view of mammals. *Proc. Natl. Acad. Sci. USA* **2019**, *116*, 13977–13982. [CrossRef] [PubMed]
26. Rask-Andersen, H.; Liu, W.; Erixon, E.; Kinnefors, A.; Pfaller, K.; Schrott-Fischer, A.; Glueckert, R. Human Cochlea: Anatomical Characteristics and their Relevance for Cochlear Implantation. *Anat. Rec.* **2012**, *295*, 1791–1811. [CrossRef] [PubMed]
27. Agrawal, S.; Schart-Morén, N.; Liu, W.; Ladak, H.M.; Rask-Andersen, H.; Li, H. The secondary spiral lamina and its relevance in cochlear implant surgery. *Upsala J. Med Sci.* **2018**, *123*, 9–18. [CrossRef]
28. Bas, E.; Dinh, C.T.; Garnham, C.; Polak, M.; Van de Water, T.R. Conservation of hearing and protection of hair cells in cochlear implant patients' with residual hearing. *Anat. Rec.* **2012**, *295*, 1909–1927. [CrossRef]
29. Cooper, N.P.; Vavakou, A.; Van Der Heijden, M. Vibration hotspots reveal longitudinal funneling of sound-evoked motion in the mammalian cochlea. *Nat. Commun.* **2018**, *9*, 3054. [CrossRef]
30. Dong, W.; Xia, A.; Raphael, P.D.; Puria, S.; Applegate, B.E.; Oghalai, J.S. Organ of Corti vibration within the intact gerbil cochlea measured by volumetric optical coherence tomography and vibrometry. *J. Neurophysiol.* **2018**, *120*, 2847–2857. [CrossRef]
31. Jawadi, Z.; Applegate, B.E.; Oghalai, J.S. Optical Coherence Tomography to Measure Sound-Induced Motions Within the Mouse Organ of Corti In Vivo. In *Methods in Molecular Biology*; Humana Press: New York, NY, USA, 2016; Volume 1427, pp. 449–462.

32. Iyer, J.S.; Yin, B.; Stankovic, K.M.; Tearney, G.J. Endomicroscopy of the human cochlea using a micro-optical coherence tomography catheter. *Sci. Rep.* **2021**, *11*, 17932. [CrossRef]
33. He, L.; Guo, J.-Y.; Liu, K.; Wang, G.-P.; Gong, S.-S. Research Progress on Flat Epithelium of the Inner Ear. *Physiol. Res.* **2020**, *69*, 775–785. [CrossRef]
34. Lukashkin, A.N.; Richardson, G.P.; Russell, I.J. Multiple roles for the tectorial membrane in the active cochlea. *Hear. Res.* **2010**, *266*, 26–35. [CrossRef]
35. Bullen, A.; Forge, A.; Wright, A.; Richardson, G.P.; Goodyear, R.J.; Taylor, R. Ultrastructural defects in stereocilia and tectorial membrane in aging mouse and human cochleae. *J. Neurosci. Res.* **2020**, *98*, 1745–1763. [CrossRef] [PubMed]
36. Goodyear, R.J.; Cheatham, M.A.; Naskar, S.; Zhou, Y.; Osgood, R.T.; Zheng, J.; Richardson, G.P. Accelerated Age-Related Degradation of the Tectorial Membrane in the Ceacam16βgal/βgal Null Mutant Mouse, a Model for Late-Onset Human Hereditary Deafness DFNB. *Front. Mol. Neurosci.* **2019**, *12*, 147. [CrossRef]
37. Salt, A.N.; Plontke, S.K. Endolymphatic Hydrops: Pathophysiology and Experimental Models. *Otolaryngol. Clin. North Am.* **2010**, *43*, 971–983. [CrossRef]
38. AlZamil, K.S.; Linthicum, F.H. Extraneous round window membranes and plugs: Possible effect on intratympanic therapy. *Ann. Otol. Rhinol. Laryngol.* **2000**, *109*, 30–32. [CrossRef] [PubMed]
39. Luers, J.C.; Hüttenbrink, K.B.; Beutner, D. Surgical anatomy of the round window-Implications for cochlear implantation. *Clin. Otolaryngol.* **2018**, *43*, 417–424. [CrossRef] [PubMed]
40. Marchioni, D.; Alicandri-Ciufelli, M.; Pothier, D.; Rubini, A.; Presutti, L. The round window region and contiguous areas: Endoscopic anatomy and surgical implications. *Eur. Arch. Oto-Rhino-Laryngol.* **2015**, *272*, 1103–1112. [CrossRef] [PubMed]
41. Şahin, B.; Orhan, K.S.; Aslıyüksek, H.; Kara, E.; Büyük, Y.; Güldiken, Y. Endoscopic evaluation of middle ear anatomic variations in autopsy series: Analyses of 204 ears. *Braz. J. Otorhinolaryngol.* **2020**, *86*, 74–82. [CrossRef]
42. Plontke, S.K.; Salt, A.N. Local drug delivery to the inner ear: Principles, practice, and future challenges. *Hear. Res.* **2018**, *368*, 18. [CrossRef]
43. Koch, R.W.; Elfarnawany, M.; Zhu, N.; Ladak, H.M.; Agrawal, S.K. Evaluation of Cochlear Duct Length Computations Using Synchrotron Radiation Phase-Contrast Imaging. *Otol. Neurotol.* **2017**, *38*, e92–e99. [CrossRef]
44. Erixon, E.; Rask-Andersen, H. How to predict cochlear length before cochlear implantation surgery. *Acta Oto-Laryngol.* **2013**, *133*, 1258–1265. [CrossRef]
45. Atturo, F.; Barbara, M.; Rask-Andersen, H. On the Anatomy of the 'Hook' Region of the Human Cochlea and How It Relates to Cochlear Implantation. *Audiol. Neurotol.* **2014**, *19*, 378–385. [CrossRef] [PubMed]
46. Jwair, S.; Prins, A.; Wegner, I.; Stokroos, R.J.; Versnel, H.; Thomeer, H.G.X.M. Scalar Translocation Comparison Between Lateral Wall and Perimodiolar Cochlear Implant Arrays-A Meta-Analysis. *Laryngoscope* **2021**, *131*, 1358–1368. [CrossRef] [PubMed]
47. Géléoc, G.S.G.; Holt, J.R. Sound Strategies for Hearing Restoration. *Science* **2014**, *344*, 1241062. [CrossRef] [PubMed]
48. Landegger, L.D.; Psaltis, D.; Stankovic, K.M. Human audiometric thresholds do not predict specific cellular damage in the inner ear. *Hear. Res.* **2016**, *335*, 83–93. [CrossRef] [PubMed]
49. Kujawa, S.G.; Liberman, M.C. Translating animal models to human therapeutics in noise-induced and age-related hearing loss. *Hear. Res.* **2019**, *377*, 44–52. [CrossRef]
50. Starovoyt, A.; Quirk, B.C.; Putzeys, T.; Kerckhofs, G.; Nuyts, J.; Wouters, J.; McLaughlin, R.A.; Verhaert, N. An Optically-Guided Cochlear Implant Sheath for Real-Time Monitoring of Electrode Insertion into the Human Cochlea. *Sci Rep.* **2022**, *12*, 19234. [CrossRef]
51. Lin, J.; Staecker, H.; Samir Jafri, M.S. Optical Coherence Tomography Imaging of the Inner Ear: A Feasibility Study With Implications for Cochlear Implantation. *Ann. Otol. Rhinol. Laryngol.* **2008**, *117*, 341–346. [CrossRef]
52. Schachern, P.A.; Paparella, M.M.; Duvall, A.J.; Choo, Y.B. The Human Round Window Membrane: An Electron Microscopic Study. *Arch. Otolaryngol. Head Neck Surg.* **1984**, *110*, 15–21. [CrossRef]
53. Sahni, R.S.; Paparella, M.M.; Schachern, P.A.; Goycoolea, M.V.; Le, C.T. Thickness of the Human Round Window Membrane in Different Forms of Otitis Media. *Arch. Otolaryngol. Head Neck Surg.* **1987**, *113*, 630–634. [CrossRef]
54. Yoda, S.; Cureoglu, S.; Shimizu, S.; Morita, N.; Fukushima, H.; Sato, T.; Harada, T.; Paparella, M.M. Round Window Membrane in Ménière's Disease: A Human Temporal Bone Study. *Otol. Neurotology.* **2011**, *32*, 147–151. [CrossRef]
55. Cho, N.H.; Wang, H.; Puria, S. Cochlear Fluid Spaces and Structures of the Gerbil High-Frequency Region Measured Using Optical Coherence Tomography (OCT). *J. Assoc. Res. Otolaryngol.* **2022**, *23*, 195–211. [CrossRef] [PubMed]
56. Kim, W.; Kim, S.; Oghalai, J.S.; Applegate, B.E. Endoscopic optical coherence tomography enables morphological and subnanometer vibratory imaging of the porcine cochlea through the round window. *Opt. Lett.* **2018**, *43*, 1966. [CrossRef] [PubMed]
57. Burwood, G.W.S.; Fridberger, A.; Wang, R.K.; Nuttall, A.L. Revealing the morphology and function of the cochlea and middle ear with optical coherence tomography. *Quant. Imaging Med. Surg.* **2019**, *9*, 858–881. [CrossRef] [PubMed]

Disclaimer/Publisher's Note: The statements, opinions and data contained in all publications are solely those of the individual author(s) and contributor(s) and not of MDPI and/or the editor(s). MDPI and/or the editor(s) disclaim responsibility for any injury to people or property resulting from any ideas, methods, instructions or products referred to in the content.

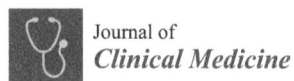

Article

Robotized Cochlear Implantation under Fluoroscopy: A Preliminary Series

Thierry Mom [1,2,*], Mathilde Puechmaille [1], Mohamed El Yagoubi [1], Alexane Lère [1], Jens-Erik Petersen [1], Justine Bécaud [1], Nicolas Saroul [1], Laurent Gilain [1], Sonia Mirafzal [3] and Pascal Chabrot [3]

[1] Department of Otolaryngology Head Neck Surgery, University Hospital Center, Hospital Gabriel Montpied, 58, Rue Montalembert, 63000 Clermont-Ferrand, France
[2] Mixt Unit of Research (UMR) 1107, National Institute of Health and Medical Research (INSERM), University of Clermont Auvergne (UCA), 63000 Clermont-Ferrand, France
[3] Department of Radiology, University Hospital Center, Hospital Gabriel Montpied, 58, Rue Montalembert, 63000 Clermont-Ferrand, France
* Correspondence: tmom@chu-clermontferrand.fr

Abstract: It is known that visual feedback by fluoroscopy can detect electrode array (EA) misrouting within the cochlea while robotized EA-insertion (rob-EAI) permits atraumatic cochlear implantation. We report here our unique experience of both fluoroscopy feedback and rob-EAI in cochlear implant surgery. We retrospectively analyzed a cohort of consecutive patients implanted from November 2021–October 2022 using rob-EAI, with the RobOtol®, to determine the quality of EA-insertion and the additional time required. Twenty-three patients (10 females, 61+/−19 yo) were tentatively implanted using robot assistance, with a rob-EAI speed < 1 mm/s. Only three cases required a successful revised insertion by hand. Under fluoroscopy (n = 11), it was possible to achieve a remote rob-EAI (n = 8), as the surgeon was outside the operative room, behind an anti-radiation screen. No scala translocation occurred. The additional operative time due to robot use was 18+/−7 min with about 4 min more for remote rob-EAI. Basal cochlear turn fibrosis precluded rob-EAI. In conclusion, Rob-EAI can be performed in almost all cases with a low risk of scala translocation, except in the case of partial cochlear obstruction such as fibrosis. Fluoroscopy also permits remote rob-EAI.

Keywords: cochlear implant; electrode-array insertion; Robot; fluoroscopy; scala translocation

1. Introduction

Cochlear implantation is a treatment employed all over the world to rehabilitate hearing in the case of severe to profound deafness [1–3] The surgical procedure is well-codified and comprises the insertion of an electrode-array (EA) within the cochlear scala tympani, where the spiral ganglion of the cochlear nerve can be electrically stimulated by the cochlear implant. Great advances in cochlear implantation have been achieved in recent years, making it possible, for example, in selected cases, to preserve residual hearing [4–6]. It has been shown that cochlear implantation can be less invasive and deleterious to the cochlea, if a thin EA is inserted at low speed [7]. Although EA-translocation from the scala tympani into the scala vestibuli could result in damage to the fine cochlear structure, controversy exists in the literature, with some teams reporting better results in well-placed EAs within the scala tympani [8–12], while others did not [13,14]. Visual feedback through fluoroscopy has shown that it is possible to detect early in real -time errors such as EA-misrouting, EA-tip foldover, or EA-tip blockage within the cochlea and to immediately correct them [15]. Recently, a robotized EA insertion (rob-EAI) technique has been shown to perform less traumatic insertion, with a lower rate of scala translocation [16,17]. Herein, we report our first experience of rob-EAI, with or without intraoperative visual feedback through fluoroscopy. To our knowledge, this intraoperative procedure associating fluoroscopy feedback together with rob-EAI has never been reported to date. We reveal the

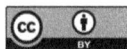

advantages and pitfalls that can be encountered when using this combination of rob-EAI with fluoroscopy feedback.

2. Materials and Methods

2.1. Chart Inclusion

From November 2021 to October 2022, all the candidate adults for a cochlear implantation were informed that a rob-EAI would be attempted, with or without fluoroscopy, depending on the availability of the hybrid operating room equipped with a robotic cone-beam C-arm system (Angio suite, Imabloc). This hybrid operating room is located in the radiology department of our institution and can host several types of procedures, e.g., cardiovascular, gynecological, and oncological procedures. This Angio suite is currently available for us once every two weeks. In all cases, preoperative imaging of the head and petrous bone was routinely prescribed but not all patients underwent this specific imaging in our institution. Because both rob-EAI and visual control of EA-insertion through fluoroscopy are routine procedures for cochlear implantation in our institution, no additional administrative procedure apart from providing clear information was required. All the patients were free to refuse the use of their personal data for scientific purposes, but none did so. This non-refusal procedure, consisting of the retrospective analysis of patients' records, was subject to the approval of our local ethics committee (00013412, "CHU de Clermont-Ferrand IRB #1", IRB number 2022 CF-079) in compliance with the French policy of individual data protection.

2.2. Surgical Procedure

2.2.1. In the Regular Operating Room of Our Otolaryngologic Department

The patient was installed on a surgical bed with a flat head support, bordered by metal rails. This is mandatory for securing the command of the robot (rob-space mouse; rob-SM) to the upper rail, just up to the vertex of the patient. The head was securely placed on a circular head support, with a frontal adhesive tape, attached to the table in the relevant position, i.e., turned to the opposite site of the ear being operated on, with a slight extension of approximatively 15–20°. In addition, to prevent any slipping of the patient's body when rotating the table, two straps were placed, one at the chest, the second at the lap. The table was then rotated 12° forward, and 5° backward before surgery, to check the stability of the patient's head on the table. Once the patient had been installed, the surgical team, consisting of a surgeon, a resident doctor and an instrument nurse, could prepare the operative field and drape both the microscope and the robot.

The surgical approach to the cochlea was a regular transmastoid route with posterior tympanotomy, achieved through microscopic control. Once the round window was clearly exposed, the cochlear implant was placed in a subperiosteal area with or without drilling a dedicated bed in the temporal bone. Then, the tip of the EA was delicately positioned at the round window, after the round window membrane had been opened.

The robot used was the RobOtol® (Collin Medical, Paris, France). This device is equipped with a robotized arm (RA) capable of moving with six degrees of freedom. The RA movements were controlled by the manually actuated rob-SM. It is important to note that this rob-SM allows RA movements in several directions but can also be locked in translation only (in the three spatial dimensions), or in rotation only. It is also possible, once an adequate axis is chosen, to fix the axis so that translation only along this axis is possible. Three types of RA movement speeds can be chosen: high speed, regular, or slow speed. When choosing slow-speed movements, insertion is never faster than 1 mm/s. It can be slowed by adjusting the hand pressure on the rob-SM button. The specific cochlear implant holder (CIHo) is unique for each brand of cochlear implant. During the surgical procedure, the RobOtol® is directed towards the head of the patient, in front of the surgeon, perpendicular to the table, and secured in the position chosen (Figure 1).

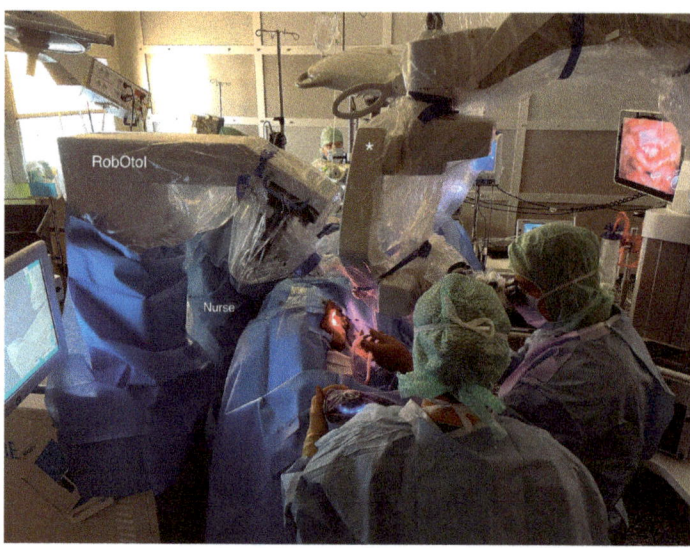

Figure 1. Intraoperative view showing the placement of the RobOtol® and microscope in the regular operating room (* marks the operating microscope).

The RA was then moved above the head so that the CIHo could be directed towards the surgical route to the round window. The cochlear implant EA was then secured to the CIHo, either by inserting the ailette in the specific fork-shaped tip of the CIHo for CI622® cochlear implants (Cochlear, Sydney, Australia), or by placing it in a specific gutter at the tip of the CIHo for the two other brands used, i.e., Flex 24® or Flex 26® (Med El, Innsbruck, Austria) and Neuro ZTI CLA or EVO (Oticon Medical, Vallauris, France). Finally, the EA could be inserted, under microscopic control, using the rob-SM at low speed, at less than 1 mm/s. Once the insertion had been achieved, the EA was detached from the CIHo, then the RA withdrawn from the mastoid, and the RobOtol® moved back from the operating field. The EA could then be rolled down within the mastoid cavity, the ground electrode, if any (depending on the brand of cochlear implant) placed in a temporal pocket muscle, after which the wound was closed layer by layer. Finally, the patient underwent a postoperative petrous bone computed tomography (CT)-scan before being discharged on the same, or on the following, day.

2.2.2. Surgical Procedure in the Angio Suite Imabloc

The patient was installed in the same way as in our regular operating room. However, the Robotol® and the robotized C-arm of the cone beam (Artis Zeego, Siemens, Erlangen, Germany) had to be positioned in the expected surgical position to check that the radiological robotized C-arm could be moved without touching the microscope or the RobOtol®. Sufficient room and careful placement are required to ensure feedback from the rob-EAI under microscope with fluoroscopy (Figure 2).

The following rob-EAI did not differ from the regular operating room, except that the surgeon took several minutes to put on a protective leaded jacket before switching on the fluoroscopy. In some cases, the surgeon could leave the hybrid room, and perform a remote EAI, with visual control of the surgical field recorded from the microscope camera together with the fluoroscopy (Figure 3).

Surgical and fluoroscopy views were projected on the same large screen facing the surgeon outside the hybrid room, protected by an anti-radiation screen (Figure 4).

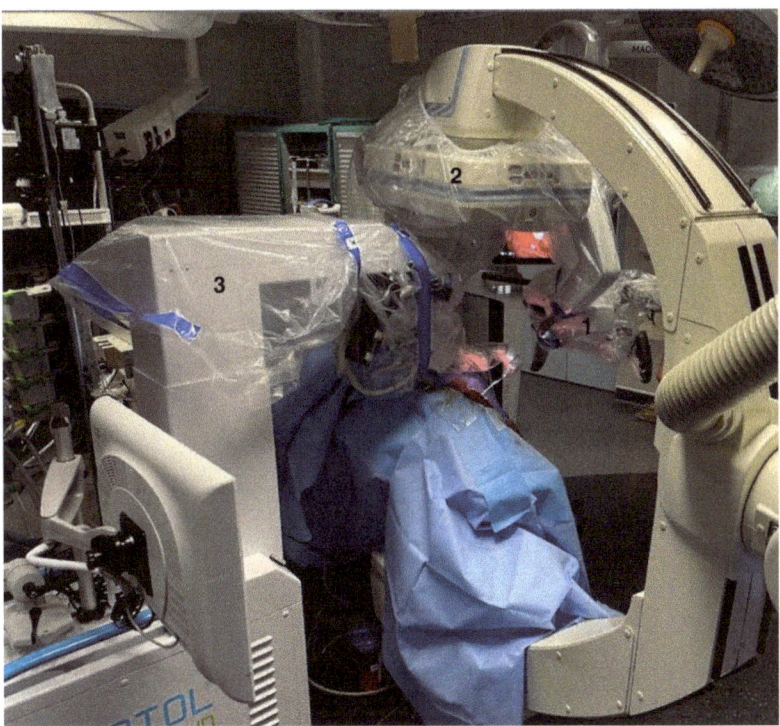

Figure 2. Intraoperative view showing the placement of the RObOtol® (3), microscope (1) and radiological robotized C-arm (2).

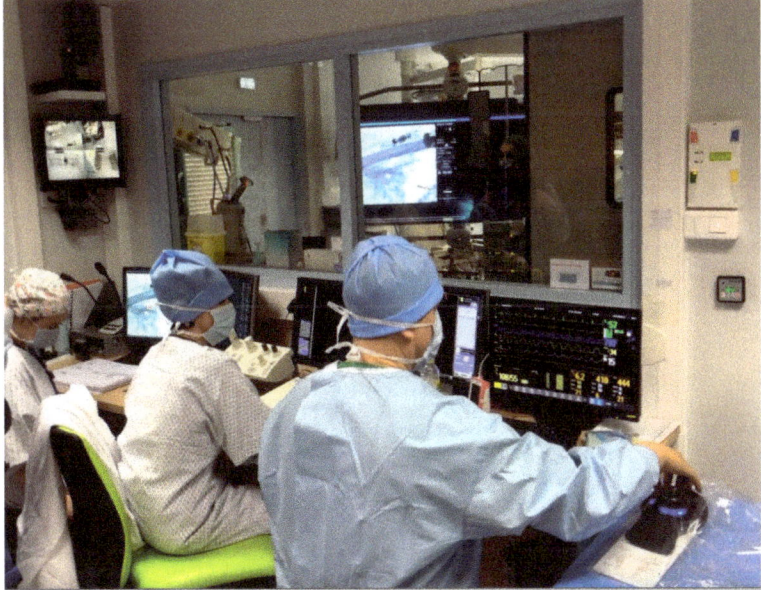

Figure 3. The surgeon can start the rob- EAI remotely outside of the Angio suite, sitting next to the anesthetists.

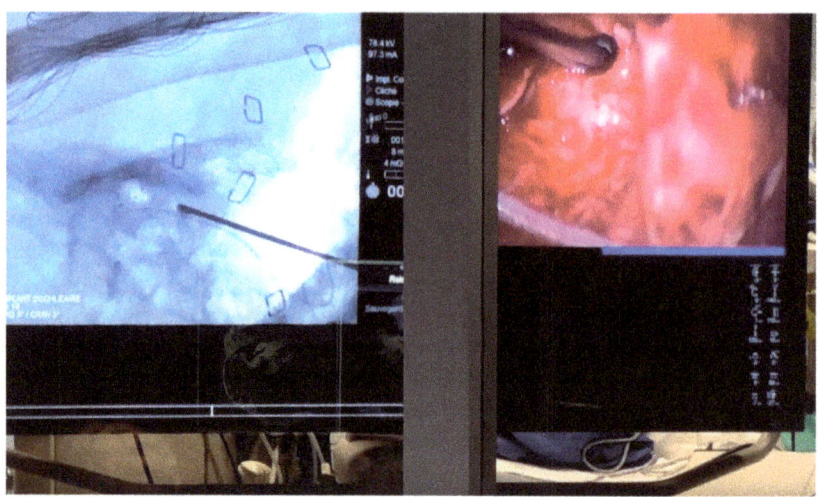

Figure 4. Simultaneous view of the surgical and fluoroscopy screen, as seen behind the protective shield at the end of a remote-EAI.

2.3. Postoperative Imaging

Patients operated in our regular operating room underwent a postoperative CT-scan of their petrous bones without contrast the same or the following day. For those operated in the Angio suite Imabloc, postoperative 3D cone beam acquisition was carried out on the operating table before the patient was awakened.

2.4. Data Collection

Patient characteristics were recorded anonymously. The additional time of installation due to the RobOtol®, and to the checking of the double installation of the RobOtol® and the robotized C-arm fluoroscope when using the hybrid room was recorded. The duration of RobOtol® use during the surgical procedure was also recorded, depending on which procedure was used, i.e., regular operative room (ROR), Angio suite Imabloc (Imabloc), or Angio suite Imabloc with remote EA-insertion (Remote-EAI). The success or failure of EA-insertion with the RobOtol® was recorded. The angle of insertion was collected for each patient. Any misrouting of the EA was noted. Particular attention was given to cases with failure of the rob-EAI to identify its cause. The postoperative petrous bone cone beams, or the postoperative petrous bone CT-scans, were analyzed by the radiology teams to determine if any translocation of the EA was suspected. When the basilar membrane was identified on the preoperative magnetic resonance imaging (MRI), the postoperative petrous bone cone beam, or the postoperative petrous bone CT-scan, was merged with the pre-operative three dimentional (3D) T2 space MRI by the radiology team to identify translocation. (coregistration fusion with advantage Workstation (ADW) 4.5, General Electric). When the basilar membrane was not identified on the preoperative MRI, only the postoperative petrous bone cone beams or the postoperative petrous bone CT-scans were analyzed, based on the aspect and location of the EA in maximum intensity projection (MIP), to determine if any translocation of the EA was suspected.

2.5. Statistics

The comparisons used an ANOVA and a post hoc Scheffé test. A value for $p \leq 0.05$ was considered significant.

3. Results

Table 1 summarizes the patients' characteristics and indicates whether the robotized EA insertion was successful. Among the 23 patients (10 females, 61+/−19 y.o.) 19 (82.6%) were implanted successfully with a rob-EAI. The rob-EAI with the RobOtol® required on 18+/−7 min average for the entire series.

Table 1. Patients' characteristics.

Patient	Sex	Age (Years)	Cochlear Implant Brand	Imabloc	Time of Robot Use (Min)	Remote EAI	Success
1	M	60	COCHLEAR CI622	no	13	no	YES
2	M	44	COCHLEAR CI622	yes	20	no	YES
3	M	83	MED-EL FLEX 24	no	18	no	YES
4	F	76	MED EL FORM 24	yes	18	YES	YES
5	F	72	COCHLEAR CI622	yes	20	no	no
6	M	79	COCHLEAR CI622	no	18	no	YES
7	M	82	COCHLEAR CI622	yes	22	YES	YES
8	F	60	COCHLEAR CI622	no	18	no	YES
9	M	57	COCHLEAR CI622	yes	19	YES	no
10	M	77	COCHLEAR CI622	Yes	25	YES	YES
11	M	74	COCHLEAR CI622	yes	21	no	YES
12	M	37	COCHLEAR CI622	yes	40	YES	YES
13	M	70	COCHLEAR CI622	no	25	no	YES
14	F	40	COCHLEAR CI622	no	8	no	YES
15	M	79	MED EL FLEX 24	no	14	no	YES
16	M	15	COCHLEAR CI622	yes	23	YES	YES
17	M	26	COCHLEAR CI622	no	N/A	no	no
18	F	66	MED EL FLEX 26	no	12	no	YES
19	F	42	COCHLEAR CI622	no	13	no	YES
20	F	74	COCHLEAR CI622	yes	15	no	YES
21	F	73	COCHLEAR CI622	yes	23	YES	YES
22	F	57	OTICON MEDICAL NZTI CLA	no	12	no	YES
23	F	54	COCHLEAR CI622	yes	9,45	YES	no

3.1. Patients Operated on in the Angio Suite Imabloc

Eleven cases were implanted under fluoroscopy feedback in the Angio suite Imabloc associated with the implementation of rob-EAI. Among all the patients implanted in the Angio suite, remote-EAI was attempted in eight cases (72.7%). Regarding the three cases where the robotized EAI failed, they were eventually successfully implanted by hand using a classical procedure. In these three cases, failure was due only to our lack of experience with this double control of EA-insertion. Patient 9 failed because the tip of the EA was not securely positioned at the round window before remote-EAI. Therefore, the EA went out of the round window at the very beginning of the remote EAI. The EA bent in a spring shape out of the cochlea. It was slowly withdrawn, manually realigned, then slowly inserted by hand. The operation on patient 5 failed because the table changed its position every time the assistant radiologist tried to position the robotized C-arm, which was not compatible with the positioning of the CIHo required. The operation on patient 23 failed because the surgeon focused on the fluoroscopy scene instead of the surgical field, therefore they did not detect the misrouting in the mastoid of the CIHo, only the late EA- bending on the fluoroscopy screen. The EA was removed, manually realigned, and then slowly inserted by hand. In one case (patient 2) the EA inserted showed an initial square shape on the fluoroscopy screen, with a limited angle of insertion at 360°. The EA was thus removed using the RobOtol® after which a second rob-EAI with a suitable round shape was inserted successfully, allowing for a full rob-EAI with a 540° angle. Nobody could have detected that the initial insertion was square-shaped if it had not been displayed on the fluoroscopy scene. Regarding the Imabloc patients, the time dedicated to the robot was 23+/−7 min, (22+/−9 min in Remote-EAI patients; 18+/−3 min with no remote EA-insertion, the difference was not significant, $p = 0.65$).

3.2. Patients Operated in the Regular Operated Room
3.2.1. Global Results

Among these 22 cases, 21 (95.4%) underwent a successful rob-EAI. The only case of failure of rob- EAI occurred in patient 17, where an extensive fibrosis of the basal turn almost precluded cochlear implantation. In this case, the deep cochlear fibrosis made smooth EAI impossible. After having clearly identified the obstruction of the entire basal turn by fibrosis, we decided to largely open the basal turn to allow the correct removal of the fibrosis. We were obliged to force the residual fibrosis obstructing the end of the basal turn with a rigid dummy EA before achieving a difficult insertion of the EA by hand. In this case the rob-EAI was of no use. The additional time due to the use of the RobOtol® was on average 15+/−4 min. Although shorter than in the Angio suite Imabloc, this duration did not significantly differ, neither with the group implanted under fluoroscopy in the Angio suite Imabloc ($p = 0.79$), nor with the remote-EAI group; $p = 0.10$).

3.2.2. Quality of rob-EAI

The angle of insertion was on average 477°+/−63 among the 22 patients with no attempt at hearing preservation. All the patients had a full insertion except one with a Mondini malformation (type 2 incomplete cochlear partition). In the sole patient (patient 19) whose hearing was tentatively preserved, the desired angle at 360° was obtained. Hearing was preserved, with a mean postoperative pure tone average (PTA) between 250 Hz–4 kHz at 88 dB versus 83 dB in the preoperative period, which was not significant. The patient spontaneously reported that she could still hear her intrinsic throat noises the same day after surgery.

Whatever the type of rob-EAI, we never succeeded in defining a unique perfect axis leading to a full insertion. In all the patients, despite having determined a likely adequate preinsertion axis of the CIHo, we had to correct it during insertion, using the rob-SM to adjust the EA trajectory.

Postoperative CT scans and preoperative MRIs of the cochlea made it possible for the radiologist to merge postoperative CT and preoperative MRI images when the basilar membrane was identified on MRI. In three cases the resolution of MRI and CT scans were sufficient to build these merged images (Figure 5).

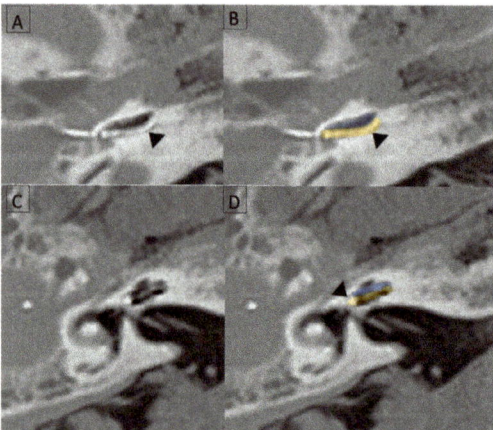

Figure 5. Images from the same patient (M8) obtained by merging preoperative MRI and postoperative CT-scans. Black arrow heads point to the EA. (**A**) postoperative CT-scan axial slice of the basal turn; (**B**) Merged images at the same level as (**A**) after identification of the scala tympani (yellow) and vestibuli (blue) on MRI; (**C**) postoperative CT-scan axial slice of the second turn; and (**D**) Merged images at the same level as (**C**) after identification of the scala tympani (yellow) and vestibuli (blue) on MRI. In this example, EA was fully inserted into the scala tympani.

It was clear that the EA was not translocated in these three cases. We did not suspect any scala translocation in the other cases, based on the comparisons of their postoperative CT-scans with the three cases with merged cochlear images.

4. Discussion

This preliminary report demonstrates for the first time that cochlear implantation with rob-EAI can be coupled with visual feedback through fluoroscopy. It confirms that a rob-EAI is feasible in most patients. To our knowledge, this is the first time that such remote EAI has been reported in cochlear implantation. To date, several teams has reported this type of EA-insertion using RobOtol® but none of them used fluoroscopy as visual feedback [7,17,18]. Recently, a cochlear implantation under fluoroscopy with the HEARO procedure has been reported [19]. In this interesting report, while the approach was robotized, the EA insertion was not, which is quite different from our procedure. In this series, we did not use intraoperative electrocochleography (EcoG). It is interesting to note that intraoperatively EcoG during a rob-EAI using the RobOtol® has been proven feasible [18]. In order to improve the chance of hearing preservation, a rob-EAI could be advantageously associated with fluoroscopy and intraoperative EcoG monitoring. This combination of different tools for a smooth and mini-invasive EAI needs further studies to highlight its interest in preserving hearing. The use of a robotized EA-insertion leads to steady and low-speed insertion that has been proven to be less deleterious to the cochlea [7,17,20]. Therefore, rob-EAI could be the preferred technique of cochlear implantation if it is capable of harmonious and steady EA-insertion at a low speed. Here, we revealed the additional advantage of using fluoroscopy, which provides visual feedback. Case 2 was particularly demonstrative of this advantage, for which the first robotized EA-insertion ended in a square-shaped insertion with a limited angle at 360° that was detected by fluoroscopy and then corrected. It should be mentioned that the RobOtol® provides no haptic feedback. We know that even with the haptic feedback of the human hand, in some cases it is very difficult to feel certain errors during EA-insertion, such as EA-tip-foldover or EA-misrouting. Hopefully, these errors can be revealed by fluoroscopy [15]. It is therefore not surprising that, with no haptic control at all, a rob-EAI can result in a divergent EA winding around the modiolus. Thus, case 2 convinced us to use fluoroscopy feedback with the RobOtol® as much as possible. Another positive point of using a hybrid room like the Angio suite Imabloc is that the RobOtol® permits remote-EAI under fluoroscopy, limiting the irradiation delivered to the operating staff. The total fluoroscopic time has been previously precisely reported [15]. Because fluoroscopy only served for control of the EA- insertion, the exposition time of patients to radiation was very low, less than 5 min. Herein, the use of the RObOtol® did not increase the time of fluoroscopy. The EA-insertion was always performed at low speed (<1 mm/s) even before we used the RobOtol®. This time was reported previously at less than 4 min [15]. The total radiation dose was calculated at 4053+/−1994 µGray m^2, including the radiation due to the final cone beam CT scan responsible for the most part of the X-ray dose. From a clinical standpoint, it is equivalent to less than four digital substrate radiographs (DSA), which is acceptable in adults. In the case of children, we had recommended to skip the final cone beam CT scan, avoiding 96% of the total radiation dose, which was thus responsible for a low irradiation, less than one DSA [15]. By contrast, the total radiation dose can become harmful to the surgeon who repeatedly performs operations, as their hands are exposed to the radiation of fluoroscopy. Alternative means of protecting the surgeon's hands from radiation do not as yet exist. While special anti-radiation gloves seem to protect against indirect scattered radiation [21], paradoxically, they could increase the dose of radiation received by direct exposure [22]. In addition, they are thicker than regular surgical gloves, which is uncomfortable for the delicate handling of micro-instruments. As soon as a remote EAI proved possible, we therefore systematically used it. However, among the eight patients who underwent remote-EAI, two cases failed. We now know, after patients 17 and 23, that when attempting a remote- EAI, it is necessary to double check that the EA tip is well secured at the entrance of the round window and focus on the surgical field rather than on the fluoroscopy scene.

For us, the additional time required to use the RobOtol® in the Angio suite Imabloc was acceptable at around 23 min, vs. 15 min in the regular operation room. This double additional refinement of EAI, i.e., rob-EAI with visual fluoroscopy feedback, which ensures optimal EAI in selected cases, makes it worthwhile to spend a bit less than 30 additional minutes in the operating room. The postoperative control of the EA- scala position, was achieved here in three cases by merging preoperative MRIs and postoperative CT-scans. When these images are of high quality, the technique appears to be very accurate, as it allows the direct visualization of the basilar membrane, in contrast to other techniques based only on CT-scans [23]. However, this merging technique requires high quality images. Today we systematically ask for high quality preoperative labyrinthine MRIs and postoperative CT-scans, in order to build-up merged pre and postoperative images of the cochlea for all patients. Thus, it is likely that no translocation occurred in our series with rob-EAI.

In the case of basal fibrosis, such as in case 17, robotized-EAI becomes very hard to achieve. The lack of haptic control makes it difficult to force the obstacle with a suitable force of insertion while avoiding any EA bending. In this situation, the haptic feedback of an experienced surgeon is much preferable and can be helped by fluoroscopy [15]. Also, because the basal fibrosis has to be partially removed and the EA forced through the fibrosis, the objective is no longer to perform a minimally invasive insertion, but to achieve it.

It must be born in mind that the RobOtol® is currently well-suited for straight EAs, but for only one perimodiolar EA (Mid-scala from Advanced Bionics®). This is a real limitation in cases where the cochlear implant team would prefer such EAs, for instance in certain cases of otosclerosis to minimize the current diffusion through the diseased bone [24]. Herein, we did not select patients with the need of perimodiolar EAI, as the Mid-scala EA from Advanced Bionics® is not currently available in our institution.

5. Conclusions

In conclusion, our preliminary cochlear implant cohort using the RobOtol® confirmed that rob-EAI is feasible in almost all cases, except those with extensive cochlear fibrosis. In addition, combining the use of a rob- EAI and fluoroscopy feedback, which permits remote EAI, can be done with safety for both the patient and the surgeon in most cases.

Author Contributions: Validation, P.C.; Investigation, T.M., M.P., M.E.Y., A.L., J.-E.P., J.B. and N.S.; Writing—original draft, T.M.; Writing—review & editing, S.M.; Visualization, L.G. and S.M. All authors have read and agreed to the published version of the manuscript.

Funding: This research received no external funding.

Institutional Review Board Statement: The study was conducted in accordance with the Declaration of Helsinki, and approved by our local ethics committee (00013412, "CHU de Clermont-Ferrand IRB #1", IRB number 2022 CF-079).

Informed Consent Statement: Informed consent was obtained from all subjects involved in the study.

Data Availability Statement: All data supporting our results are included in the text, table, and figures.

Acknowledgments: We thank the management of our University Hospital for having found and given the credits required to acquire the RobOtol®.

Conflicts of Interest: The authors declare no conflict of interest.

References

1. Clark, G.M. Electrical Stimulation of the Auditory Nerve: The Coding of Frequency, the Perception of Pitch and the Development of Cochlear Implant Speech Processing Strategies for Profoundly Deaf People. *Clin. Exp. Pharmacol. Physiol.* **1996**, *23*, 766–776. [CrossRef]
2. Zwolan, T.A.; Basura, G. Determining Cochlear Implant Candidacy in Adults: Limitations, Expansions, and Opportunities for Improvement. *Semin. Hear.* **2021**, *42*, 331–341. [CrossRef]
3. Gay, R.D.; Enke, Y.L.; Kirk, J.R.; Goldman, D.R. Therapeutics for Hearing Preservation and Improvement of Patient Outcomes in Cochlear Implantation-Progress and Possibilities. *Hear. Res.* **2022**, *426*, 108637. [CrossRef]
4. Gantz, B.J.; Turner, C.W. Combining Acoustic and Electrical Hearing. *Laryngoscope* **2010**, *113*, 1726–1730. [CrossRef]
5. James, C.J.; Fraysse, B.; Deguine, O.; Lenarz, T.; Mawman, D.; Ramos, Á.; Ramsden, R.; Sterkers, O. Combined Electroacoustic Stimulation in Conventional Candidates for Cochlear Implantation. *Audiol. Neurotol.* **2006**, *11* (Suppl. 1), 57–62. [CrossRef]

6. Balkany, T.J.; Connell, S.S.; Hodges, A.V.; Payne, S.L.; Telischi, F.F.; Eshraghi, A.A.; Angeli, S.I.; Germani, R.; Messiah, S.; Arheart, K.L. Conservation of Residual Acoustic Hearing After Cochlear Implantation. *Otol. Neurotol.* **2006**, *27*, 1083–1088. [CrossRef]
7. Torres, R.; Jia, H.; Drouillard, M.; Bensimon, J.-L.; Sterkers, O.; Ferrary, E.; Nguyen, Y. An Optimized Robot-Based Technique for Cochlear Implantation to Reduce Array Insertion Trauma. *Otolaryngol.-Head Neck Surg. Off. J. Am. Acad. Otolaryngol.-Head Neck Surg.* **2018**, *159*, 900–907. [CrossRef]
8. Finley, C.C.; Holden, T.A.; Holden, L.K.; Whiting, B.R.; Chole, R.A.; Neely, G.J.; Hullar, T.E.; Skinner, M.W. Role of Electrode Placement as a Contributor to Variability in Cochlear Implant Outcomes. *Otol. Neurotol. Off. Publ. Am. Otol. Soc. Am. Neurotol. Soc. Eur. Acad. Otol. Neurotol.* **2008**, *29*, 920–928. [CrossRef]
9. Wanna, G.B.; Noble, J.H.; Carlson, M.L.; Gifford, R.H.; Dietrich, M.S.; Haynes, D.S.; Dawant, B.M.; Labadie, R.F. Impact of Electrode Design and Surgical Approach on Scalar Location and Cochlear Implant Outcomes. *Laryngoscope* **2014**, *124* (Suppl. S6), S1–S7. [CrossRef]
10. De Seta, D.; Nguyen, Y.; Bonnard, D.; Ferrary, E.; Godey, B.; Bakhos, D.; Mondain, M.; Deguine, O.; Sterkers, O.; Bernardeschi, D.; et al. The Role of Electrode Placement in Bilateral Simultaneously Cochlear-Implanted Adult Patients. *Otolaryngol.-Head Neck Surg. Off. J. Am. Acad. Otolaryngol.-Head Neck Surg.* **2016**, *155*, 485–493. [CrossRef]
11. Shaul, C.; Dragovic, A.S.; Stringer, A.K.; O'Leary, S.J.; Briggs, R.J. Scalar Localisation of Peri-Modiolar Electrodes and Speech Perception Outcomes. *J. Laryngol. Otol.* **2018**, *132*, 1000–1006. [CrossRef]
12. Jwair, S.; Prins, A.; Wegner, I.; Stokroos, R.J.; Versnel, H.; Thomeer, H.G.X.M. Scalar Translocation Comparison Between Lateral Wall and Perimodiolar Cochlear Implant Arrays—A Meta-Analysis. *Laryngoscope* **2021**, *131*, 1358–1368. [CrossRef]
13. Riggs, W.J.; Dwyer, R.T.; Holder, J.T.; Mattingly, J.K.; Ortmann, A.; Noble, J.H.; Dawant, B.M.; Valenzuela, C.V.; O'Connell, B.P.; Harris, M.S.; et al. Intracochlear Electrocochleography: Influence of Scalar Position of the Cochlear Implant Electrode on Postinsertion Results. *Otol. Neurotol. Off. Publ. Am. Otol. Soc. Am. Neurotol. Soc. Eur. Acad. Otol. Neurotol.* **2019**, *40*, e503–e510. [CrossRef]
14. Berg, K.A.; Noble, J.H.; Dawant, B.M.; Dwyer, R.T.; Labadie, R.F.; Gifford, R.H. Speech Recognition with Cochlear Implants as a Function of the Number of Channels: Effects of Electrode Placement. *J. Acoust. Soc. Am.* **2020**, *147*, 3646. [CrossRef]
15. Perazzini, C.; Puechmaille, M.; Saroul, N.; Plainfossé, O.; Montrieul, L.; Bécaud, J.; Gilain, L.; Chabrot, P.; Boyer, L.; Mom, T. Fluoroscopy Guided Electrode-Array Insertion for Cochlear Implantation with Straight Electrode-Arrays: A Valuable Tool in Most Cases. *Eur. Arch. Oto-Rhino-Laryngol. Off. J. Eur. Fed. Oto-Rhino-Laryngol. Soc. EUFOS Affil. Ger. Soc. Oto-Rhino-Laryngol.-Head Neck Surg.* **2021**, *278*, 965–975. [CrossRef]
16. Wanna, G.B.; Noble, J.H.; Gifford, R.H.; Dietrich, M.S.; Sweeney, A.D.; Zhang, D.; Dawant, B.M.; Rivas, A.; Labadie, R.F. Impact of Intrascalar Electrode Location, Electrode Type, and Angular Insertion Depth on Residual Hearing in Cochlear Implant Patients: Preliminary Results. *Otol. Neurotol. Off. Publ. Am. Otol. Soc. Am. Neurotol. Soc. Eur. Acad. Otol. Neurotol.* **2015**, *36*, 1343–1348. [CrossRef]
17. Daoudi, H.; Lahlou, G.; Torres, R.; Sterkers, O.; Lefeuvre, V.; Ferrary, E.; Mosnier, I.; Nguyen, Y. Robot-Assisted Cochlear Implant Electrode Array Insertion in Adults: A Comparative Study With Manual Insertion. *Otol. Neurotol. Off. Publ. Am. Otol. Soc. Am. Neurotol. Soc. Eur. Acad. Otol. Neurotol.* **2021**, *42*, e438–e444. [CrossRef]
18. Gawęcki, W.; Balcerowiak, A.; Podlawska, P.; Borowska, P.; Gibasiewicz, R.; Szyfter, W.; Wierzbicka, M. Robot-Assisted Electrode Insertion in Cochlear Implantation Controlled by Intraoperative Electrocochleography—A Pilot Study. *J. Clin. Med.* **2022**, *11*, 7045. [CrossRef]
19. Jablonski, G.E.; Falkenberg-Jensen, B.; Bunne, M.; Iftikhar, M.; Greisiger, R.; Opheim, L.R.; Korslund, H.; Myhrum, M.; Sørensen, T.M. Fusion of Technology in Cochlear Implantation Surgery: Investigation of Fluoroscopically Assisted Robotic Electrode Insertion. *Front. Surg.* **2021**, *8*, 741401. [CrossRef]
20. van der Jagt, A.M.A.; Briaire, J.J.; Boehringer, S.; Verbist, B.M.; Frijns, J.H.M. Prolonged Insertion Time Reduces Translocation Rate of a Precurved Electrode Array in Cochlear Implantation. *Otol. Neurotol. Off. Publ. Am. Otol. Soc. Am. Neurotol. Soc. Eur. Acad. Otol. Neurotol.* **2022**, *43*, e427–e434. [CrossRef]
21. Cantlon, M.B.; Ilyas, A.M. Assessment of Radiation Protection in Hand-Shielding Products With Mini C-Arm Fluoroscopy. *Hand N. Y.* **2021**, *16*, 505–510. [CrossRef]
22. Guersen, J.; Donadille, L.; Rehel, J.L.; Charvais, A.; Zaknoune, R.; Cassagnes, L.; Chabrot, P.; Boyer, L. Intérêt des gants radio-atténuateurs en radiologie interventionnelle: Une évaluation expérimentale. *Radioprotection* **2011**, *46*, 387–397. [CrossRef]
23. Torres, R.; Drouillard, M.; De Seta, D.; Bensimon, J.-L.; Ferrary, E.; Sterkers, O.; Bernardeschi, D.; Nguyen, Y. Cochlear Implant Insertion Axis Into the Basal Turn: A Critical Factor in Electrode Array Translocation. *Otol. Neurotol. Off. Publ. Am. Otol. Soc. Am. Neurotol. Soc. Eur. Acad. Otol. Neurotol.* **2018**, *39*, 168–176. [CrossRef]
24. Battmer, R.; Pesch, J.; Stöver, T.; Lesinski-Schiedat, A.; Lenarz, M.; Lenarz, T. Elimination of Facial Nerve Stimulation by Reimplantation in Cochlear Implant Subjects. *Otol. Neurotol. Off. Publ. Am. Otol. Soc. Am. Neurotol. Soc. Eur. Acad. Otol. Neurotol.* **2006**, *27*, 918–922. [CrossRef]

Disclaimer/Publisher's Note: The statements, opinions and data contained in all publications are solely those of the individual author(s) and contributor(s) and not of MDPI and/or the editor(s). MDPI and/or the editor(s) disclaim responsibility for any injury to people or property resulting from any ideas, methods, instructions or products referred to in the content.

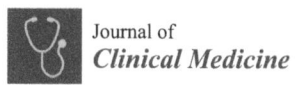

Article

Immediate-Early Modifications to the Metabolomic Profile of the Perilymph Following an Acoustic Trauma in a Sheep Model

Luc Boullaud [1,2,*], Hélène Blasco [2,3,4], Eliott Caillaud [1], Patrick Emond [2,4] and David Bakhos [1,2,4,5]

1. ENT Department and Cervico-Facial Surgery, CHU de Tours, 2 Boulevard Tonnellé, 37044 Tours, France
2. INSERM U1253, iBrain, University of Tours, 10 Boulevard Tonnellé, 37000 Tours, France
3. Department of Biochemistry and Molecular Biology, CHU de Tours, 2 Boulevard Tonnellé, 37044 Tours, France
4. Faculty of Medicine, University of Tours, 10 Boulevard Tonnellé, 37000 Tours, France
5. House Institute Foundation, Los Angeles, CA 90089, USA
* Correspondence: luc.boullaud@gmail.com; Tel.: +33-02-4747-4747

Abstract: The pathophysiological mechanisms of noise-induced hearing loss remain unknown. Identifying biomarkers of noise-induced hearing loss may increase the understanding of pathophysiological mechanisms of deafness, allow for a more precise diagnosis, and inform personalized treatment. Emerging techniques such as metabolomics can help to identify these biomarkers. The objective of the present study was to investigate immediate-early changes in the perilymph metabolome following acoustic trauma. Metabolomic analysis was performed using liquid chromatography coupled to mass spectrophotometry to analyze metabolic changes in perilymph associated with noise-induced hearing loss. Sheep ($n = 6$) were exposed to a noise designed to induce substantial hearing loss. Perilymph was collected before and after acoustic trauma. Data were analyzed using univariate analysis and a supervised multivariate analysis based on partial least squares discriminant analysis. A metabolomic analysis showed an abundance of 213 metabolites. Four metabolites were significantly changed following acoustic trauma (Urocanate ($p = 0.004$, FC = 0.48), S-(5'-Adenosyl)-L-Homocysteine ($p = 0.06$, FC = 2.32), Trigonelline ($p = 0.06$, FC = 0.46) and N-Acetyl-L-Leucine ($p = 0.09$, FC = 2.02)). The approach allowed for the identification of new metabolites and metabolic pathways involved with acoustic trauma that were associated with auditory impairment (nerve damage, mechanical destruction, and oxidative stress). The results suggest that metabolomics provides a powerful approach to characterize inner ear metabolites which may lead to identification of new therapies and therapeutic targets.

Keywords: metabolomic; perilymph; acoustic trauma; hearing loss

1. Introduction

Hearing loss affects approximately 466 million people (5% of the worldwide population), including 34 million children. Estimates show that by 2050, 900 million people (10% of the worldwide population) will suffer from a disabling hearing loss [1]. The economic cost of hearing loss is estimated to be 750 billion dollars in the USA [1,2]. Hearing loss is the most common sensory deficit and represents a major public health problem [3], negatively affecting oral language development, education, and social interaction [2]. Hearing loss can lead to reduced quality of life by limiting communication and socio-professional relationships; in adults, it leads to social isolation, socio-professional difficulties, and the appearance of a depressive state. Hearing loss has been associated with other public health problems, such as repeated falls, cognitive decline, dementia, and increased hospitalization [3,4]. In about 50% of individuals with sensorineural hearing loss (SNHL), especially post-lingual SNHL, the pathophysiological mechanisms leading to hearing loss and cell loss in the cochlea are myriad and interrelated, and the etiology often remains unknown [5]. Noise-induced hearing loss (NIHL) accounts for 1/3 of SNHL cases, and 10% of the world's population is exposed to potentially harmful sounds [6].

Several hypotheses have been raised regarding the pathophysiological mechanisms of NIHL. NIHL appears to be the result of a reactive oxygen species (ROS) accumulation in the cochlea due to oxidative stress, mechanical destruction of cells in the auditory nerve organ, and retrocochlear nerve damage [6]. However, the mechanism leading to NIHL is not well understood. Impulse noise can lead to a temporary threshold shift, whereas continuous noise can lead to permanent hearing loss [7,8]. In addition to the cochlear damage that is already known, the impaired neurotransmission associated with the loss of synaptic connections between the inner hair cells and the spiral ganglion neuron fibers, as well as metabolic imbalances, are implicated in elevated hearing thresholds and merit further research to elucidate the mechanisms of hearing loss [9].

Research regarding biomarkers in health has expanded over the past few years, along with an increased interest in omic techniques. Omic techniques comprise genomics (the study of Deoxyribonucleic Acid (DNA)), transcriptomics (the study of Ribonucleic Acids (RNA)), and proteomics and metabolomics. Metabolomics is an emerging technique which can be used to identify biomarkers by analyzing the different metabolites present in a sample. The metabolome refers to all metabolites below 1500 Daltons that provides insight into physiological or pathological states at a given time [10].

To better understand the effects of acoustic trauma on the inner ear, we performed a metabolomic analysis to provide a comprehensive overview of the perilymph fluid metabolome following noise trauma.

2. Methods

2.1. Experimental Groups and Noise Exposure

All animal procedures were approved by an ethical committee (APAFIS #2018112714344369) and all experiments were performed in accordance with current guidelines and regulations. Six sheep were included in the study (breed = Île-de-France). For the sampling of the perilymph, each animal underwent general anesthesia. General anesthesia was induced by intravenous isoflurane 3% oxygen and 10 mg/kg ketamine along with 0.05 mg/kg xylazine. An oro-tracheal intubation was performed. At the end of the procedure, the sheep were euthanized by overdosing with phenobarbital. Only female sheep (ewes) were used because the cortical bone is thinner than in rams. In each sheep, one ear served as the normal-hearing (NH) model and the contralateral ear was subjected to acoustic trauma and served as the NIHL model; as such, each sheep served as its own comparator. The choice of ear for noise exposure was randomized across sheep. The sound stimulus was 40-ms of pulsatile noise (frequency range = 1–10 kHz) repeated in a loop at an intensity of 120 dB SPL for 1 h. The stimulus was generated by computer using Adobe Audition 2.0® software (Adobe, San Jose, CA, USA), which was connected to an audiometer (Otométrics® Aurical Plus, Natus Medical Incorporated, San Carlos, CA, USA), which was connected to a headset (Peltor®, 3M, Saint Paul, MN, USA, H7A, EN352-1:1993). The sound level was measured by a sound level meter (Class 1 Type 2250, Bruel & Kjaer®, Naerum, Denmark) and the audiometer was calibrated with white noise. Figure 1 illustrates the study design.

2.2. Auditory Measurement

Bone-conduction auditory brain responses (BC-ABRs) were measured to estimate auditory thresholds using a NavPRO ONE bio-logic® Otometrics (Natus Medical Incorporated, San Carlos, CA, USA) setup. BC-ABR thresholds were measured to confirm the NH status at the beginning of the experiment, and then to quantify the hearing loss induced by the acoustic trauma. Auditory thresholds were tested from 50 to 20 dB nHL in 10 dB steps. The stimuli were "clicks" at a modulation frequency of 3000 Hz. Each ear was tested with masking of the contralateral ear by white noise. Thresholds were measured using a B71W bone transducer and transcutaneous needle electrodes. Biolink® software (Advanced Biometric, Mahone, NS, Canada) was used to analyze the response curves, focusing on the latencies and amplitudes of waves I to IV. The NH status was confirmed by the presence of wave IV at 30 dB nHL. As the BC-ABR was measured using bone conduction, measurements cannot be made for intensities >50 dB nHL. In many cases, no wave IV could be observed at 50 dB nHL, indicating that thresholds were higher than the measurement limit. In these cases, 60 dB nHL was considered to be the threshold.

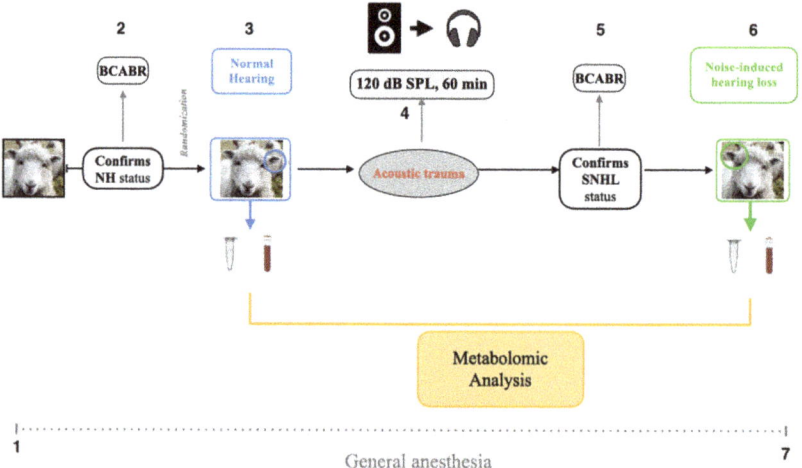

Figure 1. Study design: (1) Sheep under general anesthesia. (2) Perform BC-ABR to confirm NH status in NH ear. (3) Sample perilymph from NH ear. (4) 60 min of impulse noise exposure at 120 dB SPL. (5) Perform BC-ABR to confirm SNHL status in NIHL ear. (6) Sample perilymph from NIHL ear. (7) Sheep euthanized. The polyethylene tube represents the perilymph sample, blood tube represents the serum.

2.3. Preparation of the Samples

The perilymph was collected before sound exposure in the NH ear and after sound exposure in the contralateral NIHL ear. The round window was opened with a lumbar puncture needle (22G3 1/2 90 mm 7/10) and the perilymph was collected by capillary action using a micropipette (Microcap 15 µL, length 54 mm, Drummond Scientific Company®, Broomal, PA, USA). All samples were aliquoted into polypropylene tubes and stored at −80 °C until analysis. Metabolite extraction was performed with 400 µL of methanol added to 50 µL of perilymph.

All the samples were shaken for 5 s and incubated at −20 °C for 30 min to deproteinize the sample. After centrifugation that lasted 25 min at 5000× g rpm at 4 °C, the supernatant (350 µL) was harvested and evaporated with the SpeedVac concentrator at 40 °C. The dry residue was re-suspended in 100 µL of a methanol/water mixture (75/25) and then 5 µL of sample was injected for liquid chromatography-mass spectrometry analysis. Quality control (QC) samples were prepared by equal volume mixing of all analyzed samples (QC for each sample matrix type).

2.4. Metabolomic Analysis

The metabolomic analysis was performed using liquid chromatography coupled to high-resolution mass spectrometry (LC/HRMS) as previously described by our group [11]. The analyses were performed on a UPLC Ultimate WPS-300 system (Dionex, Germany) coupled to a Q-Exactive mass spectrometer (Thermo Fisher Scientific, Bremen, Germany) and the ionization was performed according to the positive (ESI+) and negative (ESI−) electrospray mode [11]. Liquid chromatography was performed with a hydrophilic interaction liquid chromatography (HILIC) column (1.6 µL 150 × 2.10 mm, 100 A), maintained at 40 °C. Two mobile phases were used, and the chromatographic gradients were at a flow rate of 0.3 mL/min. During acquisition, the instrument operated at a resolution of 70,000 (m/z = 200).

Metabolites identification was performed using a standard Mass Spectrometry Metabolite Library compound library (IROA Technologies™, Sea Girt, NJ, USA). Signal values were calculated with Xcalibur® software (Thermo Fisher Scientific, San Jose, CA, USA) by integrating the chromatography peaks corresponding to the selected metabolites. The coefficient of variation (CV) associated with the area of each metabolite was calculated for the control samples (QC) [CV% = (standard deviation/average) × 100]. Metabolites with a CV in the QCs greater than that of the sample and/or CV > 30% were excluded.

2.5. Statistical Analysis

In a first step, we evaluated the inter-individual variability of metabolites in perilymph during physiological conditions. Within each sheep, the CV of each metabolite was calculated for the NH ear and compared to the CV for the NIHL ear. Next, we evaluated metabolic changes induced by noise in the perilymph. The percentage of change in relative concentrations of each metabolite in the perilymph between the NIHL and NH ears was calculated and compared to the CV for the same metabolites in QC. These data were analyzed by univariate and multivariate analysis (NH vs. NIHL). All statistical analyses were performed using MetaboAnalyst software (version 5.0; www.metaboanalyst.ca/ (accessed on 25 May 2021)). The univariate analysis of metabolites levels between groups was based on the volcano plot that represents the fold-change (FC) values and the threshold of significance after the non-parametric Wilcoxon test. Significant metabolites were selected by the volcano plot based on FC thresholds < 0.8 or >1.2 and t-test p-value thresholds < 0.1. Classification was performed by unsupervised Principal Component Analysis (PCA) to visualize the distribution of samples and to highlight putative outsiders. By representing the QC and the different sheep samples, it is possible to understand the inter-individual variability among the sheep in relation to the analytical variability represented by the distribution of the QCs. Partial least squares discriminant analysis (PLS-DA), representing a supervised multivariate analysis, was also performed. The score plot provides an overview of the classified samples. The values of variable influence on projection (VIP) enable the identification of the most important metabolites involved in the discrimination in the supervised multivariate model. The performance of the model was evaluated by the permutation test. Multiple testing was taken into account by the False Discovery Rate (FDR).

2.6. Pathways Analyses

Pathways analyses were performed on the most significant metabolites highlighted in the PLS-DA analysis and in univariate analysis. Metabolic pathway enrichment analysis and pathway topology analysis were performed using the MetaboAnalyst computational platform (https://www.metaboanalyst.ca/ (accessed on 25 May 2021)). This strategy presents a single p value for each metabolic pathway. Pathway analysis was used to calculate the pathway impact, which represents a combination of the centrality and pathway enrichment results; impact values represent the relative importance of the pathway compared to the others included in the analysis. The pathway impact value was calculated as the sum of the importance measures of the metabolites normalized by the sum of importance measures of all metabolites in each pathway.

An interactive Google-Map-style visualization system was also used to present the analysis results in an intuitive way.

3. Results

In this section, we describe the sheep population used, the inducement of NIHL, and the metabolomic results.

3.1. Animal Model of Acoustic Trauma

Six sheep (all ewes) were included in the study. The characteristics of the population are presented in Table 1. The average age was 29.9 ± 3 months. The mean weight was 68 ± 11 kg. The average duration of general anesthesia was 205 ± 29.5 min.

Table 1. Characteristics of the 6 included sheep.

Sheep	Breed	Sex	Age (Months)	Weight (kg)	Duration of Anesthesia (Min)	Stimulation Sampling Time (Min)
1	IDF	F	27.5	64	240	45
2	IDF	F	27.8	52	240	80
3	IDF	F	28.4	72	180	60
4	IDF	F	30.0	82	180	50
5	IDF	F	35.5	63	210	60
6	IDF	F	29.9	72	180	45
Mean			29.9	67.5	205	56.7
SD			2.97	10.23	29.5	13.3

Legend: SD: Standard deviation, IDF: Ile-De-France, F: female.

Hearing thresholds were compared before and after the acoustic trauma. As shown in Table 2, the mean hearing threshold before noise exposure was 28.3 ± 4.1 dB nHL for the NH ear and 26.7 ± 5.2 dB nHL for the NIHL ear. The mean hearing threshold in the NIHL ear was measured after the acoustic trauma was 58.3 ± 4.1 dB nHL. A paired t-test showed a significant difference in hearing threshold before and after noise exposure [t(5) = 10.3; $p < 0.001$]. All sheep exhibited NIHL after noise exposure.

Table 2. Auditory thresholds (wave IV from BC-ABRs) for the NH model ear before perilymph sampling, and for the NIHL model ear before perilymph sampling and after acoustic trauma.

	NH Model		NIHL Model		
Sheep N°	Side	Threshold before Sampling (dB)	Side	Threshold before Sampling (dB)	Threshold after Acoustic Trauma (dB)
1	L	30	R	30	60
2	L	30	R	30	50
3	R	30	L	30	60
4	R	30	L	30	60
5	R	30	L	20	60
6	L	20	R	20	60
Mean	-	28.3		26.7	58.3
SD	-	4.1		5.2	4.1

NH, normal hearing; NIHL, noise-induced hearing loss. Legend: SD: Standard Deviation, NIHL: noise-induced hearing loss, L: Left, R: Right, dB: decibel.

3.2. Effect of Acoustic Trauma on the Perilymph Metabolome

Twelve perilymph samples were collected: six from the NH control ear and six from the NIHL ear. The mean volume of perilymph collected was 89 ± 11 µL. Perilymph from the NH ear was collected at baseline and perilymph from NIHL ear was collected following the noise exposure. The samples were analyzed using LC/HRMS to perform the metabolomic analysis, and 213 metabolites were identified. The PCA score plot based on the metabolic profiles of the QC and sheep samples did not reveal any outliers (Figure 2).

Paired univariate analysis between NH control and NIHL perilymph samples with a $p < 0.1$ and FC ratio < 0.8 or >1.2 revealed four significantly different metabolites: Urocanate ($p = 0.004$; FC = 0.48), S-(5'-Adenosyl)-L-Homocysteine ($p = 0.060$; FC = 2.32), Trigonelline ($p = 0.060$; FC = 0.46), and N-Acetyl-L-Leucine ($p = 0.090$; FC = 2.02).

Paired supervised multivariate analysis showed some discrimination between the NH and NIHL groups; however, this was not significant (accuracy 50%; permutation test $p = 0.75$). This model enabled the identification of metabolites involved in pathophysiological mechanisms associated with acoustic trauma. Some metabolites tended to increase after noise exposure: Urocanate, Oleate, 5-Oxo-L-Proline, N-Acetyl-Glucose, N-Acetylneuraminate, L-Tyrosine, Trigonelline, Leukotriene-B4, 5,6-Dihydrouracil, and

3-Ureidopropionate. Some metabolites tended to decrease after noise exposure: Deoxycarnitine, L-Carnitine, N-Acetyl-L-Leucine, S-(5′-Adenosyl)-L-Homocysteine, and Epinephrine.

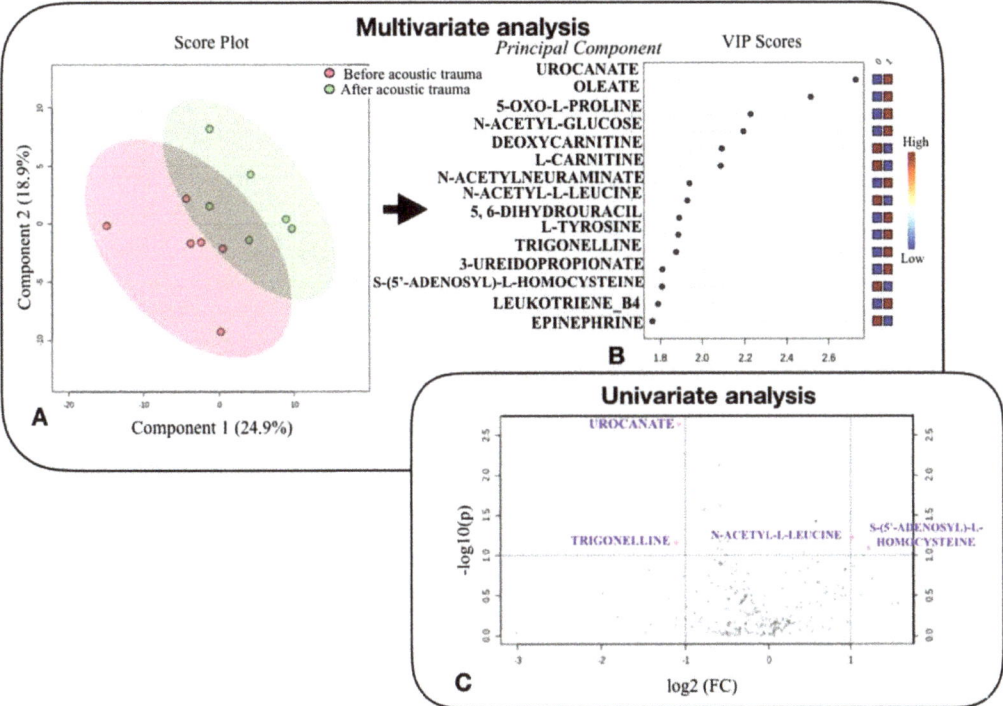

Figure 2. Statistical analysis to compare the metabolomic profile of perilymph fluid from sheep before and after acoustic trauma. (**A**): Multivariate analysis using partial least squares discriminant analysis (PLSDA) to distinguish metabolomic profile of perilymph fluid from sheep before (red circles) and after acoustic trauma (green circles). Components 1 and 2 represent a linear combination of relevant metabolites expressing maximum variance. (**B**): The rank of different metabolites (top 15) identified by PLSDA according to the VIP (Variable Influence of Projection) score on the left. The colored boxes on the right indicate the relative concentrations of the corresponding metabolite in each group studied. (**C**): Univariate analysis via a plot based on fold change and p-value, highlighting 4 metabolites. The volcano plot based on the comparison between NH control and NIHL perilymph samples, highlighting metabolites characterized by a FC > 1.2 concentration ratio and a t-test (y) < 0.1 (pink points). Note that fold changes and p-values are log transformed. The further away from (0.0) position, the more important the feature.

3.3. Analysis of Metabolic Pathways

Uni- and multi-variate metabolomic analysis of perilymph before and after acoustic trauma revealed significant metabolites of interest. Subsequently, an interpretation of the metabolic pathways involved from these metabolites was performed.

As shown in Table 3, according to all metabolites considered to be relevant after uni- and multi-variate analysis, metabolic pathway analysis revealed the involvement of 5 main pathways: phenylalanine/tyrosine/tryptophan metabolism ($p = 0.037$; impact = 0.5), β-alanine metabolism ($p = 0.015$; impact = 0.16), pantothenate and CoA biosynthesis ($p = 0.012$; impact = 0.05), pyrimidine metabolism ($p = 0.046$; Impact = 0.11), and amino and nucleotide sugar metabolism ($p = 0.044$; impact = 0.05).

Table 3. Significant metabolic pathways involved in noise-induced hearing loss via perilymph analysis. The p-value was calculated from the enrichment analysis. p-FDR is the adjusted p-value using the false discovery rate. Impact values were calculated from the path topology analysis.

Pathway	p-Value	p-FDR	Impact
Pantothenate and CoA biosynthesis	0.012	0.64	0.05
β-alanine metabolism	0.015	0.64	0.16
Phenylalanine, tyrosine, tryptophan biosynthesis	0.037	0.78	0.50
Amino sugar and nucleotide metabolism	0.044	0.78	0.11
Pyrimidine metabolism	0.046	0.78	0.05

An interactive Google-Map visualization system was implemented to facilitate data exploration. Pathway and compound identification was dynamically generated based on interactions with the visualization system (Figure 3). The main metabolic pathway identified was phenylalanine, tyrosine, and tryptophan biosynthesis.

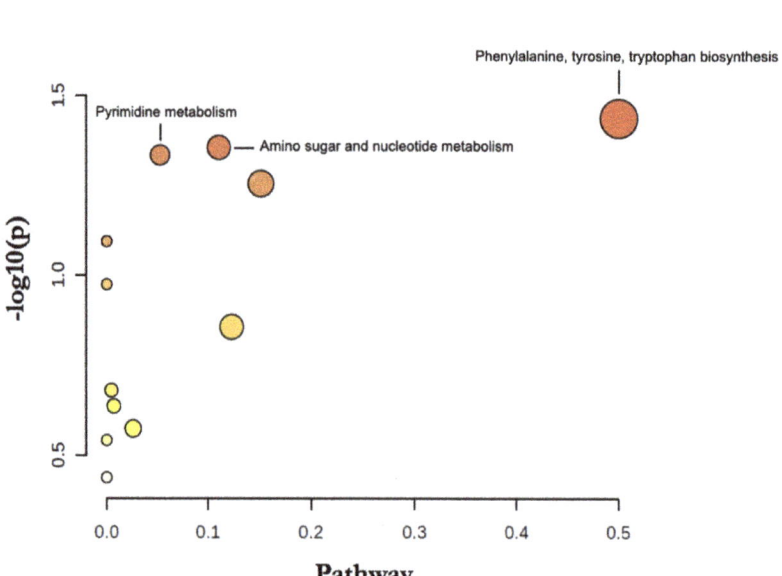

Figure 3. Metabolomic Pathway Analysis based on the 15 VIP metabolites the most discriminant in the multivariate model explaining hearing loss. The circles resume all matched pathways according to the p values from the pathway enrichment analysis and pathway impact values from the pathway topology analysis (calculated as the sum of importance measures of the matched metabolites normalized by the sum of the importance measures of all metabolites in each pathway). Each circle represents a metabolite set with its color based on its p-value (darker colors indicate more significant changes in metabolites belonging to the corresponding pathway), and its size is based on pathway impact score. The most impacted pathways are annotated.

4. Discussion

The results of our metabolomic analysis model identified 213 metabolites in sheep perilymph and provide new findings regarding NIHL. Because compounds related to cochlear neurotransmission and metabolic stress were altered by acoustic trauma, this supports the validity of the methodology. Importantly, the analysis identified several previously unknown pathways that were altered by noise exposure (pantothenate and

CoA biosynthesis, β-alanine metabolism, and pyrimidine metabolism), indicating that this emerging omic technique may provide new insights regarding metabolome changes in the perilymph triggered by acoustic trauma.

4.1. Interest in the Sheep Model

In otology research, rodents have been the most frequently used animal model [12], due to their availability and preferable housing facilities. Yet, rodents show little anatomical, biological, or metabolic similarity to humans with respect to the auditory system [12]. Anatomically, the sheep cochlea has two and a half turns, similar to humans, and has been investigated in a computed tomography study [13]. Unlike the guinea pig, the anatomy of the round window membrane of the sheep shows multiple similarities with humans [14,15]. The auditory spectrum of sheep is comparable to that of humans [16], with humans having an auditory spectrum from 20 to 20,000 Hz and sheep from 100 to 30,000 Hz [16,17]. In rodents and small animals, it is difficult to collect cochlear fluids such as perilymph given the anatomy of the inner ear. In large animals, the perilymph volume is larger and easier to sample through the round window [13,18,19]. For these reasons, sheep may be a better animal model and was therefore used in the present study.

4.2. Research Approach

Our research approach appears to be valid and effective. The acoustic trauma technique resulted in significant hearing loss. The sheep were euthanized at the end of the procedure because it is not ethical to wake up a deafened sheep given the damage to the facial nerve. As such, we did not re-measure thresholds to observe whether any hearing recuperation occurred. Two types of noise stimuli can be used to induce acoustic trauma: impulse noise and continuous noise. Impulse noise causes immediate damage and a shift in transient thresholds, whereas continuous noise causes cochlear damage with inflammatory healing, resulting in transient and permanent hearing loss over the longer term [7]. The choice of impulse noise was dictated by the objective of causing rapid lesions with significant hearing loss in order to observe consequences at the metabolic level. The choice of 120 dB SPL stimulus intensity with 1 h of exposure was motivated by the fact that synaptopathy lesions are visible from a threshold of 100 dB SPL [18] and cochlear lesions can be observed from a threshold of 115 dB SPL [20]. The impulse noise of 120 dB SPL for 1 h resulted in substantial and significant hearing loss.

4.3. Metabolomics as a Powerful Approach to Characterize Perilymph

To date, six previous studies on inner ear metabolomics have been published [18,19,21–24]. Two studies focused on the metabolomic analysis of perilymph during cochlear implantation in humans [21,22]. One study analyzed perilymph fluid following cisplatin-induced ototoxicity in guinea pigs [24]. For an analysis of the metabolomics of the perilymph following NIHL, two studies were performed using guinea pigs and found approximately 100 metabolites [19,23], far fewer than the 213 metabolites found in the present study. Another study analyzed metabolomics following NIHL using mice [18], finding 220 metabolites [18]; however, the whole inner ear was sampled (bone and perilymph), as opposed to only perilymph in the present study. The abundance of metabolites found in the present study may be attributed to metabolomic analysis technique [21], the larger volume of perilymph collected, and the use of capillarity to sample the perilymph.

4.4. Metabolomic Modifications following Acoustic Trauma

Our results suggested the implication of different pathways to explain the pathophysiological mechanisms following acoustic trauma. Indeed, following acoustic trauma, our hypotheses are mechanical destruction of hair cells, damages of the synapses and nerve, and oxidative stress due to inflammatory reactions.

4.4.1. Neurotransmission

Of particular interest is our finding is that noise had an impact on the biosynthesis of phenylalanine, tyrosine, and tryptophan that are aromatic amino acids, the precursors of the monoamine neurotransmitters, serotonin, and catecholamines (dopamine, norepinephrine, and epinephrine) [25]. This point was raised in a previous study where alterations in these amino acids were also observed in the mammalian cochlea [18]. One study has shown that aromatic amino acids suppress discharge by afferent fibers innervating hair cells [26]. Their exact function in NIHL remains to be demonstrated.

4.4.2. Oxidative Stress

The oxidative stress pathway following acoustic trauma and its counterbalance by the action of antioxidant systems are well documented [27] and are reflected in our results. First, urocanate was significantly increased after acoustic trauma. It is likely to lead to the production of ROS responsible for increased cell death [27]. This has been observed in the brain, where urocanate has been associated with an increase in glutamate synthesis [28]. An excessive release of glutamate and/or hyper activation of glutamate receptors in the cochlea results in excitotoxicity responsible for damage to hair cell synapses [9]. Our results suggest the same mechanism in the perilymph.

Our findings also suggest the involvement of the pantothenate and CoA biosynthetic pathway after sound exposure, similar to other animal studies [23]. CoA is a cofactor for a multitude of enzymatic reactions, including the oxidation of fatty acids, carbohydrates, pyruvate, lactate, ketone bodies, and amino acids [29]. Pantothenate can regulate CoA synthesis in cell membranes and protect against increased oxidative stress by reducing the level of malondialdehyde (MDA), the major product of lipid peroxidation. It can inhibit the inflammatory process by reducing the level of inflammatory reactive proteins and promoting CoA and glutathione levels [30]. An implication of S-(5'-Adenosyl)-L-Homocysteine was found in the NIHL model. Partearroyo et al. [31] studied homocysteine and hearing loss and found that homocysteine is involved in oxidative stress.

4.4.3. Mechanical Destruction

The present results suggest the mechanical destruction of cells following acoustic trauma according to the presence of ß-alanine and N-acetylneuraminate metabolites. ß-alanine is present in hair cells; its increase in the perilymph following noise exposure suggests cellular destruction [32]. N-acetylneuraminate, a derivative of sialic acid, is usually located on the terminal portion of glycoproteins and glycolipids located on the surface of the cell membrane [22]. High concentrations of this metabolite can be explained by the rupture of the cell membrane and are found during cell death and the onset of apoptosis.

4.4.4. Nerve Damage

The present results suggest nerve damage occurred, given the difference in perilymph composition in trigonelline and N-Acetyl-L-Leucine between the NH and NIHL ears. Trigonelline was significantly altered following acoustic trauma. Its role has been demonstrated in the reduction in auditory damage and in hearing loss in mice [33,34]. Trigonelline can also reduce neurodegenerative effects with the use of nerve growth factor. It reduces oxidative stress and causes neuroprotective effects and interacts with ototoxic signaling pathways [33,34]. These results are of particular interest in terms of associations between trigonelline and NIHL; to date, literature on this subject is non-existent.

We observed a decrease in N-Acetyl-L-Leucine, which is mainly known for its vestibular action. It acts by normalizing the membrane potential at the level of the vestibular nuclei, allowing for improvement in balance function, and affects the regrowth of neurons. The consumption of N-Acetyl-L-Leucine in the perilymph following acoustic trauma may be explained by its effect on nerve healing [35]. To date, there are no studies on NIHL and N-acetyl-L-leucine.

4.5. Limits to the Study

The small number of sheep tested is a limitation to this study. However, this study represents important preliminary work for future metabolomic analysis studies in larger populations.

The duration of anesthesia is another limitation of this study. The perilymph metabolome results could have been impacted by the drugs used and the duration of procedure [36]. However, considering the pharmacokinetic properties of the anesthesia medications used, this seems unlikely. Likewise, no link has been established in the literature between the anesthesia medications used and metabolites. An alternative approach would have been to randomize the perilymph sampling across ears and sheep (e.g., first sampling the perilymph in the NIHL ear after acoustic trauma and then measuring thresholds and sampling perilymph in the NH control ear). However, this approach may have induced contralateral hearing loss in the NH ear, thereby distorting the results.

It would have been interesting to know whether hearing thresholds recovered after acoustic trauma and if so, the time course of the recovery. However, this extended testing was deemed to be unethical in consideration of the welfare of the animals.

5. Conclusions

These preliminary results suggest that in case of NIHL, several metabolic pathways are involved that relate to mechanical destruction, oxidative stress, neurotransmission, and nerve damage. Metabolomic analysis is still in the early stages of development as an approach to study SNHL. The identification of specific metabolites as biomarkers or a metabolomic profile for NIHL could be used to relate hearing loss with noise exposure, especially in cases where the cause of hearing loss is unknown. Metabolomic analysis may also contribute to development of therapeutics for NIHL. Further studies are needed to confirm these results and to develop an atraumatic approach to sample the perilymph, especially in humans.

Author Contributions: Conceptualization, D.B., H.B. and P.E.; methodology, D.B, H.B. and P.E.; validation, D.B., H.B., E.C., P.E. and L.B.; formal analysis, D.B. and H.B.; investigation, L.B. and D.B.; resources, H.B. and L.B.; data curation, L.B.; writing—original draft preparation, L.B. and D.B.; writing—review and editing, D.B. and H.B.; visualization, D.B.; supervision, D.B. and H.B. All authors have read and agreed to the published version of the manuscript.

Funding: This research received no external funding.

Institutional Review Board Statement: The animal study protocol was approved by the Ethics Committee of CEEA Val de Loire N°19 (APAFIS #2018112714344369 and 21/03/2019) for studies involving animals.

Informed Consent Statement: Not applicable.

Acknowledgments: This research is supported by Fondation Pour l'Audition (FPA RD 2020-4). Thanks to John Galvin for editorial assistance.

Conflicts of Interest: The authors declare no conflict of interest.

References

1. World Health Organisation. Deafness and Hearing Impairment. Available online: http://www.who.int/mediacentre/factsheets/fs300/en/index/html (accessed on 3 June 2022).
2. Kral, A.; O'Donoghue, G.M. Profound deafness in childhood. *N. Engl. J. Med.* **2010**, *363*, 1438–1450. [CrossRef]
3. Huddle, M.G.; Goman, A.M.; Kernizan, F.C.; Folley, D.M.; Price, C.; Frick, K.D.; Lin, F.R. The Economic Impact of Adult Hearing Loss: A Systematic Review. *JAMA Otolaryngol. Head Neck Surg.* **2017**, *143*, 1040–1048. [CrossRef] [PubMed]
4. Mathers, C.; Smith, A.; Concha, M. Global burden of hearing loss in the year 2000. *Glob. Burd. Dis.* **2000**, *18*, 1–30.
5. Blamey, P.; Artieres, F.; Başkent, D.; Bergeron, F.; Beynon, A.; Burke, E.; Dillier, N.; Dowell, R.; Fraysse, B.; Gallégo, S.; et al. Factors affecting auditory performance of postlinguistically deaf adults using cochlear implants: An update with 2251 patients. *Audiol. Neurootol.* **2013**, *18*, 36–47. [CrossRef] [PubMed]
6. Le, T.N.; Straatman, L.V.; Lea, J. Current insights in noise-induced hearing loss: A literature review of the underlying mechanism, pathophysiology, asymmetry, and management options. *J. Otolaryngol. Head Neck Surg.* **2017**, *46*, 41. [CrossRef] [PubMed]

7. Hamernik, R.P.; Hsueh, K.D. Impulse noise: Some definitions, physical acoustics and other considerations. *J. Acoust. Soc. Am.* **1991**, *90*, 189–196. [CrossRef] [PubMed]
8. Le Prell, C.G.; Hammill, T.L.; Murphy, W.J. Noise-induced hearing loss and its prevention: Integration of data from animal models and human clinical trials. *J. Acoust. Soc. Am.* **2019**, *146*, 4051. [CrossRef]
9. Kujawa, S.G.; Liberman, M.C. Adding insult to injury: Cochlear nerve degeneration after "temporary" noise-induced hearing loss. *J. Neurosci.* **2009**, *29*, 14077–14085. [CrossRef]
10. Carta, F.; Lussu, M.; Bandino, F.; Noto, A.; Peppi, M.; Chuchueva, N.; Atzori, L.; Fanos, V.; Puxeddu, R. Metabolomic analysis of urine with Nuclear Magnetic Resonance spectroscopy in patients with idiopathic sudden sensorineural hearing loss: A preliminary study. *Auris Nasus Larynx* **2017**, *44*, 381–389. [CrossRef]
11. Diémé, B.; Mavel, S.; Blasco, H.; Tripi, G.; Bonnet-Brilhault, F.; Malvy, J.; Bocca, C.; Andres, C.R.; Nadal-Desbarats, L.; Emond, P. Metabolomics Study of Urine in Autism Spectrum Disorders Using a Multiplatform Analytical Methodology. *J. Proteome Res.* **2015**, *14*, 5273–5282. [CrossRef]
12. Reis, A.; Dalmolin, S.P.; Dallegrave, E. Animal models for hearing evaluations: A literature review. *Revista CEFAC* **2017**, *19*, 417–428. [CrossRef]
13. Trinh, T.T.; Cohen, C.; Boullaud, L.; Cottier, J.P.; Bakhos, D. Sheep as a large animal model for cochlear implantation. *Braz. J. Otorhinolaryngol.* **2021**, in press. [CrossRef] [PubMed]
14. Han, S.; Suzuki-Kerr, H.; Suwantika, M.; Telang, R.S.; Gerneke, D.A.; Anekal, P.V.; Bird, P.; Vlajkovic, S.M.; Thorne, P.R. Characterization of the Sheep Round Window Membrane. *J. Assoc. Res. Otolaryngol.* **2021**, *22*, 1–17. [CrossRef]
15. Soares, H.B.; Lavinsky, L. Histology of sheep temporal bone. *Braz. J. Otolhinolaryngol.* **2011**, *77*, 285–292. [CrossRef] [PubMed]
16. Péus, D.; Dobrev, I.; Prochazka, L.; Thoele, K.; Dalbert, A.; Boss, A.; Newcomb, N.; Probst, R.; Röösli, C.; Sim, J.H.; et al. Sheep as a large animal ear model: Middle-ear ossicular velocities and intracochlear sound pressure. *Hear. Res.* **2017**, *351*, 88–97. [CrossRef] [PubMed]
17. Hill, M.W.; Heavens, R.P.; Baldwin, B.A. Auditory evoked potentials recorded from conscious sheep. *Brain Res. Bull.* **1985**, *15*, 453–458. [CrossRef]
18. Ji, L.; Lee, H.J.; Wan, G.; Wang, G.P.; Zhang, L.; Sajjakulnukit, P.; Schacht, J.; Lyssiotis, C.A.; Corfas, G. Auditory metabolomics, an approach to identify acute molecular effects of noise trauma. *Sci. Rep.* **2019**, *9*, 9273. [CrossRef] [PubMed]
19. Fujita, T.; Yamashita, D.; Irino, Y.; Kitamoto, J.; Fukuda, Y.; Inokuchi, G.; Hasegawa, S.; Otsuki, N.; Yoshida, M.; Nibu, K.I. Metabolomic profiling in inner ear fluid by gas chromatography/mass spectrometry in guinea pig cochlea. *Neurosci. Lett.* **2015**, *606*, 188–193. [CrossRef]
20. Valero, M.D.; Burton, J.A.; Hauser, S.N.; Hackett, T.A.; Ramachandran, R.; Liberman, M.C. Noise-induced cochlear synaptopathy in rhesus monkeys (*Macaca mulatta*). *Hear. Res.* **2017**, *353*, 213–223. [CrossRef]
21. Mavel, S.; Lefèvre, A.; Bakhos, D.; Dufour-Rainfray, D.; Blasco, H.; Emond, P. Validation of metabolomics analysis of human perilymph fluid using liquid chromatography-mass spectroscopy. *Hear. Res.* **2018**, *367*, 129–136. [CrossRef] [PubMed]
22. Trinh, T.T.; Blasco, H.; Emond, P.; Andres, C.; Lefevre, A.; Lescanne, E.; Bakhos, D. Relationship between metabolomics profile of perilymph in Cochlear-Implanted patients and duration of hearing loss. *Metabolites* **2019**, *9*, 262. [CrossRef] [PubMed]
23. Pirttilä, K.; Videhult Pierre, P.; Haglöf, J.; Engskog, M.; Hedeland, M.; Laurell, G.; Arvidsson, T.; Pettersson, C. An LCMS-based Untargeted Metabolomics Protocol for Cochlear Perilymph: Highlighting Metabolic Effects of Hydrogen Gas on the Inner Ear of Noise Exposed Guinea Pigs. *Metabolomics* **2019**, *15*, 138. [CrossRef] [PubMed]
24. Fransson, A.E.; Kisiel, M.; Pirttilä, K.; Pettersson, C.; Videhult Pierre, P.; Laurell, G.F. Hydrogen Inhalation Protects against Ototoxicity Induced by Intravenous Cisplatin in the Guinea Pig. *Front. Cell Neurosci.* **2017**, *11*, 280. [CrossRef] [PubMed]
25. Fernstrom, J.D.; Fernstrom, M.H. Tyrosine, phenylalanine, and catecholamine synthesis and function in the brain. *J. Nutr.* **2007**, *137*, 1539S–1547S; discussion 1548S. [CrossRef] [PubMed]
26. Mroz, E.A.; Sewell, W.F. Pharmacological alterations of the activity of afferent fibers innervating hair cells. *Hear. Res.* **1989**, *38*, 141–162. [CrossRef]
27. Brosnan, M.E.; Brosnan, J.T. Histidine Metabolism and Function. *J. Nutr.* **2020**, *150* (Suppl. S1), 2570S–2575S. [CrossRef] [PubMed]
28. Hart, P.H.; Norval, M. The Multiple Roles of Urocanic Acid in Health and Disease. *J. Invest. Dermatol.* **2021**, *141*, 496–502. [CrossRef] [PubMed]
29. Tahiliani, A.G.; Beinlich, C.J. Pantothenic acid in health and disease. *Vitam. Horm.* **1991**, *46*, 165–228. [CrossRef]
30. Ma, T.; Liu, T.; Xie, P.; Jiang, S.; Yi, W.; Dai, P.; Guo, X. UPLC-MS-based urine nontargeted metabolic profiling identifies dysregulation of pantothenate and CoA biosynthesis pathway in diabetic kidney disease. *Life Sci.* **2020**, *258*, 118160. [CrossRef] [PubMed]
31. Partearroyo, T.; Vallecillo, N.; Pajares, M.A.; Varela-Moreiras, G.; Varela-Nieto, I. Cochlear Homocysteine Metabolism at the Crossroad of Nutrition and Sensorineural Hearing Loss. *Front. Mol. Neurosci.* **2017**, *10*, 107. [CrossRef]
32. Drescher, M.J.; Drescher, D.G. N-acetylhistidine, glutamate, and beta-alanine are concentrated in a receptor cell layer of the trout inner ear. *J. Neurochem.* **1991**, *56*, 658–664. [CrossRef] [PubMed]
33. Castañeda, R.; Rodriguez, I.; Nam, Y.H.; Hong, B.N.; Kang, T.H. Trigonelline promotes auditory function through nerve growth factor signaling on diabetic animal models. *Phytomedicine* **2017**, *36*, 128–136. [CrossRef]
34. Yoshinari, O.; Takenake, A.; Igarashi, K. Trigonelline ameliorates oxidative stress in type 2 diabetic Goto-Kakizaki rats. *J. Med. Food* **2013**, *16*, 34–41. [CrossRef]

- A collection of 22 CT images of non-implanted cochleae—20 from the SMIR database of cochlea data descriptors (SICAS Medical Repository, Corroux, Switzerland) [28] and 2 from our own database.

2.2. Registration Procedure

2.2.1. Determination of Cochlea Dimensions

Selection of the "basilar membrane" template for each patient was based on several measurements of the cochlea imaged by preoperative CT. These measurements were taken in a single slice at a specific orientation and position through the cochlea. In the first implementation of the method, we used the 3D multiplanar reconstruction viewer of the General Public License (GPL) software Horos v.3.3.6 (Horos project, Geneva, Switzerland) [29]. The cochlea was aligned as follows: (1) the intersection of the three planes was placed on the mid-modiolar axis; (2) the coronal plane was aligned with the middle plane of the basal turn (center of the round window, the middle of the cochlear turn at 90°, 180°, and 270°); (3) the axial plane was consequently perpendicular to the coronal plane and passed through the center of the round window and the cochlear turn at 180°; and (4) the sagittal plane was also perpendicular to the coronal plane and passed through the cochlear turn at 90° and 270°.

Aligning the planes with the theoretical position of the middle plane of the cochlear turn is crucial. In a post-implanted cochlea, the theoretical position of this plane is defined without considering the position of the electrode array. Once alignment was completed, we measured the following (Figure 1):

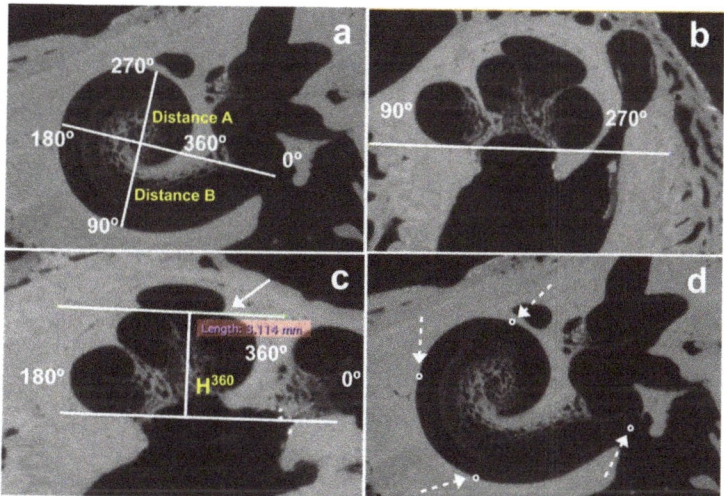

Figure 1. Measurement of distances A, B, and H^{360}. H^{360} was measured from the base of the cochlea to the highest part of the cochlear turn at 360° (white arrow). (**a**) Coronal view, (**b**) sagittal view, which has been rotated to position the basal turn inferiorly for better visualization, (**c**) axial view. (**d**) the same alignment was necessary to measure distances A and B to determine the position of the center of the round window and the lateral wall at 90°, 180°, and 270° (white discontinuous arrows).

- Distance A (A) between the center of the round window and lateral wall at 180°;
- Distance B (B) between the lateral wall at 90° and 270°;
- The height at 360° (H^{360}), measured from the base of the cochlea to the highest point of the cochlear turn at 360°.

We defined three cochlear indices from these measurements (Table 1): $A \times H^{360}$, $(A \times B) \times H^{360}$, and $(A/B) \times H^{360}$.

5. Günther, L.; Beck, R.; Xiong, G.; Potschka, H.; Jahn, K.; Bartenstein, P.; Brandt, T.; Dutia, M.; Dieterich, M.; Strupp, M.; et al. N-acetyl-L-leucine accelerates vestibular compensation after unilateral labyrinthectomy by action in the cerebellum and thalamus. *PLoS ONE* **2015**, *10*, e0120891. [CrossRef]
6. Xiao, Y.; Wen, J.; Bai, Y.; Duan, N.; Jing, G.X. Different effects of propofol and isoflurane on cochlear blood flow and hearing function in Guinea pigs. *PLoS ONE* **2014**, *9*, e96861. [CrossRef] [PubMed]

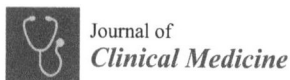

Article

Best Fit 3D Basilar Membrane Reconstruction to Routinely Assess the Scalar Position of the Electrode Array after Cochlear Implantation

Renato Torres [1,2,3,*], Jean-Yves Tinevez [4], Hannah Daoudi [1,2], Ghizlene Lahlou [1,2], Neil Grislain [2], Eugénie Breil [2], Olivier Sterkers [1,2], Isabelle Mosnier [1,2], Yann Nguyen [1,2] and Evelyne Ferrary [1,2]

1. Technologies et Thérapie Génique Pour la Surdité, Institut de l'Audition, Inserm/Institut Pasteur/Université de Paris, 75012 Paris, France; hannah.daoudi@aphp.fr (H.D.); ghizlene.lahlou@aphp.fr (G.L.); o.sterkers@gmail.com (O.S.); isabelle.mosnier@aphp.fr (I.M.); yann.nguyen@inserm.fr (Y.N.); evelyne.ferrary@inserm.fr (E.F.)
2. Unité Fonctionnelle Implants Auditifs et Explorations Fonctionnelles, Service ORL, GHU Pitié-Salpêtrière, Assistance Publique-Hôpitaux de Paris (AP-HP)/Sorbonne Université, 75013 Paris, France; neil.grislain@aphp.fr (N.G.); eugenie.breil@gmail.com (E.B.)
3. Departamento de Ciencias Fisiológicas, Facultad de Medicina, Universidad Nacional de San Agustín de Arequipa, Arequipa 04002, Peru
4. Image Analysis Hub, Institut Pasteur, Université de Paris, 75015 Paris, France; jean-yves.tinevez@pasteur.fr
* Correspondence: victor.torres-lazo@pasteur.fr

Abstract: The scalar position of the electrode array is assumed to be associated with auditory performance after cochlear implantation. We propose a new method that can be routinely applied in clinical practice to assess the position of an electrode array. Ten basilar membrane templates were generated using micro-computed tomography (micro-CT), based on the dimensions of 100 cochleae. Five surgeons were blinded to determine the position of the electrode array in 30 cadaveric cochleae. The procedure consisted of selecting the appropriate template based on cochlear dimensions, merging the electrode array reconstruction with the template using four landmarks, determining the position of the array according to the template position, and comparing the results obtained to histology data. The time taken to analyze each implanted cochlea was approximately 12 min. We found that, according to histology, surgeons were in almost perfect agreement when determining an electrode translocated to the scala vestibuli with the perimodiolar MidScala array (Fleiss' kappa (κ) = 0.82), and in moderate agreement when using the lateral wall EVO array (κ = 0.42). Our data indicate that an adapted basilar membrane template can be used as a rapid and reproducible method to assess the position of the electrode array after cochlear implantation.

Keywords: hearing loss; hearing impairment rehabilitation; scala vestibuli; scala tympani; auditory prosthesis; electrode array translocation

1. Introduction

Cochlear implantation is a surgical procedure to insert an electrode array into the cochlea. This device stimulates the ganglion auditory cells and rehabilitates hearing; however, postoperative auditory performance can vary from patient to patient. Many preoperative factors, such as the etiology of hearing loss, duration of profound deafness, use of hearing aids, and age at implantation [1,2] can affect the hearing outcome; however, the electrode array insertion is one of the few factors that can be optimized. During cochlear implantation, it is important to accomplish non-traumatic insertion of the electrode array, as this is associated with a reduction in inflammatory processes [3], preservation of residual hearing [4], and improvement in hearing performance [5–7].

Different surgical strategies have been developed to improve electrode array insertion, such as using fine and flexible electrode arrays [6], round window insertion [8], and using

hyaluronic acid after opening the cochlea to lubricate it and avoid blood c(
and perilymph leakage [9]. Most recently, robot-assisted insertion of the electr
been implemented to improve the accuracy of movement during surgery [10
development of these technical and surgical strategies, there have been a num
of incorrect location of the electrode array, with varying degrees of transl
the scala tympani to the scala vestibuli [5,6,11–13]. It is therefore essential
whether an electrode array is poorly positioned after surgery, as this will
hearing performance, requiring a technical adjustment of the cochlear impla

Different methods have been proposed to precisely determine the p
electrode array and its possible translocation. Computed tomography (CT
performed after cochlear implantation to determine the presence of any
Earlier studies have reported the use of rotational tomography [14], multisec
and cone-beam CT imaging (CBCT) [16,17]. Although different multiplanar r
have been performed to assess the position of electrode arrays, they have ma
owing to the blurring effect produced by the metallic artifacts of the electr
intracochlear structures are not visible with post-implantation imaging, anc
method is the fusion of postoperative CT imaging with preoperative magn
imaging (MRI) [18,19]. MRI is routinely performed before cochlear implant
be merged with postoperative imaging. However, the number of slices passir
cochlea is limited, and to improve image quality, the time of acquisition mu
significantly, which is not practical in a clinical scenario. To overcome the
cochlear anatomy, a method has been proposed that uses manual 3D recons
basilar membrane on preimplantation CBCT [20]. This 3D reconstruction wa
the 3D reconstruction of the electrode array from the same patient based on
the semicircular canals. Although the accuracy of this method has been v
histology, the time required to obtain a 3D reconstruction of the basilar
a limitation.

Because intracochlear structures are not visible on postoperative imag
struction models have been used to determine the position of the electrc
cochlear implantation. A rigid model was proposed as a method for estimatii
of intracochlear structures [21,22]. The high-quality rigid model obtained wa
with the CT images to determine the position of the electrode array. Howev
model, the variability of the cochlear anatomy parameters, such as its di
or the variability of the coiling of the cochlea [24,25], cannot be taken int
improve the accuracy of the method, the use of several rigid cochlear mo
a way to adapt to anatomic variations. Another proposed method used no
to determine the position of the electrode array [26,27]. This allowed th
adjusted according to the cochlear anatomy, and automatically determine
of the intracochlear structure. However, 3D reconstruction methods are tin
require considerable manual effort to handle images, and require the necessi
and training; thus, they are not included in the clinical procedure. Conseque
that allows for routine and rapid analysis of the position of the electrode a
practice is still lacking, but desirable.

In this study, we evaluated the accuracy of determining the position o
array using a 3D basilar membrane template selected to match the cochlear
30 cadaverically implanted cochleae. The position of each electrode was as
ear-nose-throat (ENT) surgeons and compared with the histology.

2. Materials and Methods

2.1. Cochlear Images Used in This Study

We based this study on an image bank that included the following:

- A set of 100 CT images from pre-implanted patients;
- Images of 30 cadaveric temporal bones, including pre- and post-impla

Table 1. Cochlear dimensions of 100 pre-implantation cochleae. The three indices (A)×H^{360}, (A×B) ×H^{360}, and (A/B)×H^{360} have a Gaussian distribution.

	Patient CT (n = 100)		Cadaveric CBCT (n = 30)		Micro-CT (n = 22)	
	Mean ± SD	Min–Max	Mean ± SD	Min–Max	Mean ± SD	Min–Max
Distance A	9.1 ± 0.30	8.0–9.6	9.1 ± 0.22	8.7–9.4	9.2 ± 0.33	8.6–9.8
Distance B	6.8 ± 0.32	5.8–7.6	6.9 ± 0.24	6.6–7.4	7.0 ± 0.31	6.5–7.5
H^{360}	2.8 ± 0.21	2.4–3.3	2.9 ± 0.17	2.6–3.3	2.9 ± 0.19	2.3–3.3
(A)×H^{360}	26 ± 2.30	20–33	26 ± 1.9	23–30	27 ± 2.4	22–29
(A×B)×H^{360}	175 ± 19.9	126–210	182 ± 17.2	159–211	194 ± 23.3	135–203
(A/B)×H^{360}	3.8 ± 0.30	3.0–4.7	3.8 ± 0.24	3.4–4.2	3.9 ± 0.29	3.1–4.4

CT: computed tomography; CBCT, cone-beam CT.

2.2.2. Determination of the Position of Four Electrode Array Landmarks

On the same slice, we then determined the 3D coordinates (x, y, z) of the four landmarks of the electrode array (Figure 2) that characterize its extent in 3D: the center of the round window, and the lateral wall at 90°, 180°, and 270°.

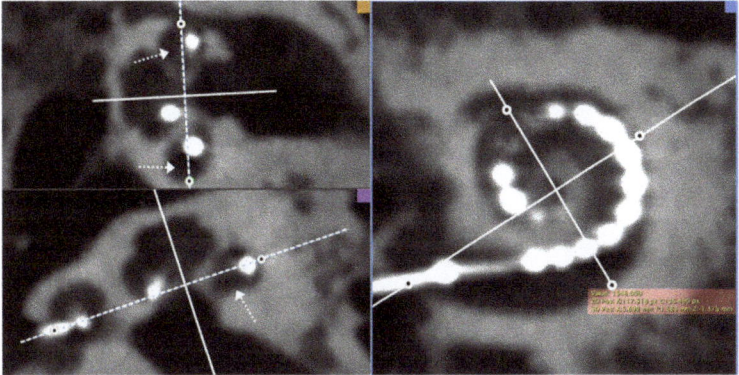

Figure 2. Determination of the 3D positions of four landmarks (the center of the round window, and the lateral wall at 90°, 180°, and 270°) on a post-implantation CBCT image. Note that the coronal plane (dashed line) is aligned with the middle of the cochlear turn regardless of the position of the electrode (white arrows). The point corresponding to the intersection between the middle cochlear turn line and the lateral wall was selected.

2.2.3. "Basilar Membrane" Segmentation

Where appropriate, the middle plane of the cochlear turn was manually segmented from the non-implanted cochleae images to obtain a 3D reconstruction, as reported in previous studies [13,20], using the GPL software ITK-SNAP v.3.4.0 (U.S. National Institutes of Health) [30]. Reconstruction of the middle plane of the cochlear turn included segmentation of the spiral lamina and basilar membrane. Throughout this paper, the term "basilar membrane" reconstruction represents reconstruction of the middle plane of the cochlear duct.

2.2.4. Electrode Array Segmentation

The electrode array was automatically segmented from CT images of the implanted cochlea. Because of its metallic composition, the array appeared as a very bright structure with pixel values well above those of the pixels in the temporal bone. We automatically segmented the electrode array volume using a threshold, as previously reported [13,20].

2.2.5. Procedure for Merging 3D Reconstruction Models

Finally, the two 3D reconstructions ("basilar membrane"/electrode array or "basilar membrane"/"basilar membrane") were registered and merged in the same scene using the four corresponding landmark points in each reconstruction (center of the round window, lateral wall at 90°, 180°, and 270°), with the point-by-point tool of the GPL software CloudCompare v.2.10.2 (https://www.cloudcompare.org) [31].

2.3. The "Basilar Membrane" Templates

Here, we describe how we built the five "basilar membrane" templates used after registration to determine the scalar position of the array. These five templates were built such that one could represent the cochlea of any patient once properly scaled. We also derived a procedure to select the best template based on the patient's cochlear dimensions as follows:

First, the cochlear dimensions and the three cochlear indices were obtained from pre-implantation CT images from 100 patients. The values obtained followed a Gaussian distribution $((A) \times H^{360}$: $p = 0.82$; $(A \times B) \times H^{360}$: $p = 0.85$; $(A/B) \times H$: $p = 0.13$; Shapiro–Wilk test). Consequently, five micro-CT cochleae were selected according to the Gaussian distribution of the patients' CT imaging (Figure 3), and this procedure was repeated for the three indices. In each case, the "basilar membrane" reconstruction and the four landmarks were obtained.

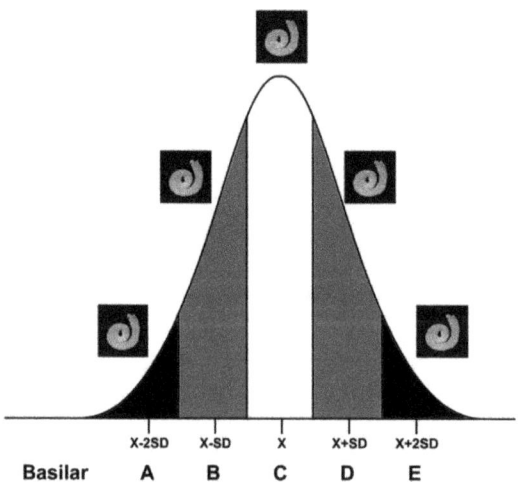

Figure 3. Five "basilar membrane" templates selected according to the normal distribution of each index—$(A) \times H^{360}$, $(A \times B) \times H^{360}$, and $(A/B) \times H^{360}$—on 100 CT images from pre-implanted patients.

Second, we reconstructed 10 "basilar membranes" from CBCT images of cadaveric temporal bones. The cochlear index was calculated based on each CBCT image, and the corresponding "basilar membrane" template was selected. Then, both "basilar membranes" were merged by means of the corresponding landmarks using the point-to-point tool in CloudCompare. Because it is quite difficult to manually segment the basilar membrane in CBCT images (hook region and beyond 540°), both "basilar membranes" (micro-CT and CBCT) were cropped from 90° to 540° at some locations.

Finally, the mean distances between the reconstruction models were calculated using the cloud/cloud distance tool of CloudCompare (Figure 4).

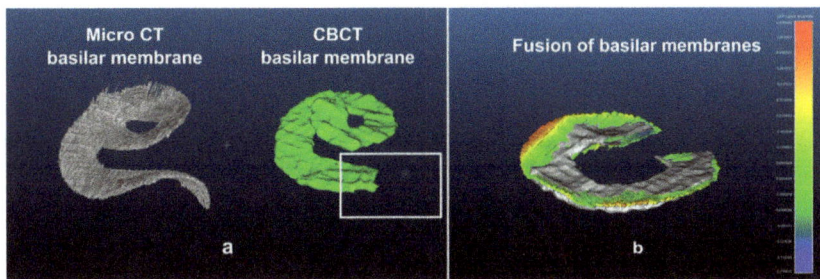

Figure 4. Comparison of basilar reconstruction segmented from micro-CT images and CBCT. The term basilar membrane represents the middle plane of the cochlear turn which includes the basilar membrane and the spiral lamina. (**a**) The hook region has not been segmented on CBCT images because of its complexity (open square); (**b**) the distance between both segmented "basilar membranes" (both cropped from 90° to 540°) was calculated. The color scale represents the distance between both basilar membranes, from green (shorter gap) to red (greater gap). In grey, both basilar membranes are superposed.

This procedure was repeated for each CBCT image and for the three cochlear indices. The distance after merging both "basilar membranes" was similar using the three indices ($(A) \times H^{360}$: 0.15 ± 0.03; $(A \times B) \times H^{360}$: 0.16 ± 0.02; $(A/B) \times H^{360}$: 0.14 ± 0.02; $p = 0.08$, Kruskal–Wallis and Bonferroni post hoc test). The $(A/B) \times H^{360}$ index was considered to be the best fit index because of its smaller distance error. We then used the GPL software Blender 2.8.0 (Blender Foundation, Amsterdam, The Netherlands) [32] to generate the five contralateral "basilar membrane" reconstructions.

2.4. Determination of the Intrascalar Position of Each Electrode

The best "basilar membrane" template was selected based on the $(A/B) \times H^{360}$ index measured on pre-implantation CBCT. The electrode array was segmented from the post-implantation CBCT and merged with the "basilar membrane" template using the four corresponding 3D points.

The scalar position of each electrode was determined according to the "basilar membrane", as the scala tympani, intermediary, and scala vestibuli electrodes. Owing to the rigidity of the "basilar membrane" reconstruction, the position of the electrode array was defined as follows:

- Scala tympani electrode: ≥50% of the electrode under the "basilar membrane".
- Intermediate electrode: ≥10% to <50% of the electrode under the "basilar membrane".
- Scala vestibuli electrode: <10% under the "basilar membrane".

2.5. Comparing the "Basilar Membrane" Reconstruction with Histology to Determine the Intrascalar Position of the Electrode Array

An ENT surgeon who did not participate in the image analysis chose 30 implanted cochleae from our histopathologic database (7 cochleae with translocations and 8 without for the HiFocus™ Mid-Scala electrode array (Advanced Bionics, Valencia, CA, USA); and 8 cochleae with translocations and 7 without for the Digisonic®SP EVO electrode array (Oticon Medical, Vallauris, France). The AB MidScala electrode array has 16 electrodes and the Oticon EVO electrode array has 20 electrodes. Each cochlea had a pre- and post-implantation CBCT. The same surgeon prepared a file with the pre- and post-operative CBCT for the 10 "basilar membrane" reconstructions corresponding to the $(A/B) \times H^{360}$ index, and gave it to the five surgeons for analysis. Any information on the histopathological study was made available to the surgeons. Two ENT surgeons were considered experts because of their experience in handling 3D reconstruction models. The other three ENT surgeons were considered non-experts because they had never handled 3D reconstruction models before this study.

Each surgeon performed the following procedure for each case:
1. Select a "basilar membrane" template according to the index value obtained on pre-implantation CBCT.
2. Obtain the reconstruction of the electrode array from the post-implantation CBCT.
3. Obtain the four corresponding points from the post-implantation CBCT.
4. Merge the electrode array reconstruction with the selected "basilar membrane" template according to the four landmarks.
5. Determine the position of each electrode.

Finally, the positions of each electrode determined by the described technique were compared with the histopathological analysis, which served as the ground-truth reference (Figure 5).

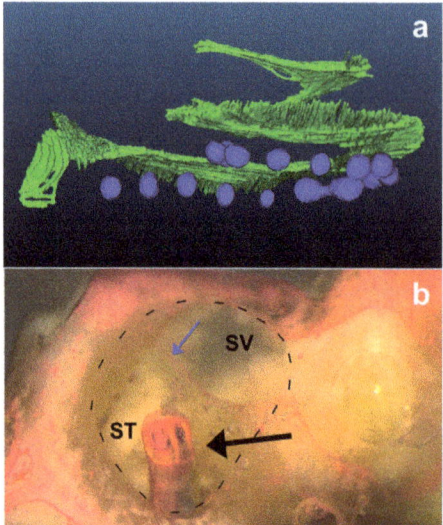

Figure 5. The middle plane of the cochlear turn reconstruction and histologic techniques were used to assess the position of each electrode array. (**a**) The "basilar membrane" reconstruction, including the basilar membrane and spiral lamina, was selected based on the dimensions of the cochlea analyzed; (**b**) the microgrinding technique shows the electrode array penetrating the scala tympani. The black discontinuous lines delimit the cochlear duct. ST: scala tympani; SV: scala vestibuli; black arrow: electrode array; blue arrow: basilar membrane.

2.6. Description of the Histopathological Analysis

All cochleae used in this study were analyzed and the results stored in our database. After electrode array insertion, the cochlea was harvested, and the apex of the cochlea and lateral semicircular canal were opened. The cochlea was then fixed with 10% formaldehyde for 24 h, dehydrated with increasing concentrations of alcohol (from 50% to 100%) for 12 h, dried at ambient air temperature for 16 h, and fixed with a crystal resin (Pebeo, Gémenos, France) until polymerization, as reported in a previous study [20]. The cochlea was then progressively ground perpendicular to the round window/modiolar axis and stopped at the level of each electrode. The cochlea was stained with Phloxine B for 15 min and visualized with a stereomicroscope (SLM 2; Karl Kaps GmbH, Wetzlar, Germany). A photograph was taken and stored in our database.

2.7. Statistical Analysis

The cochlear dimensions and index values are expressed as mean ± standard deviation. The normal distribution of the cochlear dimensions was checked using the Shapiro–Wilk test. The Fleiss' kappa coefficient was used to analyze the agreement between determining the scalar position of each electrode using a "basilar membrane" template and the histopathological study, in relation to the surgeons' experience in handling 3D reconstructions and the associated software. Data were analyzed using R statistical software v3.3.3 (R Core Team, Vienna, Austria).

3. Results

3.1. Inter-Rater Agreement in Determining the Scalar Position of Each Electrode

The entire procedure for determining the scalar position of the electrode took less than 12 min in all cases. We observed substantial agreement in determining the scalar position of each electrode of the AB MidScala electrode array, regardless of the experience of the surgeon (κ = 0.68 (0.66–0.71)). There was also substantial agreement between expert and non-expert surgeons in determining the scalar position of each electrode (κ = 0.76 (0.71–0.83) and κ = 0.67 (0.62–0.71), respectively). For the Oticon EVO electrode array, the agreement among surgeons regardless of their experience was κ = 0.39 (0.37–0.41). Experts had better agreement than non-experts in determining the scalar position of each electrode (κ = 0.46 (0.41–0.51) and κ = 0.39 (0.35–0.42), respectively). The overall agreement in determining the position of each electrode was decreased because of the higher number of electrodes in an intermediate position with the AB MidScala array (13/250 electrodes assessed by histology) than with the Oticon EVO array (50/300 electrodes) ($p < 0.001$; chi-squared test). With regard to the electrodes in the scala vestibuli, the agreement in determining the scalar position of each electrode was almost perfect for the MidScala array, regardless of the experience of the surgeon, and moderate for the Oticon EVO array (κ = 0.82 (0.79–0.84) and κ = 0.42 (0.40–0.45), respectively), (Table 2).

Table 2. Agreement of the five surgeons (two experts and three non-experts) in determining the position of each electrode based on histology. All results are expressed as Fleiss' kappa, with a target alpha of 0.05.

		All Electrodes	Scala Tympani Electrode	Intermediate Electrode	Scala Vestibuli Electrode
Advanced Bionics MidScala	Expert	0.76	0.79	0.24	0.89
	Non-expert	0.67	0.75	0.06	0.81
	Expert + Non-expert	0.68	0.76	0.12	0.82
Oticon EVO	Expert	0.46	0.55	0.24	0.60
	Non-expert	0.39	0.51	0.13	0.41
	Expert + Non-expert	0.39	0.51	0.16	0.42

3.2. Different Translocation Patterns Depending on the Type of Electrode Array

Different translocation patterns were observed depending on the type of electrode array (perimodiolar or lateral wall). With regard to the position of the array translocation, the MidScala electrode array translocated around 180° and rapidly crossed the middle plane of the cochlear duct, but beyond this point, the array remained in the scala vestibuli. Distal translocation of the array was not observed with this electrode array. In contrast, the Oticon EVO array was translocated around 180° (proximal translocations) and/or beyond 300° (distal translocations). As observed in Figure 6, the electrode array bent upward into the cochlear duct, pushing the basilar membrane, and the array remained in an intermediate position on the lateral wall.

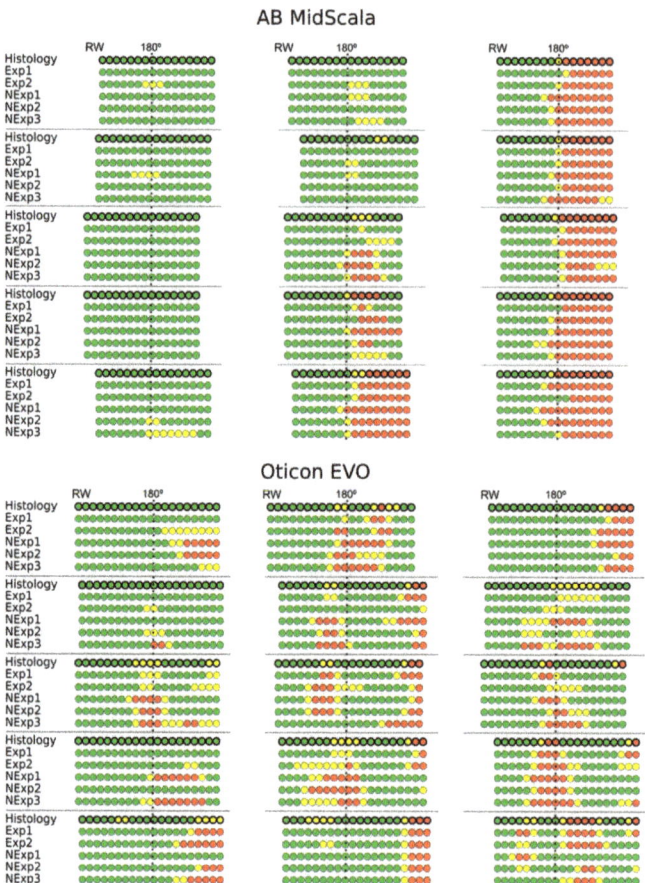

Figure 6. Assessment of the scalar position of the electrodes by five raters according to histology. The electrode array was located according to the positions of the round window (RW) and at 180° (dotted lines). Exp: expert; NExp: non-expert; scala tympani electrode: green circle; intermediate electrode: yellow circle; scala vestibuli electrode: red circle.

4. Discussion

In this study, we proposed and evaluated a rapid and reproducible technique to precisely assess the position of the electrode array according to the middle plane of the cochlear duct. To achieve this, a "basilar membrane" template was selected based on cochlear dimensions, and merged with the electrode array reconstruction to determine the position of the electrode array. In comparison with histology data, there was almost perfect agreement in determining an electrode translocated to the scala vestibuli with the AB MidScala array and a moderate agreement with the Oticon EVO array.

We selected five cochleae from a micro-CT database based on the best index obtained with the cochlear dimensions: horizontal dimensions, distances A and B; and vertical, H^{360}. Regarding the selection of H^{360} as a metric to select the "basilar membrane" template, previous reports have shown that the number of turns in the population is variable (from less than 2.5 to 3 turns) [33]. This could influence the slope of the middle plane of the cochlear turn, and two cochleae with the same full height but different numbers of turns would have marked differences in basilar membrane position. Indeed, the basilar membrane slope is higher in a cochlea with fewer turns than in one with more turns. In addition, in exceptional circumstances, the electrode array insertion depth can be greater than 540°

for all electrode array types; thus, the region of interest to detect the position of the array would range from 0° to 450° [6,12,20,34,35]. Consequently, the height of the cochlea at 360° is a more robust selection criterion for the "basilar membrane" template.

Earlier studies reported different methods to assess the position of the electrode array after cochlear implantation, such as the multiplanar reconstruction of postoperative imaging [14–16], merging pre- and post-operative imaging [18,19], rigid models [21,22], manual segmentation of the basilar membrane [20], and non-rigid models [26,27]. Each of these techniques has been used to determine the position of the electrode array; however, because of the cognitive load and time required for analysis, they are not widely included in the clinical workflow. A fundamental advantage of the proposed technique is the reduction in the time required for analysis. In addition, this method requires some measurements to be regularly performed by a surgeon, and the visual aspect offered by 3D models could provide a global insight into array insertion, as well as into the determination of the scalar position of each electrode. However, a limitation of this technique is that it uses several software tools for the analysis. Future efforts will focus on producing an all-encompassing and specialized software tool to support this method, which would further diminish the time and effort required. Furthermore, a fully automated procedure for determining the position of each electrode is achievable. This automation could mitigate the inter-rater variability and facilitate its dissemination in the clinical context.

Our data indicate a different translocation mechanism depending on the model of inserted electrode array. For the precurved AB MidScala array, translocations were observed at approximately 180°, as confirmed by other reports [13,36]. Owing to the lateral rigidity of this array, a misalignment with the direction of the scala tympani would lead to perforation of the basilar membrane and subsequent translocation, as reported in an earlier study [37]. The straight Oticon EVO array would progress in contact with the lateral wall, and the frictional forces between the array and the lateral wall would progressively increase. Consequently, the array could bend inside the scala tympani, push the basilar membrane upward, and produce detachment of the basilar membrane.

In summary, we have established a rapid and reproducible method using a 3D "basilar membrane" template selected to match the dimensions of the cochlea, which enables the scalar position of each electrode to be detected after cochlear implantation. Further studies are required to automate the entire procedure before its introduction into routine use in clinical practice.

Author Contributions: Conceptualization, R.T., Y.N. and E.F.; methodology, R.T., O.S., I.M., Y.N. and E.F.; validation, R.T., I.M., Y.N. and E.F.; formal analysis, R.T., J.-Y.T., H.D., G.L., N.G., E.B. and E.F.; investigation, R.T., H.D., G.L., N.G., E.B., Y.N. and E.F.; data curation, R.T., H.D., G.L., N.G., E.B. and E.F.; writing—original draft preparation, R.T.; writing—review and editing R.T., J.-Y.T., I.M., Y.N. and E.F.; visualization, R.T., J.-Y.T., H.D., G.L., N.G., E.B., O.S., I.M., Y.N. and E.F.; supervision, R.T., I.M., Y.N. and E.F.; project administration, Y.N. and E.F.; funding acquisition, Y.N. and E.F. All authors have read and agreed to the published version of the manuscript.

Funding: This research was funded by the Fondation pour l'Audition (Starting Grant IDA-2020), ANR Robocop ANR-19-CE19-0026-02.

Institutional Review Board Statement: Not applicable.

Informed Consent Statement: Not applicable.

Data Availability Statement: The data presented in this study are available on request from the corresponding author.

Conflicts of Interest: The authors declare no conflict of interest.

References

1. Lazard, D.S.; Vincent, C.; Venail, F.; Van de Heyning, P.; Truy, E.; Sterkers, O.; Skarzynski, P.H.; Skarzynski, H.; Schauwers, K.; O'Leary, S.; et al. Pre-, Per- and Postoperative Factors Affecting Performance of Postlinguistically Deaf Adults Using Cochlear Implants: A New Conceptual Model over Time. *PLoS ONE* **2012**, *7*, e48739. [CrossRef] [PubMed]
2. Blamey, P.; Artieres, F.; Başkent, D.; Bergeron, F.; Beynon, A.; Burke, E.; Dillier, N.; Dowell, R.; Fraysse, B.; Gallégo, S.; et al. Factors Affecting Auditory Performance of Postlinguistically Deaf Adults Using Cochlear Implants: An Update with 2251 Patients. *Audiol. Neurootol.* **2013**, *18*, 36–47. [CrossRef] [PubMed]
3. Bas, E.; Bohorquez, J.; Goncalves, S.; Perez, E.; Dinh, C.T.; Garnham, C.; Hessler, R.; Eshraghi, A.A.; Van De Water, T.R. Electrode Array-Eluted Dexamethasone Protects against Electrode Insertion Trauma Induced Hearing and Hair Cell Losses, Damage to Neural Elements, Increases in Impedance and Fibrosis: A Dose Response Study. *Hear. Res.* **2016**, *337*, 12–24. [CrossRef] [PubMed]
4. Wanna, G.B.; Noble, J.H.; Gifford, R.H.; Dietrich, M.S.; Sweeney, A.D.; Zhang, D.; Dawant, B.M.; Rivas, A.; Labadie, R.F. Impact of Intrascalar Electrode Location, Electrode Type, and Angular Insertion Depth on Residual Hearing in Cochlear Implant Patients: Preliminary Results. *Otol. Neurotol.* **2015**, *36*, 1343–1348. [CrossRef] [PubMed]
5. Holden, L.K.; Finley, C.C.; Firszt, J.B.; Holden, T.A.; Brenner, C.; Potts, L.G.; Gotter, B.D.; Vanderhoof, S.S.; Mispagel, K.; Heydebrand, G.; et al. Factors Affecting Open-Set Word Recognition in Adults with Cochlear Implants. *Ear Hear.* **2013**, *34*, 342–360. [CrossRef] [PubMed]
6. Wanna, G.B.; Noble, J.H.; Carlson, M.L.; Gifford, R.H.; Dietrich, M.S.; Haynes, D.S.; Dawant, B.M.; Labadie, R.F. Impact of Electrode Design and Surgical Approach on Scalar Location and Cochlear Implant Outcomes. *Laryngoscope* **2014**, *124* (Suppl. S6), S1–S7. [CrossRef] [PubMed]
7. O'Connell, B.P.; Hunter, J.B.; Wanna, G.B. The Importance of Electrode Location in Cochlear Implantation. *Laryngoscope Investig. Otolaryngol.* **2016**, *1*, 169–174. [CrossRef] [PubMed]
8. Jiam, N.T.; Jiradejvong, P.; Pearl, M.S.; Limb, C.J. The Effect of Round Window vs Cochleostomy Surgical Approaches on Cochlear Implant Electrode Position: A Flat-Panel Computed Tomography Study. *JAMA Otolaryngol. Head Neck Surg.* **2016**, *142*, 873–880. [CrossRef] [PubMed]
9. Laszig, R.; Ridder, G.J.; Fradis, M. Intracochlear Insertion of Electrodes Using Hyaluronic Acid in Cochlear Implant Surgery. *J. Laryngol. Otol.* **2002**, *116*, 371–372. [CrossRef] [PubMed]
10. Vittoria, S.; Lahlou, G.; Torres, R.; Daoudi, H.; Mosnier, I.; Mazalaigue, S.; Ferrary, E.; Nguyen, Y.; Sterkers, O. Robot-Based Assistance in Middle Ear Surgery and Cochlear Implantation: First Clinical Report. *Eur. Arch. Otorhinolaryngol.* **2021**, *278*, 77–85. [CrossRef] [PubMed]
11. Finley, C.C.; Holden, T.A.; Holden, L.K.; Whiting, B.R.; Chole, R.A.; Neely, G.J.; Hullar, T.E.; Skinner, M.W. Role of Electrode Placement as a Contributor to Variability in Cochlear Implant Outcomes. *Otol. Neurotol.* **2008**, *29*, 920–928. [CrossRef] [PubMed]
12. De Seta, D.; Nguyen, Y.; Bonnard, D.; Ferrary, E.; Godey, B.; Bakhos, D.; Mondain, M.; Deguine, O.; Sterkers, O.; Bernardeschi, D.; et al. The Role of Electrode Placement in Bilateral Simultaneously Cochlear-Implanted Adult Patients. *Otolaryngol. Head Neck Surg.* **2016**, *155*, 485–493. [CrossRef] [PubMed]
13. Daoudi, H.; Lahlou, G.; Torres, R.; Sterkers, O.; Lefeuvre, V.; Ferrary, E.; Mosnier, I.; Nguyen, Y. Robot-Assisted Cochlear Implant Electrode Array Insertion in Adults: A Comparative Study with Manual Insertion. *Otol. Neurotol.* **2021**, *42*, e438–e444. [CrossRef] [PubMed]
14. Aschendorff, A.; Kromeier, J.; Klenzner, T.; Laszig, R. Quality Control after Insertion of the Nucleus Contour and Contour Advance Electrode in Adults. *Ear Hear.* **2007**, *28*, 75S–79S. [CrossRef] [PubMed]
15. Verbist, B.M.; Frijns, J.H.M.; Geleijns, J.; van Buchem, M.A. Multisection CT as a Valuable Tool in the Postoperative Assessment of Cochlear Implant Patients. *Am. J. Neuroradiol.* **2005**, *26*, 424–429. [PubMed]
16. Boyer, E.; Karkas, A.; Attye, A.; Lefournier, V.; Escude, B.; Schmerber, S. Scalar Localization by Cone-Beam Computed Tomography of Cochlear Implant Carriers: A Comparative Study between Straight and Periomodiolar Precurved Electrode Arrays. *Otol. Neurotol.* **2015**, *36*, 422–429. [CrossRef] [PubMed]
17. De Seta, D.; Mancini, P.; Russo, F.Y.; Torres, R.; Mosnier, I.; Bensimon, J.L.; De Seta, E.; Heymann, D.; Sterkers, O.; Bernardeschi, D.; et al. 3D Curved Multiplanar Cone Beam CT Reconstruction for Intracochlear Position Assessment of Straight Electrodes Array. A Temporal Bone and Clinical Study. *Acta Otorhinolaryngol. Ital.* **2016**, *36*, 499–505. [CrossRef] [PubMed]
18. Sipari, S.; Iso-Mustajärvi, M.; Löppönen, H.; Dietz, A. The Insertion Results of a Mid-Scala Electrode Assessed by MRI and CBCT Image Fusion. *Otol. Neurotol.* **2018**, *39*, e1019–e1025. [CrossRef] [PubMed]
19. Dragovic, A.S.; Stringer, A.K.; Campbell, L.; Shaul, C.; O'Leary, S.J.; Briggs, R.J. Co-Registration of Cone Beam CT and Preoperative MRI for Improved Accuracy of Electrode Localization Following Cochlear Implantation. *Cochlear Implant. Int.* **2018**, *19*, 147–152. [CrossRef] [PubMed]
20. Torres, R.; Drouillard, M.; De Seta, D.; Bensimon, J.-L.; Ferrary, E.; Sterkers, O.; Bernardeschi, D.; Nguyen, Y. Cochlear Implant Insertion Axis into the Basal Turn: A Critical Factor in Electrode Array Translocation. *Otol. Neurotol.* **2018**, *39*, 168–176. [CrossRef] [PubMed]
21. Skinner, M.W.; Holden, T.A.; Whiting, B.R.; Voie, A.H.; Brunsden, B.; Neely, J.G.; Saxon, E.A.; Hullar, T.E.; Finley, C.C. In vivo estimates of the position of advanced bionics electrode arrays in the human cochlea. *Ann. Otol. Rhinol. Laryngol. Suppl.* **2007**, *197*, 2–24. [CrossRef] [PubMed]

22. Cakir, A.; Labadie, R.F.; Zuniga, M.G.; Dawant, B.M.; Noble, J.H. Evaluation of Rigid Cochlear Models for Measuring Cochlear Implant Electrode Position. *Otol. Neurotol.* **2016**, *37*, 1560–1564. [CrossRef] [PubMed]
23. Biedron, S.; Prescher, A.; Ilgner, J.; Westhofen, M. The Internal Dimensions of the Cochlear Scalae with Special Reference to Cochlear Electrode Insertion Trauma. *Otol. Neurotol.* **2010**, *31*, 731–737. [CrossRef] [PubMed]
24. Escudé, B.; James, C.; Deguine, O.; Cochard, N.; Eter, E.; Fraysse, B. The Size of the Cochlea and Predictions of Insertion Depth Angles for Cochlear Implant Electrodes. *Audiol. Neurootol.* **2006**, *11* (Suppl. S1), 27–33. [CrossRef] [PubMed]
25. Erixon, E.; Högstorp, H.; Wadin, K.; Rask-Andersen, H. Variational Anatomy of the Human Cochlea: Implications for Cochlear Implantation. *Otol. Neurotol.* **2009**, *30*, 14–22. [CrossRef] [PubMed]
26. Noble, J.H.; Labadie, R.F.; Majdani, O.; Dawant, B.M. Automatic Segmentation of Intracochlear Anatomy in Conventional CT. *IEEE Trans. Biomed. Eng.* **2011**, *58*, 2625–2632. [CrossRef] [PubMed]
27. Demarcy, T.; Vandersteen, C.; Guevara, N.; Raffaelli, C.; Gnansia, D.; Ayache, N.; Delingette, H. Automated Analysis of Human Cochlea Shape Variability from Segmented MCT Images. *Comput. Med. Imaging Graph.* **2017**, *59*, 1–12. [CrossRef] [PubMed]
28. Gerber, N.; Reyes, M.; Barazzetti, L.; Kjer, H.M.; Vera, S.; Stauber, M.; Mistrik, P.; Ceresa, M.; Mangado, N.; Wimmer, W.; et al. A Multiscale Imaging and Modelling Dataset of the Human Inner Ear. *Sci. Data.* **2017**, *4*, 170132. [CrossRef] [PubMed]
29. Horos Project. Available online: https://horosproject.org (accessed on 17 December 2019).
30. ITK-SNAP Home. Available online: http://www.itksnap.org (accessed on 3 April 2017).
31. CloudCompare—Open Source project. Available online: https://www.cloudcompare.org (accessed on 24 February 2019).
32. Blender Project—Free and Open 3D Creation Software. Available online: https://www.blender.org/ (accessed on 9 March 2019).
33. Biedron, S.; Westhofen, M.; Ilgner, J. On the Number of Turns in Human Cochleae. *Otol. Neurotol.* **2009**, *30*, 414–417. [CrossRef] [PubMed]
34. Hassepass, F.; Aschendorff, A.; Bulla, S.; Arndt, S.; Maier, W.; Laszig, R.; Beck, R. Radiologic Results and Hearing Preservation with a Straight Narrow Electrode via Round Window Versus Cochleostomy Approach at Initial Activation. *Otol. Neurotol.* **2015**, *36*, 993–1000. [CrossRef] [PubMed]
35. Tanaka Massuda, M.; Demarcy, T.; Hoen, M.; Danieli, F.; Arantes do Amaral, M.S.; Gnansia, D.; Hyppolito, M.A. Method to Quantitatively Assess Electrode Migration from Medical Images: Feasibility and Application in Patients with Straight Cochlear Implant Arrays. *Cochlear Implant. Int.* **2019**, *20*, 237–241. [CrossRef] [PubMed]
36. Dong, Y.; Briaire, J.J.; Siebrecht, M.; Stronks, H.C.; Frijns, J.H.M. Detection of Translocation of Cochlear Implant Electrode Arrays by Intracochlear Impedance Measurements. *Ear Hear.* **2021**, *42*, 1397–1404. [CrossRef] [PubMed]
37. Torres, R.; Hochet, B.; Daoudi, H.; Carré, F.; Mosnier, I.; Sterkers, O.; Ferrary, E.; Nguyen, Y. Atraumatic Insertion of a Cochlear Implant Pre-Curved Electrode Array by a Robot-Automated Alignment with the Coiling Direction of the Scala Tympani. *Audiol. Neurootol.* **2022**, *27*, 148–155. [CrossRef] [PubMed]

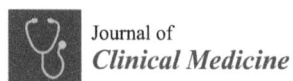

Review

Current and Emerging Therapies for Chronic Subjective Tinnitus

Ki Wan Park [1], Peter Kullar [1], Charvi Malhotra [1] and Konstantina M. Stankovic [1,2,3,*]

[1] Department of Otolaryngology-Head and Neck Surgery, Stanford University School of Medicine, 801 Welch Rd., Palo Alto, CA 94305, USA

[2] Department of Neurosurgery, Stanford University School of Medicine, 453 Quarry Rd., Palo Alto, CA 94305, USA

[3] Wu Tsai Neurosciences Institute, Stanford University, 290 Jane Stanford Way, Stanford, CA 94305, USA

* Correspondence: kstankovic@stanford.edu

Abstract: Importance: Chronic subjective tinnitus, the perception of sound without an external source for longer than six months, may be a greatly debilitating condition for some people, and is associated with psychiatric comorbidities and high healthcare costs. Current treatments are not beneficial for all patients and there is a large need for new therapies for tinnitus. Observations: Unlike rarer cases of objective tinnitus, chronic subjective tinnitus often has no obvious etiology and a diverse pathophysiology. In the absence of objective testing, diagnosis is heavily based on clinical assessment. Management strategies include hearing aids, sound masking, tinnitus retraining therapy, cognitive behavioral therapy, and emerging therapies including transcranial magnetic stimulation and electrical stimulation. Conclusions and relevance: Although current treatments are limited, emerging diagnostics and treatments provide promising avenues for the management of tinnitus symptoms.

Keywords: tinnitus; emerging therapeutics; electrical stimulation; neuromodulation; nerve block; CBT; EMDR

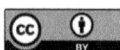

1. Introduction

Tinnitus, derived from the Latin verb *tinnire* meaning 'to ring', describes a conscious perception of an auditory sensation in the absence of a corresponding external stimulation [1]. Tinnitus is an ancient phenomenon, and an early description is found in the Babylonian Talmud which provocatively describes the curse of Titus as tinnitus caused by a gnat which "pecked at his brain" [2].

Tinnitus is classified as subjective when experienced only by the individual, or, rarely, objective when the tinnitus can also be detected by others [1]. The sensation is often described as sizzling or ringing but it can be rhythmic or pulsatile in nature [1]. Tinnitus can have a sudden onset and an acute time course although more commonly the onset is gradual and follows a chronic time course [3]. Somatosensory tinnitus can be modulated by afferents from the cervical region or temporomandibular joint [4]. The most common form of tinnitus is subjective and non-pulsatile, without other known pathological processes other than hearing loss [5]. This form, which is the subject of this review, is referred to as chronic subjective idiopathic tinnitus.

Due to the lack of objective markers of tinnitus, estimations of its prevalence rely on validated patient questionnaires, which may fail to capture the true burden of tinnitus given the heterogeneity of patient experience. It is estimated that tinnitus affects more than 740 million adults globally (14%), with over 120 million people (2%) perceiving tinnitus as a major problem [6]. Severe disturbances associated with tinnitus commonly manifest as emotional distress, insomnia, reduced concentration, and cognitive dysfunction [7–9]. Prevalence increases with age and is similar in men and women [10–12]. Children and adolescents are also commonly affected, although the prevalence varies considerably in the literature (4.7 to 46%), based on a recent systemic review [13]. However, it is estimated that only a small proportion (3.1%) have problematic tinnitus based on a prospective population-based study in the United Kingdom (UK) [14]. This form of problematic chronic tinnitus has been referred to as tinnitus disorder to reflect the associated psychological and physical impacts [15].

Financially, tinnitus also places a large economic burden on healthcare systems and may lead to a significant number of disability claims. The average cost of tinnitus-related costs per patient yearly is estimated at USD 660 in the US (2014) and GBP 717 in the UK (2017) [16,17]. In 2012, an estimated USD 1.2 billion was spent on tinnitus-related compensation by the United States Department of Veterans Affairs (VA) [18].

The primary risk factor for tinnitus development is hearing loss, and additional risk factors for severe tinnitus include stress, increased age, and head injury [19–21]. This relationship is not linear, and many people with tinnitus have audiometrically normal hearing while many with severe hearing loss do not report tinnitus [19]. Several modifiable lifestyle factors have been associated with the development of tinnitus, including noise exposure, diet, obesity, smoking, and alcohol intake [22–24]. Pharmacological agents are also an important cause of tinnitus. Aminoglycosides, platinum-based chemotherapy, and salicylates are all known ototoxic agents associated with the risk of tinnitus [25]. Tinnitus is a common feature of otological and lateral skull base disorders, such as Meniere's disease, otosclerosis, and vestibular schwannoma [10]. Tinnitus may be worsened by sleep quality and can coexist with mental health disorders including anxiety and depression [26,27]. Additionally, genetic conditions such as Williams syndrome have also been implicated in tinnitus, co-existing with hyperacusis [28]. This is thought to result from cochlear fragility and possible auditory nerve dysfunction resulting in high frequency hearing loss [28,29].

2. Etiology and Pathophysiology

There is a current consensus that the origin of subjective tinnitus is cochlear dysfunction that provokes an aberrant central neuroplastic response [30]. Jastreboff's neurophysiological model of tinnitus proposes that cochlear damage is the 'ignition' event leading to altered activity in the limbic, autonomic, and reticular systems that promote chronic tinnitus (Figure 1) [31]. Cochlear damage can include loss of outer hair cells (OHCs) and inner hair cells (IHC), loss of synapses between IHC and type 1 spiral ganglion neurons (synaptopathy), or mechanical damage to hair cells' stereocilia or the cochlea's basilar membrane [32]. It was previously believed that tinnitus could occur without cochlear damage; however, it is now evident that this damage may occur before hearing loss becomes clinically apparent [33]. For example, tinnitus patients both with and without hearing loss have been shown to have significantly different OHC function than normal subjects (as measured with distortion product otoacoustic emission (DPOAE)) [34], suggestive of OHC loss or damage that has not yet impacted audiometric thresholds. Indeed, hearing loss was undetectable in rats treated with an ototoxic drug (styrene) until >33% of OHCs were lost [35]. Additionally, the acoustic characteristics of tinnitus perception often correspond to the region of hearing loss (i.e., high-pitched tinnitus with high-frequency hearing loss) [36].

Following cochlear damage, the according reduction in auditory nerve output is proposed to initiate a neurobiological signaling cascade resulting in hyperactivity in the central auditory system encoding for tinnitus [30]. Thus, it is possible that the loss of cochlear afferent activity liberates involuntary, internally generated percepts in the brain, similar to the neural mechanism for phantom limb pain [30]. This would explain the common clinical finding that tinnitus persists even after destruction of the auditory nerve via, for example, surgery for vestibular schwannoma [37]. This theory is further bolstered by the high rate of acquired hearing loss in tinnitus patients (~90%), the rarity of tinnitus among the congenitally deaf, and that tinnitus is often suppressed by cochlear implants which functionally replace cochlear nerve output [30,38,39]. This mechanism for tinnitus is clinically relevant because treatment at the peripheral site (e.g., sound masking at the cochlea) may not correct alterations of activity in the central auditory pathway responsible for tinnitus persistence. However, restoring cochlear input via hearing-aid-mediated sound therapy can be effective in improving patients' subjective experience of tinnitus, and approximately 80% of patients with chronic tinnitus reported improvement in tinnitus annoyance and loudness in a questionnaire-based study in Japan [40].

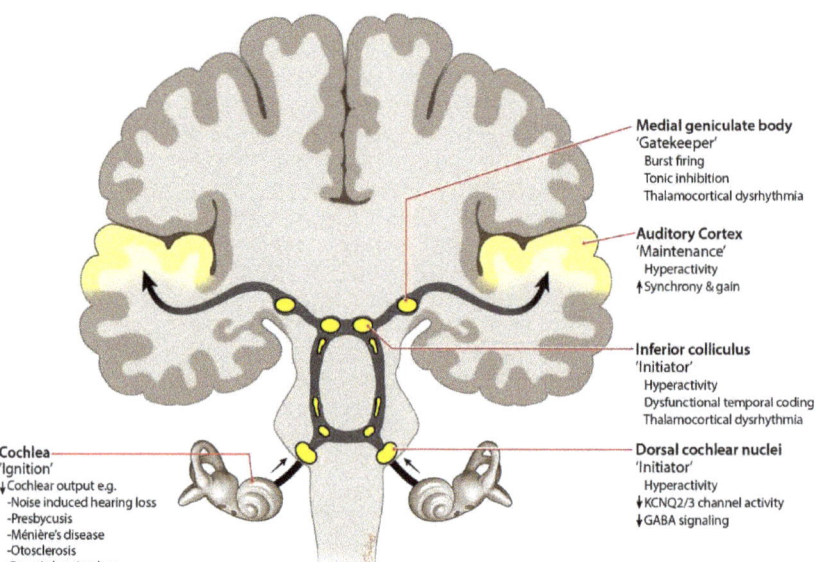

Figure 1. Auditory pathophysiology mechanisms of tinnitus. The primary pathophysiology mechanism includes reduction in cochlear output, resulting in an aberrant neuroplastic response. Abnormal dysfunctional neuronal activity in the remainder of the auditory pathway, including the ventral cochlear nucleus, inferior colliculus, medial geniculate body, and auditory cortex, is thought to be involved in tinnitus maintenance. Up arrow refers to gain, and down arrow refers to reduction. Adapted from Henton et al., 2021 [30].

Animal models of tinnitus—primarily achieved via loud sound and/or ototoxic agents following operant or reflexive conditioning to silence—have played a valuable role in understanding the pathophysiology of tinnitus [41]. Through these models, neuronal hyperactivity and hyporeactivity, neuronal gain and synchrony, and tonotopic reorganization in the brain have been associated with tinnitus symptoms [30,41]. Persistent dysfunctional neuronal activity in the ventral cochlear nucleus, inferior colliculus, medial geniculate body, and auditory cortex are thereby proposed to be responsible for tinnitus maintenance (Figure 1) [42–45]. In turn, these alterations in activity have been attributed to changes in glycinergic, GABAergic, glutaminergic, and cholinergic systems [46,47]. For example, dorsal cochlear nucleus hyperexcitability is possibly due to a reduction in potassium transport via KCNQ channels [48].

Additionally, non-auditory pathways play a critical role in the maintenance and affective response to tinnitus (Figure 2) [49]. Correspondingly, tinnitus is known to be co-morbid with depression and anxiety [50], and intracochlear-glucocorticoid-mediated glutamate release may be a link between psychological stressors and tinnitus [51]. The frontostriatal gating theory posits that the nucleus accumbens and ventromedial prefrontal cortex are important in the affective response to tinnitus [52]. Perception of tinnitus demands attentional resource, and accordingly patients with tinnitus have been shown to have poorer selective attention on auditory tasks [8]. Correspondingly, neuroimaging studies have detected changes in the attention networks [53]. The flocculus and paraflocculus, small lobes of the cerebellum, have also been implicated in tinnitus and auditory processing [54]. Animal tinnitus models have demonstrated feedback loops between the flocculus and the auditory cortex, with cochlear damage leading to upregulation of unipolar brush cells present in the cerebellum [54–56]. Similarly, neuroimaging studies have detected changes in the cerebellar regions, and a study of patients undergoing cerebellopontine tumor removal have demonstrated a correlation between flocculus volumes and tinnitus severity [57,58]. However, further investigative studies are needed before definitive conclusions can be made.

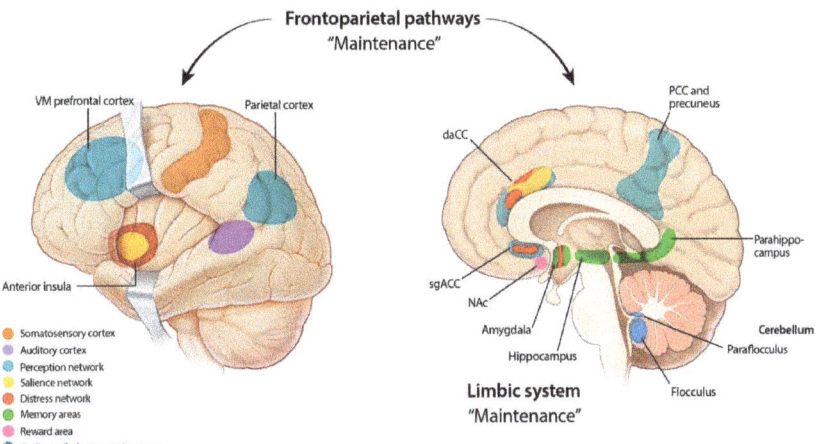

Figure 2. Non-auditory pathophysiology mechanisms of tinnitus. Non-auditory pathways play a critical role in the maintenance and affective response to tinnitus. Aberrant neuroplastic responses include the somatosensory cortex, perception networks, salience networks, distress networks, memory areas, reward areas, and audiovestibular processing areas. daCC—dorsal anterior cingulate cortex. sgACC—Subgenual anterior cingulate cortex. NAc—Nucleus accumbens. PCC—Posterior cingulate cortex. VM—Ventromedial. Adapted from Haider et al., 2018 [59].

There is growing interest in potential genetic contributions to tinnitus risk. Twin studies have estimated the heritability of tinnitus at 40–60% [60,61], although several candidate gene studies have failed to find such an association [62–64]. However, a recent (2020) large-scale, genome-wide association study (GWAS) in the UK Biobank and United States Million Veteran Program identified six genome-wide loci and 27 candidate genes associated with self-reported tinnitus among >170,000 people of European ancestry [65]. The estimated heritability was modest at 6%, but significant. This contrasts somewhat with the results of a prior GWAS that did not identify any significant candidate genes and estimated a lower heritability of 3.2%, which could be attributed to its comparatively much smaller population ($n = 167$) [66].

3. Current Options for Tinnitus

Broadly, treatment mechanisms for bothersome chronic tinnitus can be subdivided into two categories: tinnitus perception and response to tinnitus. Treatments modulating tinnitus perception, such as electrical and magnetic stimulation, aim to reduce or eliminate symptoms. On the other hand, tinnitus-response treatments aim to reduce the patient's negative affect or response to tinnitus and include cognitive behavioral therapy (CBT) and sound therapy.

The clinical guidelines for tinnitus from the AAO-HNF recommend hearing aid evaluation and CBT as options for chronic bothersome tinnitus and present sound therapy as another potential option [67]. The guidelines discourage the use of any medical drug therapy, dietary supplements, or repetitive transcranial magnetic stimulation (rTMS), given the lack of effective data at the time of the guidelines' publication in 2014. More recent guidelines from Europe (2019) and Japan (2020) continue to strongly recommend CBT, but provide poor to no recommendations against dietary supplements, sound therapy, medications, rTMS, and supplements [68,69]. New advances in both medical and surgical modalities for tinnitus have been developed which may hold promise for treating this chronic condition (Figure 3).

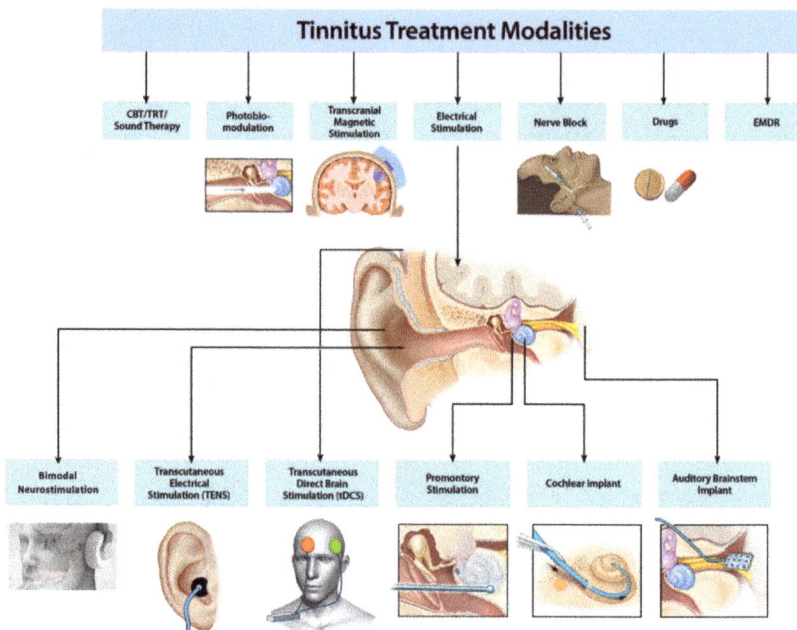

Figure 3. Schematic of current and emerging tinnitus treatments. Current and emerging treatments for tinnitus include CBT/TRT/sound therapy, transcranial magnetic stimulation (TMS), electrical stimulation (transcutaneous, promontory, cochlear implant, auditory brainstem implant), bimodal stimulation (Lenire® device from Neuromod Devices [70,71]), nerve blocks, drugs, and EMDR.

3.1. CBT

CBT, a type of psychotherapy, is used as an intervention for a wide variety of psychiatric conditions, including anxiety, depression, and the distress associated with tinnitus [72]. It aims to modulate negative thoughts associated with maladaptive behavior through reframing, using techniques like the development of positive coping skills, distraction, and relaxation. Duration of therapy for tinnitus can range from 8 to 24 weekly sessions with a trained professional [73].

To date, CBT is the only intervention for tinnitus to receive strong recommendations in clinical practice guidelines, but the benefits are primarily limited to managing tinnitus-related distress [67–69]. For example, several systemic reviews and meta-analyses have demonstrated that CBT is effective in improving patients' negative interpretations of tinnitus, but that its impact on anxiety or health-related quality of life may be less than that of audiological care, and that evidence of long-term outcomes are lacking [74–76]. A recent (2020) Cochrane review found that, compared to waiting or receiving no treatment for tinnitus, CBT meaningfully improved perception of tinnitus severity (THI score) and, to a lesser extent, measures of quality of life, anxiety, and depression [74]. Similarly, CBT provided a greater improvement on quality of life compared to usual audiological care and tinnitus retraining therapy, but there was no difference seen in depression and anxiety given the lack of long-term follow-up [74]. A randomized controlled trial (RCT) of internet-based versus in-person CBT for patients with distressing tinnitus found that both modalities were equally effective in reducing tinnitus-related distress measured with the TFI [77], although a meta-analysis of RCTs indicated that in-person CBT was more effective for tinnitus-related quality of life [75]. However, internet-based therapies may offer access to therapy for a larger subpopulation of tinnitus patients, especially in the era of the COVID pandemic. Other forms of psychotherapy have also demonstrated beneficial effects for tinnitus. For example, an RCT comparing the efficacy of mindfulness-based cognitive therapy (MBCT) and intensive relaxation therapy for chronic, distressing tinnitus found significantly greater reductions in self-reported tinnitus severity with MBCT, and persistent effects at 6 months of follow-up [78]. Improvement was observed in both tinnitus loudness and severity, along with improvements in psychological distress.

3.2. Hearing Aids

As the primary risk factor for tinnitus development is hearing loss, hearing aids are also recommended for chronic tinnitus [19]. This relationship however is not linear and many people with tinnitus have audiometrically normal hearing while many with severe hearing loss do not report tinnitus19. While hearing aids are recommended for patients with hearing loss and concurrent tinnitus in all guidelines [67–69], hearing aids for tinnitus alone is given a weak recommendation due to the lack of high-quality, robust data in the literature [69]. Several systemic reviews investigating the efficacy of hearing aids for tinnitus have found a lack of high-quality RCTs in the literature and noted equivocal results with a need for further studies [79,80].

3.3. Sound Therapy

Sound therapy aims to reduce the intensity of tinnitus by using an external sound to distract the listener [81]. This method is hypothesized to promote the habituation of tinnitus and stimulate the hypoactive neural auditory pathways impacted by hearing loss [38]. Therapy can be offered in the form of a device providing broadband low-level white noise or noise at the tinnitus frequency, or through a hearing aid to amplify external noise.

Numerous studies have investigated the efficacy of sound masking for managing tinnitus, although the results have been heterogenous. A Cochrane review investigating efficacy of the masking determined that there was weak evidence to show efficacy of sound therapy for tinnitus due to limited data and bias in the studies [82]. An RCT assessing the impact of masking, retraining therapy, educational counseling with hearing aids, or waiting (no intervention) on the perception of tinnitus severity reported similar improvement in all three intervention groups at 6 and 18 months, but no improvement in patients who waited [83].

3.4. Eye-Movement Desensitization Reprocessing

EMDR is a form of conditioning psychotherapy traditionally used for post-traumatic stress disorder and more recently applied to tinnitus, with the most recent study published in 2018 [84]. EMDR is hypothesized to reduce tinnitus distress via desensitization and reprocessing of memories and images associated with negative perceptions of tinnitus [85]. As a newer form of therapy, few studies have investigated the efficacy of EMDR for the reduction of tinnitus-related distress, although initial reports have been positive [85–87]. Prospective trials on EMDR for chronic tinnitus have found clinically significant benefits on quality-of-life tinnitus surveys [85,86]. Further, an RCT comparing bimodal therapy with tinnitus retraining therapy plus EMDR or tinnitus retraining therapy plus CBT found that both treatment modalities resulted in equivalent reductions in tinnitus severity [87].

3.5. Cochlear Implantation

Cochlear implants are surgically implanted hearing prosthetics which electrically stimulate the auditory nerve and are therapeutic options for patients with moderate to severe hearing loss, with or without tinnitus, which has not improved with hearing aids. An estimated 68–86% of adult cochlear implant candidates also experience tinnitus [88,89]. Notably, numerous studies have reported secondary improvement or even resolution of tinnitus symptoms following cochlear implantation, ranging from 34 to 92% of implantees [90–93]. Systematic reviews and meta-analyses have similarly described the beneficial effects of cochlear implantation on both quality of life and tinnitus symptoms, with Levy et al. concluding that approximately 75% of implantees across 17 studies experienced improvement in tinnitus symptoms while 15% achieved complete resolution [94,95]. The exact therapeutic mechanism is unclear, but it has been hypothesized that increased afferent input to the auditory nerve from the implant may attenuate maladaptive neural activity and initiate neuroplastic reorganization of the central auditory pathways and associated brain areas [96]. This is supported by studies reporting gradual improvement in tinnitus symptoms over the course of several months post-implantation [88].

Interestingly, however, several studies have reported worsening of tinnitus severity in a subset of patients (<5%) following cochlear implantation [95,97]. Some cochlear implantation surgeries involve the creation of a cochleostomy for electrode insertion, and this trauma may damage remaining hair cells, potentially decreasing residual hearing and worsening tinnitus. However, modification of the surgical technique to a less traumatic round window approach to insert the electrode may reduce this trauma and associated risk [98]. For example, a prospective study by Kloostra et al. assessing the post-cochlear implantation outcomes of 44 patients (66% with preoperative tinnitus) who received either a cochleostomy or round window approach found that 75% who achieved tinnitus cessation received the round window approach versus cochleostomy [99]. Thus, it is possible that a round window approach instead of a separate cochleostomy for electrode insertion may offer advantages for patients with preoperative tinnitus, although further prospective studies are needed.

Additionally, there is some evidence that the duration and chronicity of tinnitus prior to implantation impacts the likelihood of tinnitus cessation, perhaps due to entrenchment of maladaptive changes [99–101]. The abovementioned study by Kloostra et al. noted that the mean time from tinnitus onset was 32.2 years for patients who did not have cessation of tinnitus symptoms versus just 5.2 years for patients who achieved cessation [99]. Similarly, Miyamoto et al. observed that preoperative tinnitus duration of <20 years was significantly correlated with post-implantation improvement in tinnitus symptoms among 78 adult implantees [102]. While cochlear implantation remains a viable option for the treatment of tinnitus with accompanying hearing loss, there is a risk of worsening tinnitus, and thus should be used for patients who specifically want to improve their hearing ability.

4. Emerging Options for Tinnitus
4.1. Electrical Stimulation

Electrical stimulation can be divided broadly into three categories: direct cutaneous stimulation (DCT), inner ear stimulation (promontory stimulation and cochlear implants), and intraneural implants.

4.1.1. Transcranial and Transcutaneous Stimulation

Non-invasive electrical stimulation techniques to modulate neural hyperactivity in specific brain areas include transcutaneous direct current stimulation (tDCS) and transcutaneous electrical stimulation (TENS) [103]. Neuroimaging studies have reported structural abnormalities and hyperactivity in the left auditory cortex/temporoparietal region, dorsolateral prefrontal cortex (DLPFC), and limbic system associated with tinnitus perception or distress; thus, modulation of activity is primarily directed to these regions [104–108].

In studies of tDCS for tinnitus, stimulation intensity varies (i.e., 2–15 mA) but electrodes are generally placed over the temporoparietal region for several consecutive sessions. In a 2020 double-blind, placebo-controlled RCT, 24 patients with chronic tinnitus received five consecutive sessions of either tDCS (2 mA for 20 min) or a sham stimulation (n = 12 each) to the left temporoparietal region and right DLPFC [109]. The tDCS-treated patients reported significant improvements from baseline in tinnitus annoyance and severity (i.e., Tinnitus Handicap Index (THI)/Visual Analogue Scale (VAS)) and decreased alpha/beta/theta frequency, as measured by electroencephalogram, immediately following intervention. Additionally, reduced electrical activity was observed in the frontal, temporoparietal, and limbic regions of tDCS-treated patients. However, several prior RCTs and prospective studies of tDCS in patients with chronic tinnitus failed to demonstrate similarly significant effects [110–112], and a scoping review noted the transient nature of any benefit [113].

TENS involves cutaneous electrode placement, typically over the auricle or around the mastoid to target the auricular branch of the vagus nerve, or is delivered via a probe in the external auditory canal. A placebo-controlled, randomized prospective study of unilateral ($n = 20$) or bilateral ($n = 20$) cutaneous TENS for chronic tinnitus reported that scores on the THI and a survey of depression significantly improved in both TENS-treated groups compared to their pre-intervention baseline [114]. However, a significant placebo effect was observed among the sham-treated patients as well. Another RCT of cutaneous TENS for chronic tinnitus reported no significant benefit for the active intervention group as well as large placebo effects among sham-treated patients [115]. In a large study of 500 patients with tinnitus who received probe TENS to the tympanic membrane, approximately half (53%) reported some benefit in symptom reduction and 7% had complete suppression of tinnitus [116]. Placebo effects were not assessed in that study, 13 patients experienced worsening of tinnitus, and 27% of the patients who reported initial benefits reported no benefit at 3 months.

Taken together, the evidence suggests that TENS may confer transient beneficial effects for tinnitus, but may be due to a high placebo effect and have no obvious long-term benefit. Three recent systematic reviews and meta-analyses likewise concluded that that electrical stimulation may indeed provide a benefit for tinnitus, but high bias is present in most studies and further investigation into the most effective stimulation pattern and modality are needed before recommendation to patients [117–119].

4.1.2. Promontory and Round Window Stimulation

Inner ear stimulation techniques include promontory and round window biphasic stimulation [120–122]. Prospective studies assessing trans-tympanic promontory probe stimulation among small cohorts have demonstrated some significant improvements in tinnitus symptoms during or soon after intervention, but a return to baseline and loss of benefit at longer-term follow-up when stimulation is stopped. For example, in a study of ten patients with severe unilateral tinnitus who received multiple consecutive trans-tympanic needle electrode stimulation pulses to the promontory, self-reported tinnitus loudness (assessed with the VAS) and THI scores significantly improved for five patients, but VAS returned to baseline 4 weeks post-intervention [120]. Additionally, there were no changes in measures of tinnitus-specific audiological tests (i.e., minimum masking level, tinnitus loudness, and pitch) from the baseline. A small study by Wenzel et al. repurposed a cochlear implant to provide long-term (4 h per day for 3.5 years) stimulation via a non-penetrating ball electrode to the round window of patients with tinnitus and unilateral deafness ($n = 3$) [121]. At least one measure of tinnitus severity improved for all patients, although the electrode was eventually removed when the patients received conventional cochlear implants, the outcomes of which were not compared. There have also been recent efforts to develop an implantable system for suppression of tinnitus symptoms, with one ongoing open-label clinical trial testing feasibility in 16 adults with disruptive, intractable chronic tinnitus [123].

4.2. Repetitive Transcranial Magnetic Stimulation

Repetitive transcranial magnetic stimulation (rTMS) uses an electromagnetic field to noninvasively stimulate neural networks and modify dysfunctional cortical networks from outside the cranium [124]. Repetitive application of the magnetic field is proposed to induce lasting changes in targeted cortical regions and associated networks, and is routinely used for conditions such as refractory depression and obsessive–compulsive disorder [124]. Currently, it is also experimentally used for chronic tinnitus. While there is no consensus on the correct protocol for rTMS, it typically involves the placement of an electromagnetic coil over the left temporoparietal junction (TPJ), auditory cortex, or multiple sites that emits at low frequency (1 Hz) and 100−110% of resting motor threshold [113,125–127]. Participants may undergo resting state functional connectivity MRI prior to and immediately following rTMS treatment to assess structural or connectivity changes. The most common side effect of rTMS is a transient headache, but can rarely lead to a generalized seizure [128].

There is not yet consensus in the literature on the efficacy of rTMS for chronic tinnitus. In 2015, a double-blind RCT of rTMS applied to the TPJ of patients with chronic, bothersome tinnitus reported no significant functional connectivity changes or improvement from baseline THI score in those who received active ($n = 16$) or sham therapy ($n = 14$) [127]. The authors concluded that the TPJ alone may not be the ideal target for rTMS therapy for tinnitus, and successful neuromodulation may require multiple or personalized stimulation targets. Other studies have also investigated the ideal location(s) for rTMS stimulation for tinnitus. A randomized study by Khedr et al. compared the effect of rTMS delivered to the TPJ contralateral or ipsilateral to tinnitus in 62 patients with unilateral chronic tinnitus [129]. The results indicated that significantly greater improvement in THI score was achieved with contralateral stimulation than either ipsilateral or left side stimulation at 10 months, with no effect from frequency type (1 and 25 Hz), although there was no sham therapy group in that study. However, a similar RCT by Kim et al. assessing 1 Hz rTMS at the TPJ contralateral or ipsilateral to unilateral tinnitus did not find any differences between stimulation laterality, as both modalities resulted in significant improvements in THI and VAS scores at 1 month [130].

Further improvement and reliability in responses may be seen with personalized, targeted stimulation targets, as performed for depression [131]. Recent efforts from Lan et al. assessed neuroimaging indicators for optimal chronic tinnitus treatment [132]. Functional neural connections were assessed with resting state functional MRI, with preliminary results suggesting that patients with neural connections in the salience network–right frontoparietal network may respond better to rTMS [132]. However, further robust investigation is needed before rTMS can be formally recommended for chronic tinnitus.

4.3. Nerve Block

Nerve blocks have also been investigated for non-somatosensory tinnitus. A retrospective chart review assessed auriculotemporal nerve and facial nerve blocks with lidocaine in 55 patients with chronic (>6 months, $n = 40$) or sub-acute (>3 months, $n = 15$) tinnitus after trigeminal and facial nerve stimulation and other treatments (i.e., intratympanic steroids or medications) [133]. The results indicated that approximately 88% of patients experienced some improvement in scores on a modified VAS after several integrative treatments (stimulation and block). Transient facial palsy (5–15 min) was noted right after the nerve block, which spontaneously resolved.

Other nerve blocks in the literature have targeted the occipital nerve to reduce tinnitus-associated otalgia [134,135]. A retrospective study of 33 patients with tinnitus and otalgia underwent ultrasound guided occipital nerve blocks, with significant reduction in immediately after the nerve block [134]. Long-term results, however, were varied and patients in this study had several varying etiologies for otalgia including somatosensory tinnitus (temporomandibular joint pain, myofascial pain syndrome, and cervical stenosis) which limits generalizability. Further investigations and dedicated studies are needed to elucidate the benefit of nerve blocks for chronic tinnitus.

4.4. Bimodal Neuromodulation

Bimodal neuromodulation, which pairs sound and electrical stimulation of peripheral nerves, is an emerging therapy for tinnitus. Bimodal neuromodulation is thought to drive plasticity and changes in the auditory pathway (midbrain, cortex, or brainstem) involved with tinnitus in several animal studies [136,137]. Congruent with animal studies, clinical trials have also appeared promising for chronic tinnitus, with the Food and Drug Administration (FDA) granting de novo approval for the biomodulation wearable Lenire® in March of 2023 [138]. Lenire® is a Class IIa device delivering electrical stimulation to the tongue with an oral device and sound stimulation. In a randomized, blinded trial of 326 patients with chronic subjective tinnitus, the efficacy of Lenire® was tested in three separate groups with different stimulation settings. Over a 12-week period, all intervention groups had a statistically significant reduction in tinnitus symptom severity, with sustained therapeutic improvement seen at a 12-month follow-up [71]. However, there were diminishing returns on the second 6 weeks of treatment, likely due to treatment habituation. In a follow-up clinical trial, there were enhanced therapeutic benefits in tinnitus symptom severity achieved by changing stimulation parameters during the second 6-week treatment period, overcoming treatment habituation [70]. Bimodal stimulation appears promising for the treatment of chronic tinnitus, with the advantage of an FDA-approved at-home device for treatment. Further investigations will be needed to follow up long-term therapeutic benefit past 12 months, to delineate specific stimulation patterns among tinnitus populations, and to evaluate the effect of bimodal stimulation over a placebo in a real-world setting.

4.5. Pharmaceutical Therapy

Psychiatric comorbidities associated with tinnitus include depression, anxiety, and obsessive–compulsive disorder traits [26,139]. Accordingly, antidepressants and antipsychotics for chronic tinnitus have been assessed in several RCTs, but have failed to show evidence of efficacy while also reporting common adverse events with these drugs [140]. A double-blind, placebo-controlled study of trazadone for bothersome tinnitus (<1 year duration and normal audiograms) found that patients receiving trazadone (n = 43) experienced similar improvements in tinnitus severity, quality of life, or tinnitus-related discomfort as those receiving a placebo (n = 42) [141]. Similarly, an RCT of 115 non-depressed patients with chronic tinnitus did not find any significant benefit with the selective serotonin reuptake inhibitor paroxetine compared with a placebo [142]. A 2012 Cochrane review concluded there was insufficient evidence of the efficacy of antidepressants for tinnitus due to poorly randomized and low-quality studies, and further investigation was warranted [140].

Lidocaine interferes with fast-gated sodium channels and is hypothesized to inhibit hypersensitivity in the central auditory pathways [143]. Accordingly, lidocaine has been investigated as a pharmaceutical option for tinnitus, delivered either intravenously or trans-tympanically, although most beneficial effects at tinnitus suppression appear to be transient [144–147]. A double-blind, cross-over study by Baguley et al. assessed the inhibitory effects of intravenous 2% lidocaine (1.5 mg/kg) versus saline placebo in 16 patients with postoperative tinnitus following translabyrinthine resection of unilateral, sporadic vestibular schwannoma [148]. Interestingly, patients who received lidocaine had significant improvements in tinnitus loudness and distress (measured with VAS) compared to placebo patients at 5 min, but not at 20 min, post-infusion. Importantly, intravenous lidocaine is associated with several adverse events, including the risk of increased tinnitus severity. For example, in an 1983 double-blind RCT, over 30% of tinnitus patients treated with intravenous lidocaine (100 mg) reported worsened sensation of tinnitus, and there was a high rate of adverse events (e.g., disequilibrium, slurred speech, numbness, and tingling of the extremities) [146]. Subsequent small cohort studies have investigated intratympanic lidocaine injections for subjective tinnitus, with heterogenous results [149–151]. However, the AAO-HNF tinnitus treatment guidelines do not recommend intratympanic lidocaine injections due to the lack of strong efficacy evidence, or intravenous lidocaine due to the risk of adverse events [67].

Benzodiazepines have also been investigated in several RCTs but lack robust literature to support their use. Benzodiazepines are hypothesized to bind to GABA receptors and enhance inhibitory signals, thus modulating hyperactivity signals associated with tinnitus [152]. A randomized cross-over trial by Han et al. compared the effects of clonazepam and Ginkgo biloba [153]. There was significant improvement in tinnitus loudness, duration, and annoyance in the clonazepam group, but no significant differences in the Ginkgo biloba group. Accordingly, several prior systemic reviews have found no benefit in the use of Ginkgo biloba for the treatment of chronic tinnitus [154,155]. The efficacy of alprazolam, on the other hand, has been equivocal with conflicting results in the literature [156,157]. Given the lack of robust literature and side effect profile of benzodiazepines, benzodiazepines are not recommended for the treatment of subjective tinnitus alone at this time [67,69].

5. Other Limited Evidence Treatments

Photobiomodulation (PBM) or low-level laser therapy (LLLT) is an investigative treatment that utilizes low power light to modulate neural activity. The therapeutic mechanism of PBM is yet unclear but is proposed to be cellular-level stimulation of cytochrome C, synthesis of growth factors, and activation of repair mechanisms in the inner ear [158]. PBM tinnitus treatment involves the placement of a trans-meatal probe to delivery laser therapy, generally in the visible or near-infrared spectrum (532–1064 nm), at varying power levels (5–100 mW) [158]. Previous RCTs and studies of the efficacy of PBM for tinnitus have reported conflicting results [159–164]. For example, a double-blind RCT of trans-meatal LLLT (810 nm at 60 mW) for chronic, disabling tinnitus found no significant differences in any measures of tinnitus between active treatment ($n = 23$) or placebo groups ($n = 20$) [165]. A large systematic review of RCTs of LLLT for tinnitus (2022) similarly found conflicting results regarding the benefit of PBM given the heterogeneity of study designs, high levels of bias, equivocal results, and lack of long-term follow-up [166].

Migraine medications have also been investigated for treatment of chronic tinnitus. The disruption of somatosensory and auditory inputs of the trigeminal nerve have been implicated in the pathophysiology of tinnitus as the dorsal cochlear nucleus receives indirect input from the trigeminal nerve [167]. This suggests a potential connection between tinnitus and migraines [168]. Many migraine patients have auditory manifestations, including tinnitus. Thus, migraine medications may serve as an option to potentially reduce the severity of tinnitus in a subset of patients, but further robust trials are warranted at this time. One active clinical trial aims to assess the effects of nortriptyline/topiramate and verapamil/paroxetine migraine medications in reducing the severity of tinnitus [169].

6. Conclusions and Future Directions

Over the past several decades, advances in basic and clinical research have greatly improved our understanding of tinnitus. Despite these advances, the overall impact of available tinnitus treatment remains poor without consensus, and is a source of frustration for patients. In a 2018 survey of patients regarding their expectations and the outcomes of tinnitus treatment, 36% responded with having "no expectation" and 49% reported that their treatment was "not at all successful" [170]. The lack of both diagnostic and definitive treatment options remains a huge challenge in the management of chronic subjective tinnitus. The most common treatments, such as hearing aids, CBT, and masking, address patients' response to tinnitus, but viable treatment modalities for tinnitus suppression remain few.

Tinnitus research remains challenging owing to a lack of methodological standardization in both research and clinical trials, as well the need for longer-term follow-up of patients in existing trials [171]. There is a lack of strong objective measures, and a strong placebo effect present in many tinnitus trials [172]. Many validated tinnitus questionnaires exist and have favorable psychometric signatures, and thus there is no consensus or standardization for a specific questionnaire in either research or clinical use [173–175]. This lack of standardization in questionnaires remains a challenge for making accurate comparisons between treatment or research groups. There have also been recent efforts to distinguish tinnitus as a symptom and tinnitus as a disorder. Tinnitus disorder specifically reflects the associated psychological and physical impacts of the disease [15]. Standardization of these processes will prove paramount for creating a lasting impact on future tinnitus research

However, the future of tinnitus research remains bright as new technologies are rapidly emerging. In recent years, several candidate genes for tinnitus have been identified, as well as plasma metabolomic biomarkers of persistent tinnitus, which may open up exciting new avenues for diagnostics, gene-based therapeutics, and alterative therapy development [65,176]. A recent (2022) metabolomic study that compared the blood plasma levels of 466 metabolites between women with persistent tinnitus (n = 488) and controls without tinnitus (n = 5989) identified several novel biomarkers positively or inversely associated with chronic tinnitus [177]. Compounds such as triglycerides and diglycerides were positively associated with tinnitus, while other cholesterol metabolites such as cholesteryl esters and lysophosphatidylcholines were inversely associated with tinnitus. While the precise roles of these compounds in tinnitus require further investigation, lipid dysregulation may play a role in tinnitus pathogenesis, consistent with other neurodegenerative disorders such as Alzheimer's and Parkinson's disease [178,179]. Additionally, a recent study by Amanat et al. assessing genetic risk factors identified several rare synaptic genes in patients with severe tinnitus, and the authors were able to replicate these findings between two European cohorts (Spanish patients with Meniere's disease and Swedish tinnitus patients) [180]. These rare synaptic genes associated with membrane trafficking and cytoskeletal protein binding were replicated between these cohorts irrespective of their underlying hearing disorder, demonstrating the possible effect of rare variants in severe tinnitus.

Furthermore, as of November 2022, 50 clinical trials of treatments for tinnitus are registered at ClinicalTrials.gov as currently recruiting (33 of 50) or preparing to recruit. One ongoing clinical trial is enrolling patients with incapacitating unilateral tinnitus to determine the efficacy of auditory brainstem implants [181], devices originally developed for people with hearing loss due to non-functional cochlear nerves. The early results of this therapeutic application are encouraging, as a retrospective study of patients with neurofibromatosis type 2 who received auditory brainstem implants demonstrated tinnitus suppression and reduction in tinnitus severity [182]. Additionally, vagal nerve stimulator implants and deep brain stimulation are being actively investigated. Data are limited at this time, and further investigations will be needed to delineate their effects on tinnitus [183,184]. Overall, interdisciplinary research linking the genetic, diagnostic, and therapeutic modalities will be critical to develop an effective and reproducible cure for chronic subjective tinnitus.

Author Contributions: Conceptualization: K.M.S.; writing—original draft preparation, K.W.P., P.K., C.M. and K.M.S.; writing—review and editing, K.W.P., P.K., C.M. and K.M.S.; All authors have read and agreed to the published version of the manuscript.

Funding: We gratefully acknowledge support from Rick Robins and the Bertarelli Foundation Professorship (K.M.S.).

Acknowledgments: We thank Shelley Batts for critical editing of the manuscript.

Conflicts of Interest: The authors declare no conflict of interest.

References

1. Baguley, D.; McFerran, D.; Hall, D. Tinnitus. *Lancet* **2013**, *382*, 1600–1607. [CrossRef]
2. Dan, B. Titus's tinnitus. *J. Hist. Neurosci.* **2005**, *14*, 210–213. [CrossRef] [PubMed]
3. Vielsmeier, V.; Santiago Stiel, R.; Kwok, P.; Langguth, B.; Schecklmann, M. From Acute to Chronic Tinnitus: Pilot Data on Predictors and Progression. *Front. Neurol.* **2020**, *11*, 997. [CrossRef] [PubMed]
4. Ralli, M.; Greco, A.; Turchetta, R.; Altissimi, G.; de Vincentiis, M.; Cianfrone, G. Somatosensory tinnitus: Current evidence and future perspectives. *J. Int. Med. Res.* **2017**, *45*, 933–947. [CrossRef] [PubMed]
5. Shargorodsky, J.; Curhan, G.C.; Farwell, W.R. Prevalence and characteristics of tinnitus among US adults. *Am. J. Med.* **2010**, *123*, 711–718. [CrossRef]

6. Jarach, C.M.; Lugo, A.; Scala, M.; van den Brandt, P.A.; Cederroth, C.R.; Odone, A.; Garavello, W.; Schlee, W.; Langguth, B.; Gallus, S. Global Prevalence and Incidence of Tinnitus: A Systematic Review and Meta-Analysis. *JAMA Neurol.* **2022**, *79*, 888–900. [CrossRef]
7. Hallam, R.; McKenna, L.; Shurlock, L. Tinnitus impairs cognitive efficiency. *Int. J. Audiol.* **2004**, *43*, 218–226. [CrossRef]
8. Roberts, L.E.; Husain, F.T.; Eggermont, J.J. Role of attention in the generation and modulation of tinnitus. *Neurosci. Biobehav. Rev.* **2013**, *37*, 1754–1773. [CrossRef]
9. Husain, F.T.; Akrofi, K.; Carpenter-Thompson, J.R.; Schmidt, S.A. Alterations to the attention system in adults with tinnitus are modality specific. *Brain Res.* **2015**, *1620*, 81–97. [CrossRef]
10. Manche, S.K.; Madhavi, J.; Meganadh, K.R.; Jyothy, A. Association of tinnitus and hearing loss in otological disorders: A decade-long epidemiological study in a South Indian population. *Braz. J. Otorhinolaryngol.* **2016**, *82*, 643–649. [CrossRef]
11. Ahmad, N.; Seidman, M. Tinnitus in the older adult: Epidemiology, pathophysiology and treatment options. *Drugs Aging* **2004**, *21*, 297–305. [CrossRef] [PubMed]
12. Shetye, A.; Kennedy, V. Tinnitus in children: An uncommon symptom? *Arch. Dis. Child.* **2010**, *95*, 645–648. [CrossRef] [PubMed]
13. Rosing, S.N.; Schmidt, J.H.; Wedderkopp, N.; Baguley, D.M. Prevalence of tinnitus and hyperacusis in children and adolescents: A systematic review. *BMJ Open* **2016**, *6*, e010596. [CrossRef] [PubMed]
14. Humphriss, R.; Hall, A.J.; Baguley, D.M. Prevalence and characteristics of spontaneous tinnitus in 11-year-old children. *Int. J. Audiol.* **2016**, *55*, 142–148. [CrossRef]
15. De Ridder, D.; Schlee, W.; Vanneste, S.; Londero, A.; Weisz, N.; Kleinjung, T.; Shekhawat, G.S.; Elgoyhen, A.B.; Song, J.J.; Andersson, G.; et al. Tinnitus and tinnitus disorder: Theoretical and operational definitions (an international multidisciplinary proposal). *Prog. Brain Res.* **2021**, *260*, 1–25. [CrossRef]
16. Goldstein, E.; Ho, C.X.; Hanna, R.; Elinger, C.; Yaremchuk, K.L.; Seidman, M.D.; Jesse, M.T. Cost of care for subjective tinnitus in relation to patient satisfaction. *Otolaryngol. Head Neck Surg.* **2015**, *152*, 518–523. [CrossRef]
17. Stockdale, D.; McFerran, D.; Brazier, P.; Pritchard, C.; Kay, T.; Dowrick, C.; Hoare, D.J. An economic evaluation of the healthcare cost of tinnitus management in the UK. *BMC Health Serv. Res.* **2017**, *17*, 577. [CrossRef]
18. Treating and Curing Tinnitus Is Part of Our National Commitment to Veterans. Available online: https://www.ata.org/treating-and-curing-tinnitus-is-part-of-our-national-commitment-to-veterans/ (accessed on 20 June 2023).
19. Sindhusake, D.; Golding, M.; Wigney, D.; Newall, P.; Jakobsen, K.; Mitchell, P. Factors predicting severity of tinnitus: A population-based assessment. *J. Am. Acad. Audiol.* **2004**, *15*, 269–280. [CrossRef]
20. Cresswell, M.; Casanova, F.; Beaumont, R.N.; Wood, A.R.; Ronan, N.; Hilton, M.P.; Tyrrell, J. Understanding Factors That Cause Tinnitus: A Mendelian Randomization Study in the UK Biobank. *Ear Hear.* **2022**, *43*, 70–80. [CrossRef]
21. Kim, H.J.; Lee, H.J.; An, S.Y.; Sim, S.; Park, B.; Kim, S.W.; Lee, J.S.; Hong, S.K.; Choi, H.G. Analysis of the prevalence and associated risk factors of tinnitus in adults. *PLoS ONE* **2015**, *10*, e0127578. [CrossRef]
22. Veile, A.; Zimmermann, H.; Lorenz, E.; Becher, H. Is smoking a risk factor for tinnitus? A systematic review, meta-analysis and estimation of the population attributable risk in Germany. *BMJ Open* **2018**, *8*, e016589. [CrossRef] [PubMed]
23. Dawes, P.; Cruickshanks, K.J.; Marsden, A.; Moore, D.R.; Munro, K.J. Relationship between Diet, Tinnitus, and Hearing Difficulties. *Ear Hear.* **2020**, *41*, 289–299. [CrossRef] [PubMed]
24. Wang, T.C.; Chang, T.Y.; Tyler, R.; Lin, Y.J.; Liang, W.M.; Shau, Y.W.; Lin, W.Y.; Chen, Y.W.; Lin, C.D.; Tsai, M.H. Noise Induced Hearing Loss and Tinnitus-New Research Developments and Remaining Gaps in Disease Assessment, Treatment, and Prevention. *Brain Sci.* **2020**, *10*, 732. [CrossRef] [PubMed]
25. Dille, M.F.; Konrad-Martin, D.; Gallun, F.; Helt, W.J.; Gordon, J.S.; Reavis, K.M.; Bratt, G.W.; Fausti, S.A. Tinnitus onset rates from chemotherapeutic agents and ototoxic antibiotics: Results of a large prospective study. *J. Am. Acad. Audiol.* **2010**, *21*, 409–417. [CrossRef]
26. Bhatt, J.M.; Bhattacharyya, N.; Lin, H.W. Relationships between tinnitus and the prevalence of anxiety and depression. *Laryngoscope* **2017**, *127*, 466–469. [CrossRef]
27. Chen, S.; Shen, X.; Yuan, J.; Wu, Y.; Li, Y.; Tong, B.; Qiu, J.; Wu, F.; Liu, Y. Characteristics of tinnitus and factors influencing its severity. *Ther. Adv. Chronic Dis.* **2022**, *13*, 20406223221109656. [CrossRef]
28. Gothelf, D.; Farber, N.; Raveh, E.; Apter, A.; Attias, J. Hyperacusis in Williams syndrome: Characteristics and associated neuroaudiologic abnormalities. *Neurology* **2006**, *66*, 390–395. [CrossRef]
29. Barozzi, S.; Soi, D.; Corniotto, E.; Borghi, A.; Gavioli, C.; Spreatico, E.; Gagliardi, C.; Selicorni, A.; Forti, S.; Ambrosetti, U.; et al. Audiological findings in Williams syndrome: A study of 69 patients. *Am. J. Med. Genet. A* **2012**, *158A*, 759–771. [CrossRef]
30. Henton, A.; Tzounopoulos, T. What's the buzz? The neuroscience and the treatment of tinnitus. *Physiol. Rev.* **2021**, *101*, 1609–1632. [CrossRef]
31. Jastreboff, P.J.; Gray, W.C.; Gold, S.L. Neurophysiological approach to tinnitus patients. *Am. J. Otol.* **1996**, *17*, 236–240.
32. Liberman, M.C.; Dodds, L.W. Single-neuron labeling and chronic cochlear pathology. III. Stereocilia damage and alterations of threshold tuning curves. *Hear. Res.* **1984**, *16*, 55–74. [CrossRef] [PubMed]
33. Vielsmeier, V.; Lehner, A.; Strutz, J.; Steffens, T.; Kreuzer, P.M.; Schecklmann, M.; Landgrebe, M.; Langguth, B.; Kleinjung, T. The Relevance of the High Frequency Audiometry in Tinnitus Patients with Normal Hearing in Conventional Pure-Tone Audiometry. *Biomed. Res. Int.* **2015**, *2015*, 302515. [CrossRef] [PubMed]

34. Shiomi, Y.; Tsuji, J.; Naito, Y.; Fujiki, N.; Yamamoto, N. Characteristics of DPOAE audiogram in tinnitus patients. *Hear. Res.* **1997**, *108*, 83–88. [CrossRef]
35. Chen, G.D.; Tanaka, C.; Henderson, D. Relation between outer hair cell loss and hearing loss in rats exposed to styrene. *Hear. Res.* **2008**, *243*, 28–34. [CrossRef]
36. Sereda, M.; Hall, D.A.; Bosnyak, D.J.; Edmondson-Jones, M.; Roberts, L.E.; Adjamian, P.; Palmer, A.R. Re-examining the relationship between audiometric profile and tinnitus pitch. *Int. J. Audiol.* **2011**, *50*, 303–312. [CrossRef]
37. Wazen, J.J.; Foyt, D.; Sisti, M. Selective cochlear neurectomy for debilitating tinnitus. *Ann. Otol. Rhinol. Laryngol.* **1997**, *106*, 568–570. [CrossRef]
38. Jastreboff, P.J. Phantom auditory perception (tinnitus): Mechanisms of generation and perception. *Neurosci. Res.* **1990**, *8*, 221–254. [CrossRef]
39. Knipper, M.; van Dijk, P.; Schulze, H.; Mazurek, B.; Krauss, P.; Scheper, V.; Warnecke, A.; Schlee, W.; Schwabe, K.; Singer, W.; et al. The neural bases of tinnitus: Lessons from deafness and cochlear implants. *J. Neurosci.* **2020**, *40*, 7190–7202. [CrossRef]
40. Shinden, S.; Suzuki, N.; Oishi, N.; Suzuki, D.; Minami, S.; Ogawa, K. Effective sound therapy using a hearing aid and educational counseling in patients with chronic tinnitus. *Auris Nasus Larynx* **2021**, *48*, 815–822. [CrossRef]
41. Brozoski, T.J.; Bauer, C.A. Animal models of tinnitus. *Hear. Res.* **2016**, *338*, 88–97. [CrossRef]
42. Eggermont, J.J.; Roberts, L.E. The neuroscience of tinnitus. *Trends Neurosci.* **2004**, *27*, 676–682. [CrossRef] [PubMed]
43. Kalappa, B.I.; Brozoski, T.J.; Turner, J.G.; Caspary, D.M. Single unit hyperactivity and bursting in the auditory thalamus of awake rats directly correlates with behavioural evidence of tinnitus. *J. Physiol.* **2014**, *592*, 5065–5078. [CrossRef] [PubMed]
44. Vogler, D.P.; Robertson, D.; Mulders, W.H. Hyperactivity in the ventral cochlear nucleus after cochlear trauma. *J. Neurosci.* **2011**, *31*, 6639–6645. [CrossRef] [PubMed]
45. Melcher, J.R.; Levine, R.A.; Bergevin, C.; Norris, B. The auditory midbrain of people with tinnitus: Abnormal sound-evoked activity revisited. *Hear. Res.* **2009**, *257*, 63–74. [CrossRef] [PubMed]
46. Zhang, L.; Wu, C.; Martel, D.T.; West, M.; Sutton, M.A.; Shore, S.E. Remodeling of cholinergic input to the hippocampus after noise exposure and tinnitus induction in Guinea pigs. *Hippocampus* **2019**, *29*, 669–682. [CrossRef]
47. Zhang, L.; Wu, C.; Martel, D.T.; West, M.; Sutton, M.A.; Shore, S.E. Noise Exposure Alters Glutamatergic and GABAergic Synaptic Connectivity in the Hippocampus and Its Relevance to Tinnitus. *Neural Plast.* **2021**, *2021*, 8833087. [CrossRef]
48. Li, S.; Kalappa, B.I.; Tzounopoulos, T. Noise-induced plasticity of KCNQ2/3 and HCN channels underlies vulnerability and resilience to tinnitus. *Elife* **2015**, *4*, e07242. [CrossRef]
49. Davies, J.E.; Gander, P.E.; Hall, D.A. Does Chronic Tinnitus Alter the Emotional Response Function of the Amygdala? A Sound-Evoked fMRI Study. *Front. Aging Neurosci.* **2017**, *9*, 31. [CrossRef]
50. Meijers, S.M.; Rademaker, M.; Meijers, R.L.; Stegeman, I.; Smit, A.L. Correlation between Chronic Tinnitus Distress and Symptoms of Depression: A Systematic Review. *Front. Neurol.* **2022**, *13*, 870433. [CrossRef]
51. Eggermont, J.J.; Roberts, L.E. The neuroscience of tinnitus: Understanding abnormal and normal auditory perception. *Front. Syst. Neurosci.* **2012**, *6*, 53. [CrossRef]
52. Hullfish, J.; Sedley, W.; Vanneste, S. Prediction and perception: Insights for (and from) tinnitus. *Neurosci. Biobehav. Rev.* **2019**, *102*, 1–12. [CrossRef] [PubMed]
53. Carpenter-Thompson, J.R.; Schmidt, S.; McAuley, E.; Husain, F.T. Increased Frontal Response May Underlie Decreased Tinnitus Severity. *PLoS ONE* **2015**, *10*, e0144419. [CrossRef] [PubMed]
54. Brozoski, T.J.; Ciobanu, L.; Bauer, C.A. Central neural activity in rats with tinnitus evaluated with manganese-enhanced magnetic resonance imaging (MEMRI). *Hear. Res.* **2007**, *228*, 168–179. [CrossRef] [PubMed]
55. Brozoski, T.; Brozoski, D.; Wisner, K.; Bauer, C. Chronic tinnitus and unipolar brush cell alterations in the cerebellum and dorsal cochlear nucleus. *Hear. Res.* **2017**, *350*, 139–151. [CrossRef]
56. Bauer, C.A.; Wisner, K.W.; Baizer, J.S.; Brozoski, T.J. Tinnitus, unipolar brush cells, and cerebellar glutamatergic function in an animal model. *PLoS ONE* **2013**, *8*, e64726. [CrossRef]
57. Mennink, L.M.; Van Dijk, J.M.C.; Van Der Laan, B.; Metzemaekers, J.D.M.; Van Laar, P.J.; Van Dijk, P. The relation between flocculus volume and tinnitus after cerebellopontine angle tumor surgery. *Hear. Res.* **2018**, *361*, 113–120. [CrossRef]
58. Chen, J.; Fan, L.; Cai, G.; Hu, B.; Xiong, Y.; Zhang, Z. Altered Amplitude of Low-Frequency Fluctuations and Degree Centrality in Patients with Acute Subjective Tinnitus: A Resting-State Functional Magnetic Resonance Imaging Study. *J. Integr. Neurosci.* **2022**, *21*, 116. [CrossRef]
59. Haider, H.F.; Bojic, T.; Ribeiro, S.F.; Paco, J.; Hall, D.A.; Szczepek, A.J. Pathophysiology of Subjective Tinnitus: Triggers and Maintenance. *Front. Neurosci.* **2018**, *12*, 866. [CrossRef]
60. Bogo, R.; Farah, A.; Karlsson, K.K.; Pedersen, N.L.; Svartengren, M.; Skjönsberg, Å. Prevalence, Incidence Proportion, and Heritability for Tinnitus: A Longitudinal Twin Study. *Ear Hear.* **2017**, *38*, 292–300. [CrossRef]
61. Maas, I.L.; Brüggemann, P.; Requena, T.; Bulla, J.; Edvall, N.K.; Hjelmborg, J.V.B.; Szczepek, A.J.; Canlon, B.; Mazurek, B.; Lopez-Escamez, J.A.; et al. Genetic susceptibility to bilateral tinnitus in a Swedish twin cohort. *Genet. Med.* **2017**, *19*, 1007–1012. [CrossRef]
62. Pawełczyk, M.; Rajkowska, E.; Kotyło, P.; Dudarewicz, A.; Van Camp, G.; Śliwińska-Kowalska, M. Analysis of inner ear potassium recycling genes as potential factors associated with tinnitus. *Int. J. Occup. Med. Environ. Health* **2012**, *25*, 356–364. [CrossRef] [PubMed]

63. Sand, P.G.; Langguth, B.; Kleinjung, T. Deep resequencing of the voltage-gated potassium channel subunit KCNE3 gene in chronic tinnitus. *Behav. Brain Funct.* **2011**, *7*, 39. [CrossRef] [PubMed]
64. Sand, P.G.; Langguth, B.; Schecklmann, M.; Kleinjung, T. GDNF and BDNF gene interplay in chronic tinnitus. *Int. J. Mol. Epidemiol. Genet.* **2012**, *3*, 245–251.
65. Clifford, R.E.; Maihofer, A.X.; Stein, M.B.; Ryan, A.F.; Nievergelt, C.M. Novel Risk Loci in Tinnitus and Causal Inference with Neuropsychiatric Disorders among Adults of European Ancestry. *JAMA Otolaryngol. Head Neck Surg.* **2020**, *146*, 1015–1025. [CrossRef]
66. Gilles, A.; Van Camp, G.; Van de Heyning, P.; Fransen, E. A Pilot Genome-Wide Association Study Identifies Potential Metabolic Pathways Involved in Tinnitus. *Front. Neurosci.* **2017**, *11*, 71. [CrossRef]
67. Tunkel, D.E.; Bauer, C.A.; Sun, G.H.; Rosenfeld, R.M.; Chandrasekhar, S.S.; Cunningham, E.R., Jr.; Archer, S.M.; Blakley, B.W.; Carter, J.M.; Granieri, E.C.; et al. Clinical practice guideline: Tinnitus. *Otolaryngol. Head Neck Surg.* **2014**, *151*, S1–S40. [CrossRef]
68. Ogawa, K.; Sato, H.; Takahashi, M.; Wada, T.; Naito, Y.; Kawase, T.; Murakami, S.; Hara, A.; Kanzaki, S. Clinical practice guidelines for diagnosis and treatment of chronic tinnitus in Japan. *Auris Nasus Larynx* **2020**, *47*, 1–6. [CrossRef]
69. Cima, R.F.F.; Mazurek, B.; Haider, H.; Kikidis, D.; Lapira, A.; Norena, A.; Hoare, D.J. A multidisciplinary European guideline for tinnitus: Diagnostics, assessment, and treatment. *HNO* **2019**, *67*, 10–42. [CrossRef]
70. Conlon, B.; Hamilton, C.; Meade, E.; Leong, S.L.; Connor, O.C.; Langguth, B.; Vanneste, S.; Hall, D.A.; Hughes, S.; Lim, H.H. Different bimodal neuromodulation settings reduce tinnitus symptoms in a large randomized trial. *Sci. Rep.* **2022**, *12*, 10845. [CrossRef]
71. Conlon, B.; Langguth, B.; Hamilton, C.; Hughes, S.; Meade, E.; Connor, C.O.; Schecklmann, M.; Hall, D.A.; Vanneste, S.; Leong, S.L.; et al. Bimodal neuromodulation combining sound and tongue stimulation reduces tinnitus symptoms in a large randomized clinical study. *Sci. Transl. Med.* **2020**, *12*, eabb2830. [CrossRef]
72. Nakao, M.; Shirotsuki, K.; Sugaya, N. Cognitive-behavioral therapy for management of mental health and stress-related disorders: Recent advances in techniques and technologies. *Biopsychosoc. Med.* **2021**, *15*, 16. [CrossRef]
73. Jun, H.J.; Park, M.K. Cognitive behavioral therapy for tinnitus: Evidence and efficacy. *Korean J. Audiol.* **2013**, *17*, 101–104. [CrossRef]
74. Fuller, T.; Cima, R.; Langguth, B.; Mazurek, B.; Vlaeyen, J.W.; Hoare, D.J. Cognitive behavioural therapy for tinnitus. *Cochrane Database Syst. Rev.* **2020**, *1*, CD012614. [CrossRef] [PubMed]
75. Landry, E.C.; Sandoval, X.C.R.; Simeone, C.N.; Tidball, G.; Lea, J.; Westerberg, B.D. Systematic Review and Network Meta-analysis of Cognitive and/or Behavioral Therapies (CBT) for Tinnitus. *Otol. Neurotol.* **2020**, *41*, 153–166. [CrossRef] [PubMed]
76. Martinez-Devesa, P.; Perera, R.; Theodoulou, M.; Waddell, A. Cognitive behavioural therapy for tinnitus. *Cochrane Database Syst. Rev.* **2010**, *9*, CD005233. [CrossRef]
77. Beukes, E.W.; Andersson, G.; Allen, P.M.; Manchaiah, V.; Baguley, D.M. Effectiveness of Guided Internet-Based Cognitive Behavioral Therapy vs Face-to-Face Clinical Care for Treatment of Tinnitus: A Randomized Clinical Trial. *JAMA Otolaryngol. Head Neck Surg.* **2018**, *144*, 1126–1133. [CrossRef] [PubMed]
78. McKenna, L.; Marks, E.M.; Hallsworth, C.A.; Schaette, R. Mindfulness-Based Cognitive Therapy as a Treatment for Chronic Tinnitus: A Randomized Controlled Trial. *Psychother. Psychosom.* **2017**, *86*, 351–361. [CrossRef]
79. Hesse, G. Evidence and evidence gaps in tinnitus therapy. *GMS Curr. Top. Otorhinolaryngol. Head Neck Surg.* **2016**, *15*, Doc04. [CrossRef]
80. Hoare, D.J.; Edmondson-Jones, M.; Sereda, M.; Akeroyd, M.A.; Hall, D. Amplification with hearing aids for patients with tinnitus and co-existing hearing loss. *Cochrane Database Syst. Rev.* **2014**, *1*, CD010151. [CrossRef]
81. Vernon, J. Attemps to relieve tinnitus. *J. Am. Audiol. Soc.* **1977**, *2*, 124–131.
82. Hobson, J.; Chisholm, E.; El Refaie, A. Sound therapy (masking) in the management of tinnitus in adults. *Cochrane Database Syst. Rev.* **2012**, *11*, CD006371. [CrossRef]
83. Henry, J.A.; Stewart, B.J.; Griest, S.; Kaelin, C.; Zaugg, T.L.; Carlson, K. Multisite Randomized Controlled Trial to Compare Two Methods of Tinnitus Intervention to Two Control Conditions. *Ear Hear.* **2016**, *37*, e346–e359. [CrossRef] [PubMed]
84. Wilson, G.; Farrell, D.; Barron, I.; Hutchins, J.; Whybrow, D.; Kiernan, M.D. The use of eye-movement desensitization reprocessing (EMDR) therapy in treating post-traumatic stress disorder: A systematic narrative review. *Front. Psychol.* **2018**, *9*, 923. [CrossRef] [PubMed]
85. Rikkert, M.; van Rood, Y.; de Roos, C.; Ratter, J.; van den Hout, M. A trauma-focused approach for patients with tinnitus: The effectiveness of eye movement desensitization and reprocessing—A multicentre pilot trial. *Eur. J. Psychotraumatol.* **2018**, *9*, 1512248. [CrossRef] [PubMed]
86. Phillips, J.S.; Erskine, S.; Moore, T.; Nunney, I.; Wright, C. Eye movement desensitization and reprocessing as a treatment for tinnitus. *Laryngoscope* **2019**, *129*, 2384–2390. [CrossRef] [PubMed]
87. Luyten, T.R.; Jacquemin, L.; Van Looveren, N.; Declau, F.; Fransen, E.; Cardon, E.; De Bodt, M.; Topsakal, V.; Van de Heyning, P.; Van Rompaey, V.; et al. Bimodal Therapy for Chronic Subjective Tinnitus: A Randomized Controlled Trial of EMDR and TRT Versus CBT and TRT. *Front. Psychol.* **2020**, *11*, 2048. [CrossRef]
88. Quaranta, N.; Wagstaff, S.; Baguley, D.M. Tinnitus and cochlear implantation. *Int. J. Audiol.* **2004**, *43*, 245–251. [CrossRef]
89. Aschendorff, A.; Pabst, G.; Klenzner, T.; Laszig, R. Tinnitus in Cochlear Implant Users: The Freiburg Experience. *Int. Tinnitus J.* **1998**, *4*, 162–164.

90. Poncet-Wallet, C.; Mamelle, E.; Godey, B.; Truy, E.; Guevara, N.; Ardoint, M.; Gnansia, D.; Hoen, M.; Saai, S.; Mosnier, I.; et al. Prospective Multicentric Follow-Up Study of Cochlear Implantation in Adults with Single-Sided Deafness: Tinnitus and Audiological Outcomes. *Otol. Neurotol.* **2020**, *41*, 458–466. [CrossRef]
91. Ito, J. Tinnitus suppression in cochlear implant patients. *Otolaryngol.–Head Neck Surg.* **1997**, *117*, 701–703. [CrossRef]
92. Miyamoto, R.T.; Bichey, B.G. Cochlear implantation for tinnitus suppression. *Otolaryngol. Clin. N. Am.* **2003**, *36*, 345–352. [CrossRef] [PubMed]
93. Di Nardo, W.; Cantore, I.; Cianfrone, F.; Melillo, P.; Scorpecci, A.; Paludetti, G. Tinnitus modifications after cochlear implantation. *Eur. Arch. Otorhinolaryngol.* **2007**, *264*, 1145–1149. [CrossRef] [PubMed]
94. Arts, R.A.; George, E.L.; Stokroos, R.J.; Vermeire, K. Review: Cochlear implants as a treatment of tinnitus in single-sided deafness. *Curr. Opin. Otolaryngol. Head Neck Surg.* **2012**, *20*, 398–403. [CrossRef] [PubMed]
95. Levy, D.A.; Lee, J.A.; Nguyen, S.A.; McRackan, T.R.; Meyer, T.A.; Lambert, P.R. Cochlear Implantation for Treatment of Tinnitus in Single-sided Deafness: A Systematic Review and Meta-analysis. *Otol. Neurotol.* **2020**, *41*, e1004–e1012. [CrossRef] [PubMed]
96. Punte, A.K.; Vermeire, K.; Hofkens, A.; De Bodt, M.; De Ridder, D.; Van de Heyning, P. Cochlear implantation as a durable tinnitus treatment in single-sided deafness. *Cochlear Implants Int.* **2011**, *12* (Suppl. S1), S26–S29. [CrossRef]
97. Arts, R.A.; Netz, T.; Janssen, A.M.; George, E.L.; Stokroos, R.J. The occurrence of tinnitus after CI surgery in patients with severe hearing loss: A retrospective study. *Int. J. Audiol.* **2015**, *54*, 910–917. [CrossRef]
98. Richard, C.; Fayad, J.N.; Doherty, J.; Linthicum, F.H., Jr. Round window versus cochleostomy technique in cochlear implantation: Histologic findings. *Otol. Neurotol.* **2012**, *33*, 1181–1187. [CrossRef]
99. Kloostra, F.J.J.; Verbist, J.; Hofman, R.; Free, R.H.; Arnold, R.; van Dijk, P. A Prospective Study of the Effect of Cochlear Implantation on Tinnitus. *Audiol. Neurootol.* **2018**, *23*, 356–363. [CrossRef]
100. Olze, H.; Szczepek, A.J.; Haupt, H.; Forster, U.; Zirke, N.; Grabel, S.; Mazurek, B. Cochlear implantation has a positive influence on quality of life, tinnitus, and psychological comorbidity. *Laryngoscope* **2011**, *121*, 2220–2227. [CrossRef]
101. Olze, H.; Szczepek, A.J.; Haupt, H.; Zirke, N.; Graebel, S.; Mazurek, B. The impact of cochlear implantation on tinnitus, stress and quality of life in postlingually deafened patients. *Audiol. Neurootol.* **2012**, *17*, 2–11. [CrossRef]
102. Miyamoto, R.T.; Wynne, M.K.; McKnight, C.; Bichey, B. Electrical Suppression of Tinnitus via Cochlear Implants. *Int. Tinnitus J.* **1997**, *3*, 35–38. [PubMed]
103. Kuo, M.-F.; Paulus, W.; Nitsche, M.A. Therapeutic effects of non-invasive brain stimulation with direct currents (tDCS) in neuropsychiatric diseases. *Neuroimage* **2014**, *85*, 948–960. [CrossRef]
104. Mühlnickel, W.; Elbert, T.; Taub, E.; Flor, H. Reorganization of auditory cortex in tinnitus. *Proc. Natl. Acad. Sci. USA* **1998**, *95*, 10340–10343. [CrossRef]
105. Rauschecker, J.P.; Leaver, A.M.; Mühlau, M. Tuning out the noise: Limbic-auditory interactions in tinnitus. *Neuron* **2010**, *66*, 819–826. [CrossRef]
106. Schlee, W.; Schecklmann, M.; Lehner, A.; Kreuzer, P.M.; Vielsmeier, V.; Poeppl, T.B.; Langguth, B. Reduced variability of auditory alpha activity in chronic tinnitus. *Neural Plast.* **2014**, *2014*, 436146. [CrossRef] [PubMed]
107. Arnold, W.; Bartenstein, P.; Oestreicher, E.; Römer, W.; Schwaiger, M. Focal metabolic activation in the predominant left auditory cortex in patients suffering from tinnitus: A PET study with [18F] deoxyglucose. *ORL J. Otorhinolaryngol. Relat. Spec.* **1996**, *58*, 195–199. [CrossRef] [PubMed]
108. Langguth, B.; Eichhammer, P.; Kreutzer, A.; Maenner, P.; Marienhagen, J.; Kleinjung, T.; Sand, P.; Hajak, G. The impact of auditory cortex activity on characterizing and treating patients with chronic tinnitus—First results from a PET study. *Acta Oto-Laryngol.* **2006**, *126*, 84–88. [CrossRef] [PubMed]
109. Souza, D.D.S.; Almeida, A.A.; Andrade, S.; Machado, D.; Leitao, M.; Sanchez, T.G.; Rosa, M. Transcranial direct current stimulation improves tinnitus perception and modulates cortical electrical activity in patients with tinnitus: A randomized clinical trial. *Neurophysiol. Clin.* **2020**, *50*, 289–300. [CrossRef]
110. Cavalcanti, K.; Brasil-Neto, J.P.; Allam, N.; Boechat-Barros, R. A Double-blind, Placebo-controlled Study of the Effects of Daily tDCS Sessions Targeting the Dorsolateral Prefrontal Cortex on Tinnitus Handicap Inventory and Visual Analog Scale Scores. *Brain Stimul.* **2015**, *8*, 978–980. [CrossRef]
111. Pal, N.; Maire, R.; Stephan, M.A.; Herrmann, F.R.; Benninger, D.H. Transcranial Direct Current Stimulation for the Treatment of Chronic Tinnitus: A Randomized Controlled Study. *Brain Stimul.* **2015**, *8*, 1101–1107. [CrossRef]
112. Forogh, B.; Mirshaki, Z.; Raissi, G.R.; Shirazi, A.; Mansoori, K.; Ahadi, T. Repeated sessions of transcranial direct current stimulation for treatment of chronic subjective tinnitus: A pilot randomized controlled trial. *Neurol. Sci.* **2016**, *37*, 253–259. [CrossRef] [PubMed]
113. Shekhawat, G.S.; Stinear, C.M.; Searchfield, G.D. Modulation of Perception or Emotion? A Scoping Review of Tinnitus Neuromodulation Using Transcranial Direct Current Stimulation. *Neurorehabil. Neural Repair* **2015**, *29*, 837–846. [CrossRef] [PubMed]
114. Tutar, B.; Atar, S.; Berkiten, G.; Ustun, O.; Kumral, T.L.; Uyar, Y. The effect of transcutaneous electrical nerve stimulation (TENS) on chronic subjective tinnitus. *Am. J. Otolaryngol.* **2020**, *41*, 102326. [CrossRef] [PubMed]
115. Kapkin, O.; Satar, B.; Yetiser, S. Transcutaneous electrical stimulation of subjective tinnitus. A placebo-controlled, randomized and comparative analysis. *ORL J. Otorhinolaryngol. Relat. Spec.* **2008**, *70*, 156–161. [CrossRef]
116. Steenerson, R.L.; Cronin, G.W. Treatment of tinnitus with electrical stimulation. *Otolaryngol.–Head Neck Surg.* **1999**, *121*, 511–513. [CrossRef] [PubMed]

117. Assouly, K.K.S.; Dullaart, M.J.; Stokroos, R.J.; van Dijk, B.; Stegeman, I.; Smit, A.L. Systematic Review on Intra- and Extracochlear Electrical Stimulation for Tinnitus. *Brain Sci.* **2021**, *11*, 1394. [CrossRef]
118. Yang, T.; Zhang, J.; Wang, B.; Zhang, W.; Xu, M.; Yang, S.; Liu, H. Electrical stimulation to treat tinnitus: A meta-analysis and systemic review of randomized controlled trials. *Ther. Adv. Chronic Dis.* **2021**, *12*, 20406223211041069. [CrossRef]
119. Chen, S.; Du, M.; Wang, Y.; Li, Y.; Tong, B.; Qiu, J.; Wu, F.; Liu, Y. State of the art: Non-invasive electrical stimulation for the treatment of chronic tinnitus. *Ther. Adv. Chronic Dis.* **2023**, *14*, 20406223221148061. [CrossRef]
120. Perez, R.; Shaul, C.; Vardi, M.; Muhanna, N.; Kileny, P.R.; Sichel, J.Y. Multiple electrostimulation treatments to the promontory for tinnitus. *Otol. Neurotol.* **2015**, *36*, 366–372. [CrossRef]
121. Wenzel, G.I.; Sarnes, P.; Warnecke, A.; Stover, T.; Jager, B.; Lesinski-Schiedat, A.; Lenarz, T. Non-penetrating round window electrode stimulation for tinnitus therapy followed by cochlear implantation. *Eur. Arch. Otorhinolaryngol.* **2015**, *272*, 3283–3293. [CrossRef]
122. Zeng, F.G.; Djalilian, H.; Lin, H. Tinnitus treatment with precise and optimal electric stimulation: Opportunities and challenges. *Curr. Opin. Otolaryngol. Head Neck Surg.* **2015**, *23*, 382–387. [CrossRef] [PubMed]
123. ClinicalTrials.gov. Novel Tinnitus Implant System for the Treatment of Chronic Severe Tinnitus. ClinicalTrials.gov Identifier: NCT03988699. Available online: https://clinicaltrials.gov/ct2/show/results/NCT03988699 (accessed on 9 November 2022).
124. Lefaucheur, J.P.; Andre-Obadia, N.; Antal, A.; Ayache, S.S.; Baeken, C.; Benninger, D.H.; Cantello, R.M.; Cincotta, M.; de Carvalho, M.; De Ridder, D.; et al. Evidence-based guidelines on the therapeutic use of repetitive transcranial magnetic stimulation (rTMS). *Clin. Neurophysiol.* **2014**, *125*, 2150–2206. [CrossRef] [PubMed]
125. Kreuzer, P.M.; Poeppl, T.B.; Vielsmeier, V.; Schecklmann, M.; Langguth, B.; Lehner, A. The more the merrier? Preliminary results regarding treatment duration and stimulation frequency of multisite repetitive transcranial magnetic stimulation in chronic tinnitus. *Prog. Brain Res.* **2021**, *262*, 287–307. [CrossRef] [PubMed]
126. Noh, T.S.; Kyong, J.S.; Chang, M.Y.; Park, M.K.; Lee, J.H.; Oh, S.H.; Kim, J.S.; Chung, C.K.; Suh, M.W. Comparison of Treatment Outcomes Following Either Prefrontal Cortical-only or Dual-site Repetitive Transcranial Magnetic Stimulation in Chronic Tinnitus Patients: A Double-blind Randomized Study. *Otol. Neurotol.* **2017**, *38*, 296–303. [CrossRef] [PubMed]
127. Roland, L.T.; Peelle, J.E.; Kallogjeri, D.; Nicklaus, J.; Piccirillo, J.F. The effect of noninvasive brain stimulation on neural connectivity in Tinnitus: A randomized trial. *Laryngoscope* **2016**, *126*, 1201–1206. [CrossRef]
128. Durmaz, O.; Ates, M.A.; Senol, M.G. Repetitive Transcranial Magnetic Stimulation (rTMS)-Induced Trigeminal Autonomic Cephalalgia. *Noro Psikiyatr. Ars.* **2015**, *52*, 309–311. [CrossRef]
129. Khedr, E.M.; Abo-Elfetoh, N.; Rothwell, J.C.; El-Atar, A.; Sayed, E.; Khalifa, H. Contralateral versus ipsilateral rTMS of temporoparietal cortex for the treatment of chronic unilateral tinnitus: Comparative study. *Eur. J. Neurol.* **2010**, *17*, 976–983. [CrossRef]
130. Kim, B.G.; Kim, D.Y.; Kim, S.K.; Kim, J.M.; Baek, S.H.; Moon, I.S. Comparison of the outcomes of repetitive transcranial magnetic stimulation to the ipsilateral and contralateral auditory cortex in unilateral tinnitus. *Electromagn. Biol. Med.* **2014**, *33*, 211–215. [CrossRef]
131. Cole, E.J.; Stimpson, K.H.; Bentzley, B.S.; Gulser, M.; Cherian, K.; Tischler, C.; Nejad, R.; Pankow, H.; Choi, E.; Aaron, H.; et al. Stanford Accelerated Intelligent Neuromodulation Therapy for Treatment-Resistant Depression. *Am. J. Psychiatry* **2020**, *177*, 716–726. [CrossRef]
132. Lan, L.; Liu, Y.; Wu, Y.; Xu, Z.G.; Xu, J.J.; Song, J.J.; Salvi, R.; Yin, X.; Chen, Y.C.; Cai, Y. Specific brain network predictors of interventions with different mechanisms for tinnitus patients. *EBioMedicine* **2022**, *76*, 103862. [CrossRef]
133. Sirh, S.J.; Sirh, S.W.; Mun, H.Y.; Sirh, H.M. Integrative Treatment for Tinnitus Combining Repeated Facial and Auriculotemporal Nerve Blocks with Stimulation of Auditory and Non-auditory Nerves. *Front. Neurosci.* **2022**, *16*, 758575. [CrossRef] [PubMed]
134. Skinner, C.; Kumar, S. Ultrasound-Guided Occipital Nerve Blocks to Reduce Tinnitus-Associated Otalgia: A Case Series. *A A Pract.* **2022**, *16*, e01552. [CrossRef] [PubMed]
135. Matsushima, J.I.; Sakai, N.; Uemi, N.; Ifukube, T. Effects of greater occipital nerve block on tinnitus and dizziness. *Int. Tinnitus J.* **1999**, *5*, 40–46. [PubMed]
136. Marks, K.L.; Martel, D.T.; Wu, C.; Basura, G.J.; Roberts, L.E.; Schvartz-Leyzac, K.C.; Shore, S.E. Auditory-somatosensory bimodal stimulation desynchronizes brain circuitry to reduce tinnitus in guinea pigs and humans. *Sci. Transl. Med.* **2018**, *10*, eaal3175. [CrossRef] [PubMed]
137. Koehler, S.D.; Shore, S.E. Stimulus-timing dependent multisensory plasticity in the guinea pig dorsal cochlear nucleus. *PLoS ONE* **2013**, *8*, e59828. [CrossRef]
138. FDA Grants Lenire®Tinnitus Treatment Device De Novo Approval. Available online: https://www.lenire.com/lenire-granted-fda-approval/ (accessed on 20 August 2023).
139. McCormack, A.; Edmondson-Jones, M.; Fortnum, H.; Dawes, P.D.; Middleton, H.; Munro, K.J.; Moore, D.R. Investigating the association between tinnitus severity and symptoms of depression and anxiety, while controlling for neuroticism, in a large middle-aged UK population. *Int. J. Audiol.* **2015**, *54*, 599–604. [CrossRef]
140. Baldo, P.; Doree, C.; Molin, P.; McFerran, D.; Cecco, S. Antidepressants for patients with tinnitus. *Cochrane Database Syst. Rev.* **2012**, *9*, CD003853. [CrossRef]
141. Dib, G.C.; Kasse, C.A.; Alves de Andrade, T.; Gurgel Testa, J.R.; Cruz, O.L. Tinnitus treatment with Trazodone. *Braz. J. Otorhinolaryngol.* **2007**, *73*, 390–397. [CrossRef]

142. Robinson, S.K.; Viirre, E.S.; Bailey, K.A.; Gerke, M.A.; Harris, J.P.; Stein, M.B. Randomized placebo-controlled trial of a selective serotonin reuptake inhibitor in the treatment of nondepressed tinnitus subjects. *Psychosom. Med.* **2005**, *67*, 981–988. [CrossRef]
143. Scholz, A. Mechanisms of (local) anaesthetics on voltage-gated sodium and other ion channels. *Br. J. Anaesth.* **2002**, *89*, 52–61. [CrossRef]
144. Kalcioglu, M.T.; Bayindir, T.; Erdem, T.; Ozturan, O. Objective evaluation of the effects of intravenous lidocaine on tinnitus. *Hear. Res.* **2005**, *199*, 81–88. [CrossRef] [PubMed]
145. Den Hartigh, J.; Hilders, C.G.; Schoemaker, R.C.; Hulshof, J.H.; Cohen, A.F.; Vermeij, P. Tinnitus suppression by intravenous lidocaine in relation to its plasma concentration. *Clin. Pharmacol. Ther.* **1993**, *54*, 415–420. [CrossRef] [PubMed]
146. Duckert, L.G.; Rees, T.S. Treatment of tinnitus with intravenous lidocaine: A double-blind randomized trial. *Otolaryngol. Head Neck Surg.* **1983**, *91*, 550–555. [CrossRef]
147. Otsuka, K.; Pulec, J.L.; Suzuki, M. Assessment of intravenous lidocaine for the treatment of subjective tinnitus. *Ear Nose Throat J.* **2003**, *82*, 781–784. [CrossRef]
148. Baguley, D.M.; Jones, S.; Wilkins, I.; Axon, P.R.; Moffat, D.A. The inhibitory effect of intravenous lidocaine infusion on tinnitus after translabyrinthine removal of vestibular schwannoma: A double-blind, placebo-controlled, crossover study. *Otol. Neurotol.* **2005**, *26*, 169–176. [CrossRef] [PubMed]
149. Haginomori, S.; Makimoto, K.; Araki, M.; Kawakami, M.; Takahashi, H. Effect of lidocaine injection of EOAE in patients with tinnitus. *Acta Otolaryngol.* **1995**, *115*, 488–492. [CrossRef]
150. Elzayat, S.; El-Sherif, H.; Hegazy, H.; Gabr, T.; El-Tahan, A.R. Tinnitus: Evaluation of Intratympanic Injection of Combined Lidocaine and Corticosteroids. *ORL J. Otorhinolaryngol. Relat. Spec.* **2016**, *78*, 159–166. [CrossRef]
151. Sakata, H.; Kojima, Y.; Koyama, S.; Furuya, N.; Sakata, E. Treatment of cochlear tinnitus with transtympanic infusion of 4% lidocaine into the tympanic cavity. *Int. Tinnitus J.* **2001**, *7*, 46–50.
152. Sieghart, W. Pharmacology of benzodiazepine receptors: An update. *J. Psychiatry Neurosci.* **1994**, *19*, 24–29. [CrossRef]
153. Han, S.S.; Nam, E.C.; Won, J.Y.; Lee, K.U.; Chun, W.; Choi, H.K.; Levine, R.A. Clonazepam quiets tinnitus: A randomised crossover study with Ginkgo biloba. *J. Neurol. Neurosurg. Psychiatry* **2012**, *83*, 821–827. [CrossRef]
154. Hilton, M.P.; Zimmermann, E.F.; Hunt, W.T. Ginkgo biloba for tinnitus. *Cochrane Database Syst. Rev.* **2013**, *3*, CD003852. [CrossRef] [PubMed]
155. Sereda, M.; Xia, J.; Scutt, P.; Hilton, M.P.; El Refaie, A.; Hoare, D.J. Ginkgo biloba for tinnitus. *Cochrane Database Syst. Rev.* **2022**, *11*, CD013514. [CrossRef] [PubMed]
156. Johnson, R.M.; Brummett, R.; Schleuning, A. Use of alprazolam for relief of tinnitus. A double-blind study. *Arch. Otolaryngol. Head Neck Surg.* **1993**, *119*, 842–845. [CrossRef]
157. Jalali, M.M.; Kousha, A.; Naghavi, S.E.; Soleimani, R.; Banan, R. The effects of alprazolam on tinnitus: A cross-over randomized clinical trial. *Med. Sci. Monit.* **2009**, *15*, PI55–PI60.
158. Dompe, C.; Moncrieff, L.; Matys, J.; Grzech-Lesniak, K.; Kocherova, I.; Bryja, A.; Bruska, M.; Dominiak, M.; Mozdziak, P.; Skiba, T.H.I.; et al. Photobiomodulation-Underlying Mechanism and Clinical Applications. *J. Clin. Med.* **2020**, *9*, 1724. [CrossRef]
159. Demirkol, N.; Usumez, A.; Demirkol, M.; Sari, F.; Akcaboy, C. Efficacy of Low-Level Laser Therapy in Subjective Tinnitus Patients with Temporomandibular Disorders. *Photomed. Laser Surg.* **2017**, *35*, 427–431. [CrossRef]
160. Dehkordi, M.A.; Einolghozati, S.; Ghasemi, S.M.; Abolbashari, S.; Meshkat, M.; Behzad, H. Effect of low-level laser therapy in the treatment of cochlear tinnitus: A double-blind, placebo-controlled study. *Ear Nose Throat J.* **2015**, *94*, 32–36.
161. Goodman, S.S.; Bentler, R.A.; Dittberner, A.; Mertes, I.B. The effect of low-level laser therapy on hearing. *ISRN Otolaryngol.* **2013**, *2013*, 916370. [CrossRef]
162. Gungor, A.; Dogru, S.; Cincik, H.; Erkul, E.; Poyrazoglu, E. Effectiveness of transmeatal low power laser irradiation for chronic tinnitus. *J. Laryngol. Otol.* **2008**, *122*, 447–451. [CrossRef]
163. Mollasadeghi, A.; Mirmohammadi, S.J.; Mehrparvar, A.H.; Davari, M.H.; Shokouh, P.; Mostaghaci, M.; Baradaranfar, M.H.; Bahaloo, M. Efficacy of low-level laser therapy in the management of tinnitus due to noise-induced hearing loss: A double-blind randomized clinical trial. *ScientificWorldJournal* **2013**, *2013*, 596076. [CrossRef]
164. Teggi, R.; Bellini, C.; Piccioni, L.O.; Palonta, F.; Bussi, M. Transmeatal low-level laser therapy for chronic tinnitus with cochlear dysfunction. *Audiol. Neurootol.* **2009**, *14*, 115–120. [CrossRef] [PubMed]
165. Nakashima, T.; Ueda, H.; Misawa, H.; Suzuki, T.; Tominaga, M.; Ito, A.; Numata, S.; Kasai, S.; Asahi, K.; Vernon, J.A.; et al. Transmeatal low-power laser irradiation for tinnitus. *Otol. Neurotol.* **2002**, *23*, 296–300. [CrossRef] [PubMed]
166. Talluri, S.; Palaparthi, S.M.; Michelogiannakis, D.; Khan, J. Efficacy of photobiomodulation in the management of tinnitus: A systematic review of randomized control trials. *Eur. Ann. Otorhinolaryngol. Head Neck Dis.* **2022**, *139*, 83–90. [CrossRef] [PubMed]
167. Balmer, T.S.; Trussell, L.O. Trigeminal Contributions to the Dorsal Cochlear Nucleus in Mouse. *Front. Neurosci.* **2021**, *15*, 715954. [CrossRef]
168. Lee, A.; Abouzari, M.; Akbarpour, M.; Risbud, A.; Lin, H.W.; Djalilian, H.R. A proposed association between subjective nonpulsatile tinnitus and migraine. *World J. Otorhinolaryngol. Head Neck Surg.* **2023**, *9*, 107–114. [CrossRef]
169. Djalilian, H. Treatment of Tinnitus with Migraine Medications. Available online: https://classic.clinicaltrials.gov/ct2/show/NCT04404439 (accessed on 20 June 2023).
170. Husain, F.T.; Gander, P.E.; Jansen, J.N.; Shen, S. Expectations for Tinnitus Treatment and Outcomes: A Survey Study of Audiologists and Patients. *J. Am. Acad. Audiol.* **2018**, *29*, 313–336. [CrossRef]

171. Simoes, J.P.; Daoud, E.; Shabbir, M.; Amanat, S.; Assouly, K.; Biswas, R.; Casolani, C.; Dode, A.; Enzler, F.; Jacquemin, L.; et al. Multidisciplinary Tinnitus Research: Challenges and Future Directions from the Perspective of Early Stage Researchers. *Front. Aging Neurosci.* **2021**, *13*, 647285. [CrossRef]
172. Duckert, L.G.; Rees, T.S. Placebo effect in tinnitus management. *Otolaryngol. Head Neck Surg.* **1984**, *92*, 697–699. [CrossRef]
173. Meikle, M.B.; Henry, J.A.; Griest, S.E.; Stewart, B.J.; Abrams, H.B.; McArdle, R.; Myers, P.J.; Newman, C.W.; Sandridge, S.; Turk, D.C.; et al. The tinnitus functional index: Development of a new clinical measure for chronic, intrusive tinnitus. *Ear Hear.* **2012**, *33*, 153–176. [CrossRef]
174. Jacquemin, L.; Mertens, G.; Van de Heyning, P.; Vanderveken, O.M.; Topsakal, V.; De Hertogh, W.; Michiels, S.; Van Rompaey, V.; Gilles, A. Sensitivity to change and convergent validity of the Tinnitus Functional Index (TFI) and the Tinnitus Questionnaire (TQ): Clinical and research perspectives. *Hear. Res.* **2019**, *382*, 107796. [CrossRef]
175. Adamchic, I.; Langguth, B.; Hauptmann, C.; Tass, P.A. Psychometric evaluation of visual analog scale for the assessment of chronic tinnitus. *Am. J. Audiol.* **2012**, *21*, 215–225. [CrossRef] [PubMed]
176. Zeleznik, O.A.; Welling, D.B.; Stankovic, K.; Frueh, L.; Balasubramanian, R.; Curhan, G.C.; Curhan, S.G. Association of Plasma Metabolomic Biomarkers with Persistent Tinnitus: A Population-Based Case-Control Study. *JAMA Otolaryngol. Head Neck Surg.* **2023**, *149*, 404–415. [CrossRef] [PubMed]
177. Zeleznik, O.; Welling, B.; Stankovic, K.; Frueh, L.; Balasubramanian, R.; Curhan, G.; Curhan, S. A Population-Based Study of Plasma Metabolomic Profiles of Persistent Tinnitus Identifies Candidate Biomarkers. *medRxiv* **2022**. [CrossRef]
178. Chew, H.; Solomon, V.A.; Fonteh, A.N. Involvement of Lipids in Alzheimer's Disease Pathology and Potential Therapies. *Front. Physiol.* **2020**, *11*, 598. [CrossRef] [PubMed]
179. Alecu, I.; Bennett, S.A.L. Dysregulated Lipid Metabolism and Its Role in alpha-Synucleinopathy in Parkinson's Disease. *Front. Neurosci.* **2019**, *13*, 328. [CrossRef]
180. Amanat, S.; Gallego-Martinez, A.; Sollini, J.; Perez-Carpena, P.; Espinosa-Sanchez, J.M.; Aran, I.; Soto-Varela, A.; Batuecas-Caletrio, A.; Canlon, B.; May, P.; et al. Burden of rare variants in synaptic genes in patients with severe tinnitus: An exome based extreme phenotype study. *EBioMedicine* **2021**, *66*, 103309. [CrossRef]
181. Van den Berge, M.J.C.; van Dijk, J.M.C.; Metzemaekers, J.D.M.; Maat, B.; Free, R.H.; van Dijk, P. An auditory brainstem implant for treatment of unilateral tinnitus: Protocol for an interventional pilot study. *BMJ Open* **2019**, *9*, e026185. [CrossRef]
182. Roberts, D.S.; Otto, S.; Chen, B.; Peng, K.A.; Schwartz, M.S.; Brackmann, D.E.; House, J.W. Tinnitus Suppression After Auditory Brainstem Implantation in Patients with Neurofibromatosis Type-2. *Otol. Neurotol.* **2017**, *38*, 118–122. [CrossRef]
183. Tyler, R.; Cacace, A.; Stocking, C.; Tarver, B.; Engineer, N.; Martin, J.; Deshpande, A.; Stecker, N.; Pereira, M.; Kilgard, M.; et al. Vagus Nerve Stimulation Paired with Tones for the Treatment of Tinnitus: A Prospective Randomized Double-blind Controlled Pilot Study in Humans. *Sci. Rep.* **2017**, *7*, 11960. [CrossRef]
184. van Zwieten, G.; Devos, J.V.P.; Kotz, S.A.; Ackermans, L.; Brinkmann, P.; Dauven, L.; George, E.L.J.; Janssen, A.M.L.; Kremer, B.; Leue, C.; et al. A Protocol to Investigate Deep Brain Stimulation for Refractory Tinnitus: From Rat Model to the Set-Up of a Human Pilot Study. *Audiol. Res.* **2022**, *13*, 49–63. [CrossRef]

Disclaimer/Publisher's Note: The statements, opinions and data contained in all publications are solely those of the individual author(s) and contributor(s) and not of MDPI and/or the editor(s). MDPI and/or the editor(s) disclaim responsibility for any injury to people or property resulting from any ideas, methods, instructions or products referred to in the content.

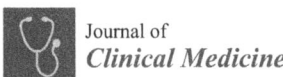

Review

Current Advances in Gene Therapies of Genetic Auditory Neuropathy Spectrum Disorder

Anissa Rym Saidia [1], Jérôme Ruel [1,2], Amel Bahloul [1], Benjamin Chaix [3], Frédéric Venail [1,3] and Jing Wang [1,3,*]

1. Institute for Neurosciences of Montpellier (INM), University Montpellier, INSERM, 34295 Montpellier, France
2. Cognitive Neuroscience Laboratory, Aix-Marseille University, CNRS, UMR 7291, 13331 Marseille, France
3. Department of ENT and Head and Neck Surgery, University Hospital of Montpellier, 34295 Montpellier, France
* Correspondence: jing.wang@inserm.fr; Tel.: +33-499-63-60-48

Abstract: Auditory neuropathy spectrum disorder (ANSD) refers to a range of hearing impairments characterized by an impaired transmission of sound from the cochlea to the brain. This defect can be due to a lesion or defect in the inner hair cell (IHC), IHC ribbon synapse (e.g., pre-synaptic release of glutamate), postsynaptic terminals of the spiral ganglion neurons, or demyelination and axonal loss within the auditory nerve. To date, the only clinical treatment options for ANSD are hearing aids and cochlear implantation. However, despite the advances in hearing-aid and cochlear-implant technologies, the quality of perceived sound still cannot match that of the normal ear. Recent advanced genetic diagnostics and clinical audiology made it possible to identify the precise site of a lesion and to characterize the specific disease mechanisms of ANSD, thus bringing renewed hope to the treatment or prevention of auditory neurodegeneration. Moreover, genetic routes involving the replacement or corrective editing of mutant sequences or defected genes to repair damaged cells for the future restoration of hearing in deaf people are showing promise. In this review, we provide an update on recent discoveries in the molecular pathophysiology of genetic lesions, auditory synaptopathy and neuropathy, and gene-therapy research towards hearing restoration in rodent models and in clinical trials.

Keywords: gene therapy; auditory neuropathy; auditory synaptopathy; hidden hearing loss; genetic deafness; hearing restoration

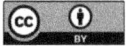

1. Introduction

Hearing in mammals relies on the ability of the sensory hair cells to convert sound-evoked mechanical stimuli into electrochemical signals. The hair-bundle deflection induces rapid opening of sensory transduction channels, leading to the generation of an influx of cations into the IHC. This results in a depolarization potential, allowing an influx of calcium through voltage-dependent calcium channels. The coupling of Ca^{2+} channels at the presynaptic site of the ribbon synapse triggers high-rate synaptic vesicle fusion and the release of neurotransmitter glutamate from the synaptic cleft. The release of glutamate in the synapse activates Ca^{2+}-sensitive AMPA receptors (Figure 1). This initiates the generation of neural spikes in spiral ganglion neuron (SGN) fibers, which encodes information about sound stimuli that is sent to the central nervous system. A dysfunction at any level of this complex transduction machinery may disturb the coding of acoustic features, particularly of temporal cues. The potential sites of damage are diverse, including the IHCs, IHC ribbon synapses, or synaptopathy, (e.g., pre-synaptic release of glutamate or postsynaptic terminals dendrites of the spiral ganglion neurons), or can be due to demyelination and axonal loss of the auditory nerve fibers and their targets in the cochlear nucleus (i.e., neuropathy, Figure 1). These auditory pathologies are named auditory neuropathy spectrum disorder (ANSD), in which the activity of outer hair cells (OHCs) is maintained (Figure 1) [1–4].

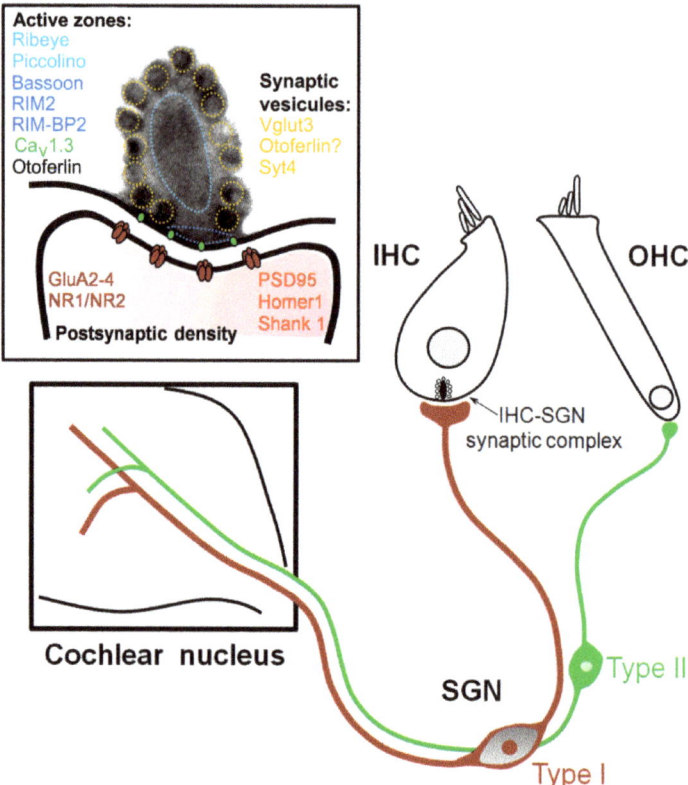

Figure 1. Inner hair cell (IHC)–spiral ganglion synaptic complex. The IHC is connected to all type I spiral ganglion neurons (SGNs) forming the radial afferent system (red) going to the cochlear nuclei. The OHC synapses with small endings from type II spiral ganglion neurons, forming the spiral afferent system (green). Molecular composition of a mature ribbon of the inner hair–cell synaptic complex ensuring the temporal precision of peripheral sound encoding. The mature ribbon synapse between the sensory inner hair cells (IHCs) and postsynaptic spiral ganglion neurons (SGNs) involves the spatial confinement of several molecular components: presynaptic density merge to one single ribbon anchor and, postsynaptically, one continuous elongated postsynaptic density composed by functional synaptic AMPA-preferring glutamate receptors, but also some silent NMDA receptors. Font color indicates association with the correspondingly colored pre-/postsynaptic localization.

The clinical profiles of ANSD are quite heterogeneous, depending on the variety of etiologies. ANSD can result from syndromic and non-syndromic genetic abnormalities, as well as environmental causes (e.g., hypoxia, noise-exposure, cytotoxic oncologic drugs) and aging. ANSD is one of the common causes of hearing loss, affecting between 1.2% and 10% of those with hearing loss [5]. Audiologically, ANSD is characterized by mild to profound sensory neural hearing loss, with impaired or absent compound action potentials (CAP) and auditory brainstem responses (ABRs, Figure 2) and deteriorated speech audiometry in quiet [6]; these are associated with normal otoacoustic emissions (OAE, Figure 2) or cochlear microphonics (CM), indicating normal OHC function. Additionally, the absence of the middle-ear stapedial reflex and of the contralateral suppression of otoacoustic emissions are usually observed [1,5,7,8].

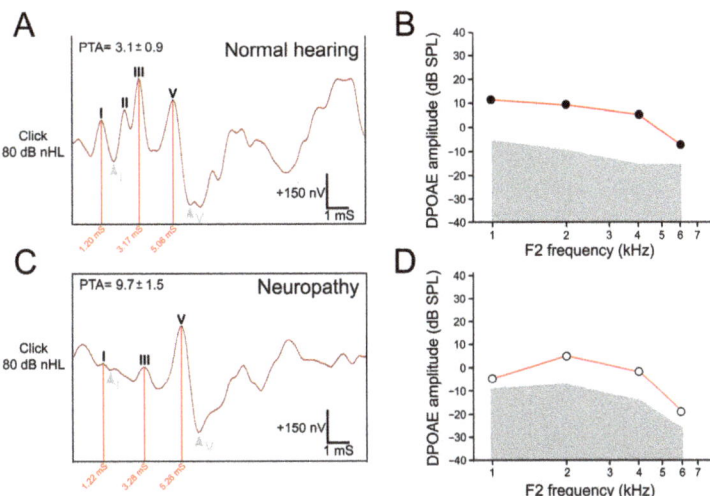

Figure 2. Auditory brainstem responses (ABRs) and distortion product of otoacoustic emissions (DPOAEs) recorded from one normal hearing control (**A**,**B**) and one patient with speech understanding difficulties (**C**,**D**). (**A**) ABRs were recorded at 80 dB nHL (decibels normal hearing level) with normal amplitudes, latencies, and morphology. (**B**) No abnormalities were detected in the DPOAEs. (**C**) A patient with speech understanding difficulties showed a clear decrease in the amplitude of waves I, II, and III. The I-V interval was 4.04 vs. 3.86 for the patient and a normal hearing subject, respectively. (**D**) DPOAEs were still present in this patient. PTAs: mean of pure-tone audiometry thresholds recorded at 250, 500, 1000, 2000, 3000, and 4000 Hz. Note that PTA is within the normal range in the patient with speech understanding difficulties. The audiologic results of this patient suggest a hidden auditory neuropathy.

Electrocochleography (ECochG) and tests of neural adaptation remain a powerful diagnostic tool to help identify the site of a lesion. For example, the absence of the summating potential in ECochG indicates the loss of IHC mechanoelectrical transduction or of the IHCs themselves. Furthermore, ECochG can also be used to distinguish auditory synaptopathy from auditory neuropathy. Indeed, patients with auditory synaptopathy displayed enhanced adaptation to frequency specific sounds [9]. By contrast, patients with auditory neuropathy showed normal adaptation for low-frequency sounds but abnormally enhanced adaptation to high-frequency sounds [9]. In patients with auditory synaptopathy, abnormal loudness adaptation is likely related to the disorder affecting IHC-ribbon synapses in the organ of Corti along the basilar membrane [9]. In the cases of auditory neuropathy, loss of nerve fibers is equally distributed throughout the cochlea, and thus the observed neural conduction disorder is probably independent of the origin of the fibers along the basilar membrane [2]. The normal adaptation observed in the low-frequency region is therefore unexpected and may reflect the compensation by central auditory structures involved in loudness perception, reducing the auditory nerve input in a frequency-specific manner [10,11].

Hidden hearing loss (HHL) or supraliminal hearing disorders are probably a specific type of ANSD caused by, e.g., noise exposure, aging, or peripheral neuropathy and characterized by normal pure-tone hearing thresholds together with deficits in sound-evoked auditory nerve activity (Figure 2). Patients with HHL display normal speech audiometry thresholds in quiet, well-synchronized ABRs, but with impaired speech discrimination in noisy environments [12].

Currently, clinical options for the hearing rehabilitation of patients suffering from ANSD are hearing aids that can amplify sound for mild or moderate deafness, or cochlear implants for severe deafness [12]. The advantage of the latter is that they can bypass non-functional sensory hair cells by directly stimulating the remnant auditory neural structures within the deafened cochlea. Actually, the data published in the literature on the long-time outcomes of hearing rehabilitation with hearing aids in children with ANSD are partially contradictory [13–15]. Some report good hearing rehabilitation [13–15], while others describe a lack of hearing and communication benefits from hearing aids in children with ANSD [1,16]. Cochlear implants, which electronically stimulate the SGNs, might provide effective auditory rehabilitation for patients with auditory synaptopathy because the generation and propagation of spikes is maintained. Generally, patients with lesions affecting the auditory nerve show poor performance with cochlear implants, probably due to altered neural transmission of the electrical signal from the cochlear implant [12]. However, in patients with OPA1-related auditory neuropathy one year after implantation, improvement in speech perception and synchronous activation of auditory pathways was observed [17], probably by either bypassing the site of lesion (which could be located in the terminal dendrites) and/or by the electrical stimuli inducing well-defined temporal SGN activation. However, to date, data on the outcome of auditory neuropathy rehabilitation are limited [5,18].

The past decade has seen significant advances in the understanding of the molecular pathogenic mechanisms that contribute to hearing impairments induced by environmental and genetic factors. This, in turn, has brought renewed hope to concepts of replacing or correcting the mutant sequences or defected genes in order to prevent auditory neurodegeneration or to promote regeneration of auditory synapse and nerve fibers. This review begins by outlining our current understanding of the molecular pathways that mediate genetic ANSD. The following sections discuss recent discoveries in gene therapies using newly designed genetic therapeutic tools for replacing the mutant sequences or defected genes for restoring hearing by rescuing cochlear function through the regeneration of synapses and/or auditory nerve fibers. These tools provide promising perspectives for the future restoration of hearing in deaf people.

2. Pathogenic Mechanisms of Auditory Neuropathy

Syndromic auditory neuropathy affects multiple cranial and peripheral nerves, while non-syndromic auditory neuropathies are limited to the auditory nerve. Most cases of non-syndromic auditory neuropathy result from impaired synaptic transfer [5].

2.1. Non-Syndromic Auditory Synaptopathies

Genetic auditory synaptopathies generally only cause deafness, such as the mutations in the *CACNA1D* gene encoding the Cav1.3L-type Ca^{2+} channel, the *OTOF* gene encoding Otoferlin, the *SLC17A8* gene encoding Vglut3, or the *DIAPH3* gene encoding the diaphanous formin 3.

2.1.1. Otoferlin DFNB9

The OTOF gene encodes otoferlin, which is a critical calcium sensor for synaptic exocytosis in cochlear IHCs [19,20]. Otoferlin is also involved in vesicular reformation, re-supply, and tethering at the active zone, making otoferlin a multi-tasking protein [20,21]. Mutations in the gene encoding otoferlin are responsible for autosomal recessive profound prelingual deafness, DFNB9 [22]. To date, about 220 pathogenic variants in *OTOF* have been identified [23]. The majority of these mutations are assumed to be nonsense or truncation mutations that provoke the inactivation of otoferlin [24]. Patients with variants in *OTOF* displayed milder hearing loss, as well as progressive and temperature-sensitive hearing loss, while OAEs were preserved [22,25–27]. Children harboring biallelic mutations of the *OTOF* gene displayed profound hearing loss, absence of ABRs and CAP, but preservation of DPOAEs and the amplitude of CM [28]. Otoferlin knock-out mice, which are profoundly deaf due to a failure of sound-evoked neurotransmitter release at the IHC synapse, are likely to be an appropriate animal model for DFNB9 [29,30]. In these mice, Ca^{2+}-triggered exocytosis in IHCs is almost abolished [29,30]; synaptic vesicles were found near the membrane at the active zone, suggesting that an absence of vesicles did not limit signal transduction, but that a late step of exocytosis was disrupted [30].

2.1.2. VGLUT3-DFNA25

Vesicular glutamate transporters (VGLUTs) are responsible for glutamate loading into synaptic vesicles, which is essential in order to achieve synaptic transmission [31]. VGLUT3 is expressed in small subsets of neurons in the central nervous system [31,32]. In mice, VGLUT3 is expressed in the IHCs [33,34] and the OHCs [35]. The genetic ablation of *Slc17a8* in mice results in the absence of CAP or ABRs to acoustic stimuli, while ABRs could be elicited by electrical stimuli, and robust otoacoustic emissions were recorded in these mice [33,34]. This thus reflects a failure in activation of the ascending auditory pathway, while the activity in OHCs is unaffected [33,34,36,37]. Patients with a 12q22-q24 deletion in the *SLC17A8* gene at the DFNA25 locus display congenital and non-syndromic autosomal dominant deafness [33,38,39]. The deafness in patients was characterized as high-frequency, progressive sensorineural hearing loss, with good hearing rescue through cochlear implantation, thus reinforcing the hypothesis of synaptopathy [33,39]. $VGLUT3^{A224V/A224V}$ mice harboring the p.A221V mutation (p.A221V in humans corresponds to p.A224V in mice) in the *Slc17a8* gene displayed progressive hearing loss with intact OHC function [40]. The summating potential was, however, reduced, indicating the alteration of the IHC receptor potential. Scanning electron microscopy examinations revealed the collapse of IHC stereocilia bundles, leaving those from OHCs unaffected. In addition, IHC ribbon synapses underwent structural and functional modifications at later stages. These results suggest that DFNA25 stems from a failure in mechano-transduction followed by a change in synaptic transmission [40].

2.1.3. Cav1.3-SANDD

Calcium influx at the base of the IHCs near the ribbon synapse is mediated via the L-type calcium (Ca^{2+}) channel Cav1.3, which is the main voltage-gated Ca^{2+} channel in IHCs and essential for hearing. Cav1.3 translates sound-induced depolarization into neurotransmitter glutamate release at the synaptic site, resulting in signal transmission to the auditory nerve [41]. Cav1.3-encoding by the *CACNA1D* gene is widely distributed across different cells such as OHCs, IHCs, cardiomyocytes, neuroendocrine cells, and neurons. A Cav1.3. mutation in *CACNA1D* may cause both sinoatrial node dysfunction and deafness (termed SANDD syndrome) in mice and in humans, in humans closely resembling that of $Cacna1d^{-/-}$ mice [41,42]. $Ca_v1.3$ is required for normal hearing and cardiac pace making in humans, and loss of function in only a subset of channels is sufficient to cause SANDD syndrome [42]. Loss-of-function mutations in the *CACNA1D* gene causes impaired synaptic neurotransmission at the IHC ribbon synapse in KO mice [41,43]. Cav1.3 protects the sensory hair cells during cochlear aging through reducing calcium-mediated oxidative stress in C57BL/6J male mice [44] and plays important roles in inner ear differentiation [45].

2.1.4. CABP2-DFNB93

Calcium-binding protein 2 (CABP2) is a potent modulator of IHC voltage-gated calcium channels CaV1.3. CABP2 regulates Ca^{2+} influx at the presynaptic site [46,47] and thus also the vesicular release of glutamate. Pathologic mutations in *CABP2* lead to autosomal-recessive, moderate-to-severe non-syndromic hearing impairment DFNB93 [48–51]. DFNB93 patients displayed an auditory synaptopathy phenotype with normal OAEs [52]. Using a knock-out mouse model, Picher et al. [52] demonstrated that DFNB93 hearing impairment may result from an enhanced steady-state inactivation of CaV1.3 channels at the IHC synapse, thus limiting their availability to trigger synaptic transmission, resulting in elevated auditory thresholds [52]. This, however, does not seem to interfere with cochlear development and does not cause the early degeneration of hair cells or their synaptic complex [52,53]. These results suggested an extended window for gene therapy.

2.1.5. DIAPH3-AUNA1

Auditory neuropathy, non-syndromic, autosomal dominant 1 (AUNA1) is a form of delayed-onset, progressive human deafness resulting from a point mutation in the 5' untranslated region of the Diaphanous homolog 3 (*DIAPH3*) gene. The *DIAPH3* mutation leads to the overexpression of the DIAPH3 protein, a formin family member involved in cytoskeleton dynamics [54]. Patients with AUNA1 displayed absent or altered ABR, while OHC functions are still maintained [1,55], thus indicating auditory neuropathy. Transgenic mice overexpressing Diap3 exhibit a progressive threshold shift but maintained a distortion product of otoacoustic emissions (DPOAEs) [54,56]. Morphological assessments revealed a selective and early onset alteration of the IHC cuticular plate and fused stereocilia with the eventual loss of the capacity of IHC to transmit incoming sensory stimuli [54,56]. Furthermore, a significant reduction in the number of IHC ribbon synapses was observed over 24 weeks in mutant mice, although this reduction did not correlate temporally with the onset and progression of hearing loss or of stereocilia bundle anomalies [54]. Together, these results suggest an important function of Diap3 in regulating the assembly and/or maintenance of actin filaments in IHC stereocilia, as well as a potential role at the IHC ribbon synapse.

2.2. Syndromic Auditory Neuropathy

Genetic neuropathies frequently affect other neurons, thus leading to syndromic phenotypes such as Charcot–Marie–Tooth disease, autosomal dominant optic atrophy, Leber's hereditary optic neuropathy, Friedreich's ataxia, Mohr–Tranebjaerg syndrome, Refsum disease, or Wolfram syndrome [57–60].

2.2.1. Charcot–Marie–Tooth

Autosomal-dominant Charcot–Marie–Tooth (CMT) is the most common hereditary peripheral polyneuropathy characterized by the degeneration of peripheral nerves. CMT can be classified into two major categories: TMC type 1 (demyelinating neuropathies) and type 2 (axonal form of neuropathies) [61,62]. CMT patients carry mutations in the MPZ genes for myelin protein zero or PMP22 coding for proteins essential for the formation and adhesion of myelin [2,63,64]. CMT type 1 A (CMT1A) is the predominant subtype, which is a demyelinating peripheral neuropathy characterized by distal muscle weakness, sensory loss, areflexia, and slow motor- and sensory-nerve conduction velocities [1,62,63]. Hearing impairment is also a relatively common symptom of CMT1A. Compared to controls, CMT1A patients had a significantly decreased speech perception capacity in a noisy environment, as well as decreased temporal and spectral resolution, thus suggesting that demyelination of auditory-nerve fibers in CMT1A causes defective cochlear neurotransmission [65]. Patients with CMT type 1 and 2 showed a delayed or reduced amplitude ABR, as well as an impaired speech intelligibility, which are electrophysiological evidence of auditory neuropathy [62].

2.2.2. Autosomal-Dominant Optic Atrophy

Autosomal-dominant optic atrophy (DOA) is the most frequent form of hereditary optic neuropathy [66], with a reported frequency of 1:10,000, and is caused by heterozygous variants in the *OPA1* gene encoding a mitochondrial-dynamin-related large GTPase [67–69]. OPA1 is involved in many mitochondrial functions, notably in the maintenance of the respiratory chain and cell membrane potential [70–72], cristae organization, control of apoptosis [72,73], and mitochondrial DNA maintenance [74–76]. DOA was initially described as a non-syndromic moderate-to-severe loss of visual acuity, with an insidious onset in early childhood caused by a progressive loss of retinal ganglion cells [77]. In the last decade, the clinical spectrum of DOA has been extended to a wide variety of symptoms, including deafness, ataxia, neuropathy, and myopathy, and is now called dominant optic atrophy plus (DOA*plus*) [74,78,79]. Deafness is the second-most prevalent clinical feature in DOA*plus*, affecting about 20% of all DOA patients [17,74,78–80].

The association of DOA and deafness is classically related to the R445H mutation in exon 14, but other *OPA1* mis-sense variants have already been reported in the literature [79,81]. Here, hearing loss starts in childhood or early adulthood [79,82]. Although the majority of studies broadly qualify the hearing disorder as 'sensorineural hearing loss', some authors have proposed auditory neuropathy as the pathophysiological mechanism underlying the hearing impairment in OPA1-DOA [17,70,83,84]. Audiological examination of OPA1 hearing impaired patients harboring missense mutations showed impaired speech perception and absence or profound alteration of ABRs but preservation of OAE and even enhanced CM potentials reflecting normal OHC function [28].

2.2.3. Leber Hereditary Optic Neuropathy

Leber hereditary optic neuropathy (LHON) is the most common mitochondrial genetic disease. It is characterized by bilateral, subacute, painless loss of vision, and over 95% of LHON cases are caused by one of three mitochondrial DNA (mtDNA) point mutations: 3460G>A, 11778G>A, and 14484T>C or mutation in the *TMEM126A* gene coding a mitochondrial protein. Severe axonal degeneration with demyelination of the optic nerve had been indicated by histological necropsy studies [85]. Patients with Leber hereditary optic neuropathy also show signs of auditory neuropathy [86,87].

2.2.4. Friedreich's Ataxia

Friedreich's ataxia (FRDA) is the most frequent autosomal-recessive inherited ataxia caused by mutations in the FXN gene coding for the mitochondrial protein Frataxin involved in regulating iron accumulation in the mitochondria. FRDA is due to an abnormal repetition of the GAA triplet (100 to 2000 GAA triplets) in the *FXN* gene [88]. In addition to impaired balance and coordination of voluntary movements, Friedreich's ataxia is associated with hearing impairment, including difficulty understanding speech in background noise; auditory thresholds were, however, unchanged [88–91], nor was OHC function [92]. Most affected individuals show abnormalities in auditory neural and brainstem responses as a result of auditory neuropathy [92–94]. Of FRDA patients, 8 to 13% show sensorineural hearing loss, as revealed in a pure-tone audiogram [95].

2.2.5. Mohr–Tranebjaerg Syndrome

Mohr–Tranebjaerg syndrome, in which deafness with progressive dystonia and visual impairment are associated, can be classified as a non-isolated auditory neuropathy. Indeed, observation of post-mortem samples shows neuronal loss with preservation of OHCs [96]. Here, again, mutations (DDP1 for deafness-dystonia) of TIMM8A/DDP1, which codes for a polypeptide of 97 amino acids located in the mitochondria, are at the origin of this syndrome.

3. Gene Therapies for Genetic Synaptopathies and Neuropathies

Gene therapy is an experimental technique that uses genes to treat or prevent disease by introducing a desired foreign gene or gene-regulatory element, such as RNA interference, into the target cells to replace or repair the defective gene [97]. Future gene therapy could promise the restoration of hearing in some forms of monogenic deafness where cochlear morphology is preserved for a period of time that allows intervention to restore hearing. Several viral vectors (e.g., adenovirus (Ad), adeno-associated virus (AAV), lentivirus) have already been used to transduce the inner ear [98,99]. The most recent studies have focused on optimizing AAV-based vector systems (Table 1), due to their efficiency in transducing cells of the sensory epithelium.

3.1. Restoration of Neurotransmission in IHC Synapses

3.1.1. DFNB9

Otoferlin knock-out mice, which are profoundly deaf due to a failure of sound-evoked neurotransmitter release at the IHC synapse, are likely to be an appropriate animal model for DFNB9 [29,30]. AAV-mediated gene transfer of the gene encoding otoferlin is technically challenging, due to the limited DNA packaging capacity of AAVs (≈4.7 kb). This limit makes it impossible to package large genes such as *Otof* (cDNA ~6 kb). To overcome this problem, Reisinger et al. [100] investigated the possibility of restoring hearing using the AAV-mediated gene transfer of the synaptotagmin1 gene into mouse hair cells deficient in otoferlin. Up to the fourth post-natal day in the mouse, calcium-triggered exocytosis depends on synaptotagmin 1 [101], whereas synaptotagmin1/2 are not expressed in adult IHCs [102]. Thus, extending synaptotagmin 1 expression over a longer term may rescue the loss of otoferlin in DFNB9. Unfortunately, the strategy failed to restore the Ca^{2+} influx-triggered exocytosis in IHCs of $Otof^{-/-}$ mice [100].

Akil et al. [103] adapted a reported dual AAV-vector method for the delivery of large cDNAs [104]. They used two different recombinant vectors, one containing the 5′ and the other the 3′ portions. They showed that a single delivery of the two vectors through the round-window membrane into the cochlea of $Otof^{-/-}$ mutant mice on P10, P17, or P30 restored production of the full-length protein and partially restored hearing in deaf $Otof^{-/-}$ mice [103].

More recently, Rankovic et al. [105] used a new gene therapeutic method of overloaded AAVs for packaging the full-length *Otof*. Indeed, they packaged the full-length *Otof* into several naturally occurring as well as more recently developed and highly potent synthetic AAV serotypes. Using a p5-7 postnatal AAV injection through the round-window membrane, they tested the efficiency of these overloaded AAVs to induce the expression of functional otoferlin in IHCs of the mouse cochlear explants in cultures as well as in vivo adult mice. They achieved specific expression of otoferlin ≈30% of all IHCs and partial restoration of hearing in $Otof^{-/-}$ mutant mice. These results indicate the feasibility of using the AAV vector to package large genes such as *Otof* to restore hearing function (Table 1, Figure 3).

3.1.2. DFNA25

Mutations in the *SLC17A8* gene coding VGLUT3 cause autosomal dominant deafness linked to auditory synaptopathy. Null mice, with a targeted deletion of exon 2 of the *Slc17a8* gene, displayed an absence of acoustic-stimuli-induced ABRs, while ABRs induced by electrical stimuli were preserved, together with intact OAEs [33,34]. A successful restoration of hearing was demonstrated in this *Slc17a8*-null mouse model by reinstating the expression of Vglut3 via postnatal AAV-mediated delivery, illustrated by the restoration of synaptic transmission and hearing [36]. A recent study showed that AAV8 expressing Vglut3 in the cochleae of 5-, 8-, and 20-week-old Vglut3-null mice resulted in exogenous expression of Vglut3 in all IHCs and successful restoration of hearing for at least 12 weeks via canalostomic injection of AAV-*Vglut3* [106] (Table 1).

DFNA25 patients harboring mutations in the *SLC17A8* gene [33,38,39] exhibited progressive sensorineural hearing loss at high frequencies, and this also was characterized as synaptopathy [33,39]. Thus far, however, AAV-mediated gene transfer to correct mutated sequences and to rescue hearing in DFNA25 rodent models has not been attempted.

3.1.3. DFNB93

Human pathological mutations in the *CABP2* gene have been shown to cause moderate-to-severe, non-syndromic autosomal recessive hearing impairment DFNB93 characterized as auditory synaptopathy [48–50,52]. A recent interesting study showed the efficiency of round-window membrane injection of AAV2/1- and AAV-PHP.eB-mediated expression of *CABP2* in IHCs of P5-7 postnatal $Cabp^{-/-}$ mice in restoring IHC Cav1.3 function and improved hearing of $Cabp^{-/-}$ mice [51] (Table 1, Figure 3).

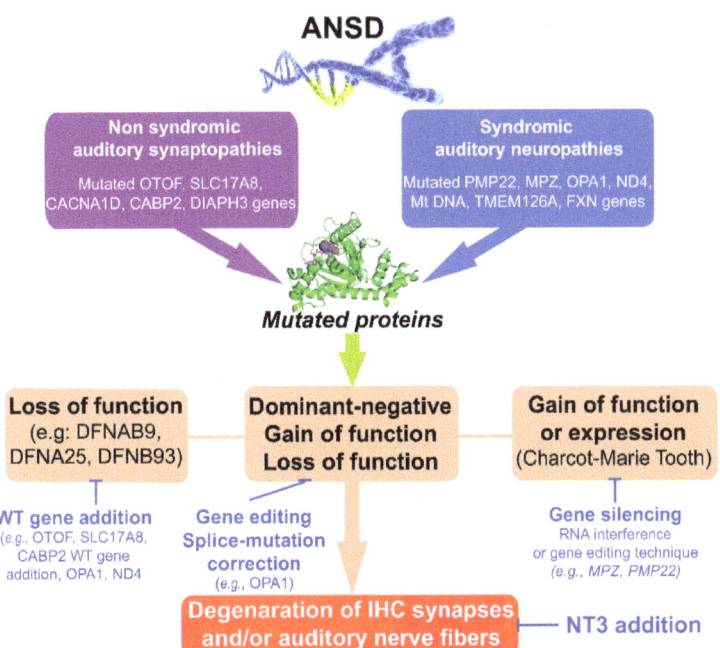

Figure 3. Summary diagram of the design gene therapies discussed in this review. Genetic syndromic auditory neuropathy affects multiple nerves, while non-syndromic auditory synaptopathy is limited to IHC ribbon synapses. These auditory phenotypes may result from loss of function, dominant negative effects, or gain-of-function expression mechanisms. Hearing rescue strategies may be designed to target the different levels of disease mechanisms, i.e., (i) WT gene addition to rescue loss function phenotype; (ii) gene or mRNA editing to correct dominant-negative, gain-of-function, or loss of function mutations; (iii) gene silencing to correct gain-of-function or expression; and (iv) NT3 gene or protein addition to enhance the repair and/or regeneration of auditory synapses and nerve fibers. The mutated protein shown here is the OPA1 protein involved in dominant optic atrophy (DOA).

3.2. Hearing Restoration in Syndromic Auditory Neuropathy

3.2.1. Charcot–Marie–Tooth

Charcot-Marie-Tooth (CMT) type 1A (demyelinating neuropathies) is caused by a *PMP22* gene duplication. The 1.4 Mb tandem intra-chromosomal duplication on chromosome 17p11.2-p12 produces three gene copies, each translated into PMP22 protein [61,107–109]. Gene-therapeutic approaches to treat CMT1A have been designed to reduce *PMP22* overexpression at the DNA or mRNA level. For this purpose, an *RNA-interference (RNAi)* [110] AAV2/9 vector expressing murine *PMP22*-targeting shRNA [111] and miR-318-downregulated *PMP22* mRNA [112] have been tested in mouse and rat CMT1A models. These therapeutic approaches normalized MPZ and PMP22 protein levels and improved myelination, function, locomotor activity, and electrophysiological parameters [111–114]. Furthermore, subcutaneous administration of *PMP22*-targeting antisense in a *CMT1A* rat also reduced the mRNA levels of *Pmp22* and improved functional and morphological abnormalities of CMT1A rodent models in a dose-depended manner [115]. However, as for the RNAi technique, antisense therapy requires repeated dosing. CRISPR/Cas9-mediated deletion of the TATA-box promoter of the *PMP22* gene in mice using non-viral intraneural injections also downregulated *Pmp22* mRNA and improved nerve pathology [116]. However, off-target effects of gene editing approaches remain a concern, and mRNA editing techniques such as spliceosome-mediated RNA trans-splicing may be an alternative approach [117].

Finally, supplementation of neurotrophin-3 (NT-3), a neurotrophic factor crucial for Schwann-cell autocrine survival and regeneration, has been proposed to treat CMT1A [118].

Subcutaneous administration of the NT-3 peptide in nude mice harboring CMT1A xenografts, Trembler^J mice with a peripheral myelin protein 22-point mutation, and CMT1A patients resulted in improved axonal regeneration in animal models for CMT1A and provided beneficial effects in patients [119]. Subsequently, the same lab showed that injection of AAV1 packaged *NT-3* cDNA into muscle can act as a secretory organ for widespread distribution of *NT-3* in Trembler^J mice with demyelinating CMT. This therapeutic approach raised measurable NT-3 secretion levels in blood sufficiently to provide an improvement in motor function, histopathology, and electrophysiology of peripheral nerves of *AAV1-NT-3* cDNA-treated Trembler^J mice [120]. These studies of the intramuscular delivery of rAAV1 NT-3 may serve as a template for other nerve diseases involving impaired nerve regeneration. Currently, AAV1 carrying the human NT-3 cDNA scAAV1.tMCK.NTF3 is in a phase I/IIa clinical trial (NCT03520751) using bilateral intramuscular injections in CMT1A patients (Table 1, Figure 3).

Despite the promise of gene therapeutic tools designed to treat CMT1A, their effects on hearing have not yet been assessed.

3.2.2. Autosomal-Dominant Optic Atrophy

It is well known that haploinsufficiency is responsible for isolated DOA, whereas dominant-negative or deleterious gain-of-function types might be responsible for DOA*plus* [121]. Thus, increasing OPA1 expression represents a promising therapeutic approach to treat OPA1-associated diseases. One of these gene therapy approaches is to increase *OPA1 gene* expression at the DNA level. To do so, Sarzi et al. [122] explored the possibility of restoring visual function by intravitreal injections of an AAV2 carrying the human variant #1 OPA1 cDNA, which gives rise to both the long and short OPA1 isoforms. Their results showed that AAV2-mediated WT *OPA1* supplementation therapy might be sufficient to prevent retinal ganglion cell degeneration, although without rescuing visual function [122]. Recently, Jüschke et al. [123] identified a novel OPA1 mutation, c.1065+5G>A, in patients with DOA. This mutation leads to the skipping of OPA1 exon 10 and reducing the OPA1 protein expression by ≈50%. Proper OPA1 function depends, however, on the fine balance of different L- and S-OPA1 isoforms. These authors proposed a promising strategy to convert misspliced OPA1 transcripts into correctly spliced OPA1 transcripts and thus increase the fraction of functional OPA1 transcripts without changing the processing of isoforms. To this end, they engineered U1 splice factors retargeted to different locations in OPA1 exon 10 or intron 10. They showed that application of U1 designed to bind to intron 10 at position +18 led to significant silencing of the effect of the mutation (skipping of exon 10) and increased the expression level of normal transcripts in DOA-patient-derived fibroblasts [123]. This study provides a proof-of-concept for the feasibility of splice-mutation correction as a treatment option for DOA.

Another potential genetic therapeutic option for DOA could be CRISPR–Cas9 gene editing. Using this technique, Sladen et al. [124] successfully achieved correction of an OPA1 c.1334G>A: p.R445H mutant in 57% of isolated DOA-patient-derived pluripotent stem cells (iPSCs). Correction of OPA1 led to restoration of mitochondrial homeostasis, network and basal respiration and ATP production, and reduced susceptibility to apoptotic stimuli in patients' iPSCs (Table 1, Figure 3).

Altogether, these promising studies pave the way for exploring gene therapy for auditory functional changes in mouse models carrying human *OPA1* mutations.

3.2.3. Leber Hereditary Optic Neuropathy (LHON)

Gene therapies have been designed to treat LHON, consistent with compensation of the mitochondrial complex 1 defect. This approach is based on delivering a functional WT gene ND4 to the nucleus of retinal ganglion cells and then importing it into the mitochondria by adding a mitochondrial targeting sequence to restore respiratory chain activity [125,126]. This strategy has been tested in several rodent LHON models via AAV-mediated intravitreal gene delivery. The different teams showed that intravitreal injection was safe and presented no ocular complications related to the treatment itself. They also showed mitochondrial internalization of AAV, together with the expression of its genetic content and the complementation of the pathogenic phenotype [127–133] (Table 1, Figure 3).

Table 1. Gene therapies for genetic synaptopathies and neuropathies that have been discussed in this review.

Diseases	Defective Genes	Therapeutic Strategies	Benefic Effects	Clinical Trials
DFNB9	OTOF	AAV-synaptotagmin 1 [100]	Embryonic inner ear and organotypic culture: Failed to rescue Ca^{2+}-influx-triggered exocytosis	DB-OTO phase 1/2 clinical trial in pediatric patients
		Dual AAV-*Otof* [103]	P10-RWM injection Total and sustained rescue ABR threshold shifts Amplitude wave I: 39% of the WT (P10injection), 50% of the WT (P17 injection) Ribbon number twice higher> non treated, but <WT	
		Single overloaded AAV-*Otof* [105]	P5-7 RWM injection: Expression of otoferlin in 30% of IHCs Partial restoration of hearing Poor preservation of wave I	
DFNA25	SLC17A8	AAV1- *Slc17a8* [36]	P1-P2 RW injection: 100% recovery ABR thresholds 40% sustained ABR recovery	
		AAV8- *Slc17a8* [106]	5 w, 8 w, and 20 w canalostomic injection: 5 w injection: restore Vglut3 expression and hearing Partially restore the number of synapses 8 w injection: partial rescue of hearing 20 w injection: rescue less than 50% of ABR threshold	
DFNB93	CABP2	AAV2/1 and PHP.eB-*CABP2* [51]	P5-7 RW injection: Improve at least 20dB in all frequencies in 67% of the injected mice	
CMT	MPZ PMP22	*RNA-interference* (RNAi) [110] AAV2/9 -*Pmp22* shRNA [111] miR-318 [112] CRISPR/Cas9 [116] PMP22 antisense [115]	Intraneural injections: Normalize MPZ and PMP22 protein levels Improve myelination, function, locomotor activity, and electrophysiological parameters Subcutaneous injection: Reduce the mRNA levels of *Pmp22*, improve functional and morphological abnormalities of CMT1A	phase I/IIa clinical trial (NCT03520751)
		NT-3 supplementation [119]	Subcutaneous injection: Improve axonal regeneration	
		AAV1-*NT-3* cDNA [120]	Intramuscular injection: Improve motor function, histopathology, and electrophysiology of peripheral nerves	
DAO	OPA	AAV2-*OPA1* [122].	Intravitreal gene delivery Reduce retinal ganglion cell degeneration without rescuing an efficient visual acuity	
		U1 splice factors [123] (bind to intron 10 at position +18 of OPA1)	In vitro: patient-derived and control fibroblasts Silence the effect of the mutation, increase the expression level of normal transcripts	
		CRISPR/Cas9–iPSCs (c.1334G>A: p.R445H) [124]	In vitro: Restore mitochondrial homeostasis, re-establish the mitochondrial network, basal respiration, and ATP production levels	
LHON	Mt DNA TMEM126A	rAAV5-NDI1 [128]	Stereotaxic injections: infusion into the optical layer of the SC Rescue vision loss induced by complex I deficiency	Phase 1 clinical trial of scAAV2-P1ND4v2 of ND4-LHON (NCT02161380)
		AAV2-NDI1 [131]	Intravitreal gene delivery: Mitochondrial internalization of AAVV Reduce RGC death and optic nerve atrophy Preserve retinal function (manganese, Mn2 þ)-enhanced magnetic resonance imaging (MEMRI) and optokinetic responses	
		AAV2-ND4 [125,127,129,133]	Restore the activity of the respiratory chain and rescuing retinal ganglion cell degeneration	Phase 3 pivotal clinical study of rAAV2/2-ND4: REFLECT (NCT03293524)

Abbreviation used in the table: RWM: round window membrane. w: weeks.

4. Conclusions

This review of the literature described pathogenic mechanisms mediating genetic ANSD, as well as genetic therapies that are currently in development. The discovery of the gene responsible for ANSD ushered in a new and exciting time for drug discovery and therapeutic genetic modulation. New discoveries are continuing to drive innovation in the development of innovative treatments for both non-syndromic and syndromic ANSD. In recent years, substantial progress has been made in developing gene therapeutic tools to regenerate auditory synapses and neurons, or to replace defective genes through gene therapies. Nevertheless, regardless of advances in capabilities for gene delivery, the complex nature of regeneration and repair processes and the wide range of molecular and cellular targets underscore the need for precisely controlled systems capable of delivering a wide range of biomaterials such as genes, siRNAs, RNAs, and DNAs.

One exciting approach relies on the use of genome-editing technologies based on programmable nucleases, including CRISPR–Cas9 [134]. These new technologies allow us to remove or correct deleterious mutations or insert protective mutations in diseased cells and tissues. The injection of CRISPR–Cas9 complexes into the ears of neonatal Beethoven mutant mice improved auditory function [135], thus providing a potential therapeutic option for deaf patients carrying monogenic mutations. CRISPR/Cas9-mediated deletion of the TATA-box promoter of the *PMP22* gene in a Charcot–Marie–Tooth mouse model using non-viral intraneural injections also downregulated *PMP22*mRNA and improved nerve pathology [116]. However, off-target effects of gene editing approaches remain a concern.

An alternative approach to correcting gene mutations is using spliceosome-mediated RNA *trans*-splicing, or SMaRT. This technique targets the mRNA sequence to correct the mutations. The proof-of-concept of SMaRT has already been established in several models of genetic diseases caused by recessive mutations [117]. This innovative technology has not yet been investigated in the inner ear but offers hope of a single treatment for restoring hearing in patients carrying recessive gene mutations.

The bench-to-bedside transition for AAV-mediated gene therapy took its first steps in 2008, when the efficacy of gene therapy was demonstrated to treat Leber congenital amaurosis. Three successful clinical trials were completed regarding the safety of subretinal injection of 65 kDa retinal pigment epithelium-specific protein (RPE65) expressed by an AAV vector for Leber congenital amaurosis [136–139]. Published studies of clinical trials of genes designed to compensate for the mitochondrial complex 1 defect with the functional wild-type gene with intravitreal injection of AAV2-ND4 in ND4-LHON patients reported clinically meaningful beneficial effects beyond the expected natural history of the disease [125]. AAV2-ND4 successfully restored the activity of the respiratory chain and rescued retinal ganglion cell degeneration [125].

These trials have paved the way for the first FDA-approved gene therapy products to treat ANSD. DB-OTO, a lead gene therapy product candidate directed by Decibel Therapeutics company to treat otoferlin mutation-induced DFNB9, has received clearance from the U.S. FDA to initiate a phase 1/2 clinical trial in pediatric patients [140]. OTOF-GT, a lead gene therapy candidate developed by Sensorion biotech, has also been granted rare pediatric disease designation from the U.S. FDA [141] for treating pediatric DFNB9 patients. To date, there have been multiple clinical trials studying AAV-mediated gene therapy in optic neuropathies. However, there have been no trials involving auditory neuropathies, although the gene therapy of monogenic disease using AAV has become feasible. The discrepancy between the progress of optic and auditory neuropathy gene therapies has mostly been attributed to the earlier preclinical success and the increased accessibility for treatments of the eye relative to the cochlea. In addition, heterogeneity is the major challenge in the treatment of genetic ANSD, as several factors affect treatment efficacy, such as therapeutic window, targets, targeting molecules, and protein function.

Future therapies to restore synaptic transmission or to regenerate auditory nerve fibers must consider multiple targets that account for the complexity of disease-causing factors and pathogenetic mechanisms. Looking back on the historical, functional, and molecular achievements made in this field, each were made possible by technological developments defining a new epoch. In order to overcome the somewhat static current status in terms of clinical trials, we now need to refine the protocol of these trials and search for more predictive animal models of deafness on which they are based. Additionally, there is also a need to develop more reliable clinical diagnostic tools for early identification of ANSD, as well as to carefully evaluate the degree of degeneration of auditory synapses and nerve fibers. Clinical trials of biologic agents to treat ANSD need valid clinical outcome measures and biomarkers.

Author Contributions: Conceptualization, J.W. and J.R.; Investigation, A.R.S.; Resources, B.C. and F.V.; Writing—original draft preparation, J.W.; Review and editing, J.W., J.R., A.R.S. and A.B.; funding acquisition, J.W. and F.V. All authors have read and agreed to the published version of the manuscript.

Funding: This work was supported by the Fondation Recherche Médicale (REP202110014234) and Fondation Gueules Cassées (65-2022). F.V. is a winner of the Early Career Research Award of Fondation pour l'Audition.

Institutional Review Board Statement: Not applicable.

Informed Consent Statement: Not applicable.

Data Availability Statement: All data analysed during this study are included in this published article.

Acknowledgments: The author would like to thank Joseph Vecchi for his editing work.

Conflicts of Interest: The authors declare no conflict of interest.

References

1. Starr, A.; Picton, T.W.; Sininger, Y.; Hood, L.J.; Berlin, C.I. Auditory Neuropathy. *Brain* **1996**, *119*, 741–753. [CrossRef] [PubMed]
2. Starr, A.; Michalewski, H.J.; Zeng, F.-G.; Fujikawa-Brooks, S.; Linthicum, F.; Kim, C.S.; Winnier, D.; Keats, B. Pathology and Physiology of Auditory Neuropathy with a Novel Mutation in the MPZ Gene (Tyr145->Ser). *Brain* **2003**, *126*, 1604–1619. [CrossRef] [PubMed]
3. Amatuzzi, M.G.; Northrop, C.; Liberman, M.C.; Thornton, A.; Halpin, C.; Herrmann, B.; Pinto, L.E.; Saenz, A.; Carranza, A.; Eavey, R.D. Selective Inner Hair Cell Loss in Premature Infants and Cochlea Pathological Patterns from Neonatal Intensive Care Unit Autopsies. *Arch. Otolaryngol.-Head Neck Surg.* **2001**, *127*, 629–636. [CrossRef] [PubMed]
4. Blegvad, B.; Hvidegaard, T. Hereditary Dysfunction of the Brain Stem Auditory Pathways as the Major Cause of Speech Retardation. *Scand. Audiol.* **1983**, *12*, 179–187. [CrossRef] [PubMed]
5. Moser, T.; Starr, A. Auditory Neuropathy—Neural and Synaptic Mechanisms. *Nat. Rev. Neurol.* **2016**, *12*, 135–149. [CrossRef] [PubMed]
6. Iliadou, V.V.; Ptok, M.; Grech, H.; Pedersen, E.R.; Brechmann, A.A.; Deggouj, N.N.; Kiese-Himmel, C.; Sliwinska-Kowalska, M.; Nickisch, A.; Demanez, L.; et al. A European Perspective on Auditory Processing Disorder-Current Knowledge and Future Research Focus. *Front. Neurol.* **2017**, *8*, 622. [CrossRef]
7. Starr, A.; McPherson, D.; Patterson, J.; Don, M.; Luxford, W.; Shannon, R.; Sininger, Y.; Tonakawa, L.; Waring, M. Absence of Both Auditory Evoked Potentials and Auditory Percepts Dependent on Timing Cues. *Brain* **1991**, *114*, 1157–1180. [CrossRef]
8. Starr, A.; Sininger, Y.; Nguyen, T.; Michalewski, H.J.; Oba, S.; Abdala, C. Cochlear Receptor (Microphonic and Summating Potentials, Otoacoustic Emissions) and Auditory Pathway (Auditory Brain Stem Potentials) Activity in Auditory Neuropathy. *Ear Hear.* **2001**, *22*, 91–99. [CrossRef]
9. Wynne, D.P.; Zeng, F.-G.; Bhatt, S.; Michalewski, H.J.; Dimitrijevic, A.; Starr, A. Loudness Adaptation Accompanying Ribbon Synapse and Auditory Nerve Disorders. *Brain* **2013**, *136 Pt 5*, 1626–1638. [CrossRef]
10. Zeng, F.G.; Shannon, R.V. Loudness-Coding Mechanisms Inferred from Electric Stimulation of the Human Auditory System. *Science* **1994**, *264*, 564–566. [CrossRef]
11. Zeng, F.-G. An Active Loudness Model Suggesting Tinnitus as Increased Central Noise and Hyperacusis as Increased Nonlinear Gain. *Hear. Res.* **2013**, *295*, 172–179. [CrossRef] [PubMed]
12. De Siati, R.D.; Rosenzweig, F.; Gersdorff, G.; Gregoire, A.; Rombaux, P.; Deggouj, N. Auditory Neuropathy Spectrum Disorders: From Diagnosis to Treatment: Literature Review and Case Reports. *JCM* **2020**, *9*, 1074. [CrossRef] [PubMed]
13. Pelosi, S.; Wanna, G.; Hayes, C.; Sunderhaus, L.; Haynes, D.S.; Bennett, M.L.; Labadie, R.F.; Rivas, A. Cochlear Implantation versus Hearing Amplification in Patients with Auditory Neuropathy Spectrum Disorder. *Otolaryngol.-Head Neck Surg.* **2013**, *148*, 815–821. [CrossRef] [PubMed]

14. Walker, E.; McCreery, R.; Spratford, M.; Roush, P. Children with Auditory Neuropathy Spectrum Disorder Fitted with Hearing Aids Applying the American Academy of Audiology Pediatric Amplification Guideline: Current Practice and Outcomes. *J. Am. Acad. Audiol.* **2016**, *27*, 204–218. [CrossRef] [PubMed]
15. Humphriss, R.; Hall, A.; Maddocks, J.; Macleod, J.; Sawaya, K.; Midgley, E. Does Cochlear Implantation Improve Speech Recognition in Children with Auditory Neuropathy Spectrum Disorder? A Systematic Review. *Int. J. Audiol.* **2013**, *52*, 442–454. [CrossRef] [PubMed]
16. Ching, T.Y.C.; Day, J.; Dillon, H.; Gardner-Berry, K.; Hou, S.; Seeto, M.; Wong, A.; Zhang, V. Impact of the Presence of Auditory Neuropathy Spectrum Disorder (ANSD) on Outcomes of Children at Three Years of Age. *Int. J. Audiol.* **2013**, *52* (Suppl. S2), S55–S64. [CrossRef] [PubMed]
17. Santarelli, R.; Rossi, R.; Scimemi, P.; Cama, E.; Valentino, M.L.; La Morgia, C.; Caporali, L.; Liguori, R.; Magnavita, V.; Monteleone, A.; et al. OPA1-Related Auditory Neuropathy: Site of Lesion and Outcome of Cochlear Implantation. *Brain* **2015**, *138*, 563–576. [CrossRef] [PubMed]
18. Roush, P.; Frymark, T.; Venediktov, R.; Wang, B. Audiologic Management of Auditory Neuropathy Spectrum Disorder in Children: A Systematic Review of the Literature. *Am. J. Audiol.* **2011**, *20*, 159–170. [CrossRef]
19. Johnson, C.P.; Chapman, E.R. Otoferlin Is a Calcium Sensor That Directly Regulates SNARE-Mediated Membrane Fusion. *J. Cell Biol.* **2010**, *191*, 187–197. [CrossRef]
20. Michalski, N.; Goutman, J.D.; Auclair, S.M.; Boutet de Monvel, J.; Tertrais, M.; Emptoz, A.; Parrin, A.; Nouaille, S.; Guillon, M.; Sachse, M.; et al. Otoferlin Acts as a Ca^{2+} Sensor for Vesicle Fusion and Vesicle Pool Replenishment at Auditory Hair Cell Ribbon Synapses. *Elife* **2017**, *6*, e31013. [CrossRef]
21. Pangršič, T.; Reisinger, E.; Moser, T. Otoferlin: A Multi-C2 Domain Protein Essential for Hearing. *Trends Neurosci.* **2012**, *35*, 671–680. [CrossRef] [PubMed]
22. Yasunaga, S.; Grati, M.; Cohen-Salmon, M.; El-Amraoui, A.; Mustapha, M.; Salem, N.; El-Zir, E.; Loiselet, J.; Petit, C. A Mutation in OTOF, Encoding Otoferlin, a FER-1-like Protein, Causes DFNB9, a Nonsyndromic Form of Deafness. *Nat. Genet.* **1999**, *21*, 363–369. [CrossRef] [PubMed]
23. Vona, B.; Doll, J.; Hofrichter, M.A.H.; Haaf, T.; Varshney, G.K. Small Fish, Big Prospects: Using Zebrafish to Unravel the Mechanisms of Hereditary Hearing Loss. *Hear. Res.* **2020**, *397*, 107906. [CrossRef] [PubMed]
24. Santarelli, R.; del Castillo, I.; Cama, E.; Scimemi, P.; Starr, A. Audibility, Speech Perception and Processing of Temporal Cues in Ribbon Synaptic Disorders Due to OTOF Mutations. *Hear. Res.* **2015**, *330*, 200–212. [CrossRef] [PubMed]
25. Choi, B.Y.; Ahmed, Z.M.; Riazuddin, S.; Bhinder, M.A.; Shahzad, M.; Husnain, T.; Riazuddin, S.; Griffith, A.J.; Friedman, T.B. Identities and Frequencies of Mutations of the Otoferlin Gene (OTOF) Causing DFNB9 Deafness in Pakistan. *Clin. Genet.* **2009**, *75*, 237–243. [CrossRef] [PubMed]
26. Rodríguez-Ballesteros, M.; Reynoso, R.; Olarte, M.; Villamar, M.; Morera, C.; Santarelli, R.; Arslan, E.; Medá, C.; Curet, C.; Völter, C.; et al. A Multicenter Study on the Prevalence and Spectrum of Mutations in the Otoferlin Gene (OTOF) in Subjects with Nonsyndromic Hearing Impairment and Auditory Neuropathy. *Hum. Mutat.* **2008**, *29*, 823–831. [CrossRef]
27. Varga, R.; Avenarius, M.R.; Kelley, P.M.; Keats, B.J.; Berlin, C.I.; Hood, L.J.; Morlet, T.G.; Brashears, S.M.; Starr, A.; Cohn, E.S.; et al. OTOF Mutations Revealed by Genetic Analysis of Hearing Loss Families Including a Potential Temperature Sensitive Auditory Neuropathy Allele. *J. Med. Genet.* **2006**, *43*, 576–581. [CrossRef]
28. Santarelli, R.; Scimemi, P.; La Morgia, C.; Cama, E.; Del Castillo, I.; Carelli, V. Electrocochleography in Auditory Neuropathy Related to Mutations in the OTOF or OPA1 Gene. *Audiol. Res.* **2021**, *11*, 639–652. [CrossRef]
29. Pangrsic, T.; Lasarow, L.; Reuter, K.; Takago, H.; Schwander, M.; Riedel, D.; Frank, T.; Tarantino, L.M.; Bailey, J.S.; Strenzke, N.; et al. Hearing Requires Otoferlin-Dependent Efficient Replenishment of Synaptic Vesicles in Hair Cells. *Nat. Neurosci.* **2010**, *13*, 869–876. [CrossRef]
30. Roux, I.; Safieddine, S.; Nouvian, R.; Grati, M.; Simmler, M.-C.; Bahloul, A.; Perfettini, I.; Le Gall, M.; Rostaing, P.; Hamard, G.; et al. Otoferlin, Defective in a Human Deafness Form, Is Essential for Exocytosis at the Auditory Ribbon Synapse. *Cell* **2006**, *127*, 277–289. [CrossRef]
31. El Mestikawy, S.; Wallén-Mackenzie, A.; Fortin, G.M.; Descarries, L.; Trudeau, L.-E. From Glutamate Co-Release to Vesicular Synergy: Vesicular Glutamate Transporters. *Nat. Rev. Neurosci.* **2011**, *12*, 204–216. [CrossRef] [PubMed]
32. Zhang, G.; Li, X.; Cao, H.; Zhao, H.; Geller, A.I. The Vesicular Glutamate Transporter-1 Upstream Promoter and First Intron Each Support Glutamatergic-Specific Expression in Rat Postrhinal Cortex. *Brain Res.* **2011**, *1377*, 1–12. [CrossRef] [PubMed]
33. Ruel, J.; Emery, S.; Nouvian, R.; Bersot, T.; Amilhon, B.; Van Rybroek, J.M.; Rebillard, G.; Lenoir, M.; Eybalin, M.; Delprat, B.; et al. Impairment of SLC17A8 Encoding Vesicular Glutamate Transporter-3, VGLUT3, Underlies Nonsyndromic Deafness DFNA25 and Inner Hair Cell Dysfunction in Null Mice. *Am. J. Hum. Genet.* **2008**, *83*, 278–292. [CrossRef] [PubMed]
34. Seal, R.P.; Akil, O.; Yi, E.; Weber, C.M.; Grant, L.; Yoo, J.; Clause, A.; Kandler, K.; Noebels, J.L.; Glowatzki, E.; et al. Sensorineural Deafness and Seizures in Mice Lacking Vesicular Glutamate Transporter 3. *Neuron* **2008**, *57*, 263–275. [CrossRef]
35. Weisz, C.J.C.; Williams, S.-P.G.; Eckard, C.S.; Divito, C.B.; Ferreira, D.W.; Fantetti, K.N.; Dettwyler, S.A.; Cai, H.-M.; Rubio, M.E.; Kandler, K.; et al. Outer Hair Cell Glutamate Signaling through Type II Spiral Ganglion Afferents Activates Neurons in the Cochlear Nucleus in Response to Nondamaging Sounds. *J. Neurosci.* **2021**, *41*, 2930–2943. [CrossRef]
36. Akil, O.; Seal, R.P.; Burke, K.; Wang, C.; Alemi, A.; During, M.; Edwards, R.H.; Lustig, L.R. Restoration of Hearing in the VGLUT3 Knockout Mouse Using Virally Mediated Gene Therapy. *Neuron* **2012**, *75*, 283–293. [CrossRef]

37. Kim, K.X.; Payne, S.; Yang-Hood, A.; Li, S.-Z.; Davis, B.; Carlquist, J.; V.-Ghaffari, B.; Gantz, J.A.; Kallogjeri, D.; Fitzpatrick, J.A.J.; et al. Vesicular Glutamatergic Transmission in Noise-Induced Loss and Repair of Cochlear Ribbon Synapses. *J. Neurosci.* **2019**, *39*, 4434–4447. [CrossRef]
38. Petek, E.; Windpassinger, C.; Mach, M.; Rauter, L.; Scherer, S.W.; Wagner, K.; Kroisel, P.M. Molecular Characterization of a 12q22-Q24 Deletion Associated with Congenital Deafness: Confirmation and Refinement of the DFNA25 Locus. *Am. J. Med. Genet. Part A* **2003**, *117*, 122–126. [CrossRef]
39. Ryu, N.; Sagong, B.; Park, H.-J.; Kim, M.-A.; Lee, K.-Y.; Choi, J.Y.; Kim, U.-K. Screening of the SLC17A8 Gene as a Causative Factor for Autosomal Dominant Non-Syndromic Hearing Loss in Koreans. *BMC Med. Genet.* **2016**, *17*, 6. [CrossRef]
40. Joshi, Y.; Petit, C.P.; Miot, S.; Guillet, M.; Sendin, G.; Bourien, J.; Wang, J.; Pujol, R.; El Mestikawy, S.; Puel, J.-L.; et al. VGLUT3-p.A211V Variant Fuses Stereocilia Bundles and Elongates Synaptic Ribbons. *J. Physiol.* **2021**, *599*, 5397–5416. [CrossRef]
41. Brandt, A.; Striessnig, J.; Moser, T. CaV1.3 Channels Are Essential for Development and Presynaptic Activity of Cochlear Inner Hair Cells. *J. Neurosci.* **2003**, *23*, 10832–10840. [CrossRef] [PubMed]
42. Baig, S.M.; Koschak, A.; Lieb, A.; Gebhart, M.; Dafinger, C.; Nürnberg, G.; Ali, A.; Ahmad, I.; Sinnegger-Brauns, M.J.; Brandt, N.; et al. Loss of Ca(v)1.3 (*CACNA1D*) Function in a Human Channelopathy with Bradycardia and Congenital Deafness. *Nat. Neurosci.* **2011**, *14*, 77–84. [CrossRef] [PubMed]
43. Platzer, J.; Engel, J.; Schrott-Fischer, A.; Stephan, K.; Bova, S.; Chen, H.; Zheng, H.; Striessnig, J. Congenital Deafness and Sinoatrial Node Dysfunction in Mice Lacking Class D L-Type Ca^{2+} Channels. *Cell* **2000**, *102*, 89–97. [CrossRef] [PubMed]
44. Qi, F.; Zhang, R.; Chen, J.; Zhao, F.; Sun, Y.; Du, Z.; Bing, D.; Li, P.; Shao, S.; Zhu, H.; et al. Down-Regulation of Cav1.3 in Auditory Pathway Promotes Age-Related Hearing Loss by Enhancing Calcium-Mediated Oxidative Stress in Male Mice. *Aging* **2019**, *11*, 6490–6502. [CrossRef] [PubMed]
45. Eckrich, S.; Hecker, D.; Sorg, K.; Blum, K.; Fischer, K.; Münkner, S.; Wenzel, G.; Schick, B.; Engel, J. Cochlea-Specific Deletion of Cav1.3 Calcium Channels Arrests Inner Hair Cell Differentiation and Unravels Pitfalls of Conditional Mouse Models. *Front. Cell. Neurosci.* **2019**, *13*, 225. [CrossRef]
46. Haeseleer, F.; Imanishi, Y.; Sokal, I.; Filipek, S.; Palczewski, K. Calcium-Binding Proteins: Intracellular Sensors from the Calmodulin Superfamily. *Biochem. Biophys. Res. Commun.* **2002**, *290*, 615–623. [CrossRef]
47. Christel, C.; Lee, A. Ca^{2+}-Dependent Modulation of Voltage-Gated Ca^{2+} Channels. *Biochim. Biophys. Acta* **2012**, *1820*, 1243–1252. [CrossRef]
48. Tabatabaiefar, M.A.; Alasti, F.; Shariati, L.; Farrokhi, E.; Fransen, E.; Nooridaloii, M.R.; Chaleshtori, M.H.; Van Camp, G. DFNB93, a Novel Locus for Autosomal Recessive Moderate-to-Severe Hearing Impairment. *Clin. Genet.* **2011**, *79*, 594–598. [CrossRef]
49. Schrauwen, I.; Helfmann, S.; Inagaki, A.; Predoehl, F.; Tabatabaiefar, M.A.; Picher, M.M.; Sommen, M.; Zazo Seco, C.; Oostrik, J.; Kremer, H.; et al. A Mutation in CABP2, Expressed in Cochlear Hair Cells, Causes Autosomal-Recessive Hearing Impairment. *Am. J. Hum. Genet.* **2012**, *91*, 636–645. [CrossRef]
50. Bademci, G.; Foster, J.; Mahdieh, N.; Bonyadi, M.; Duman, D.; Cengiz, F.B.; Menendez, I.; Diaz-Horta, O.; Shirkavand, A.; Zeinali, S.; et al. Comprehensive Analysis via Exome Sequencing Uncovers Genetic Etiology in Autosomal Recessive Nonsyndromic Deafness in a Large Multiethnic Cohort. *Genet. Med.* **2016**, *18*, 364–371. [CrossRef]
51. Oestreicher, D.; Picher, M.M.; Rankovic, V.; Moser, T.; Pangrsic, T. Cabp2-Gene Therapy Restores Inner Hair Cell Calcium Currents and Improves Hearing in a DFNB93 Mouse Model. *Front. Mol. Neurosci.* **2021**, *14*, 689415. [CrossRef] [PubMed]
52. Picher, M.M.; Gehrt, A.; Meese, S.; Ivanovic, A.; Predoehl, F.; Jung, S.; Schrauwen, I.; Dragonetti, A.G.; Colombo, R.; Van Camp, G.; et al. Ca^{2+}-Binding Protein 2 Inhibits Ca^{2+}-Channel Inactivation in Mouse Inner Hair Cells. *Proc. Natl. Acad. Sci. USA* **2017**, *114*, E1717–E1726. [CrossRef] [PubMed]
53. Yang, T.; Hu, N.; Pangršič, T.; Green, S.; Hansen, M.; Lee, A. Functions of CaBP1 and CaBP2 in the Peripheral Auditory System. *Hear. Res.* **2018**, *364*, 48–58. [CrossRef] [PubMed]
54. Schoen, C.J.; Burmeister, M.; Lesperance, M.M. Diaphanous Homolog 3 (Diap3) Overexpression Causes Progressive Hearing Loss and Inner Hair Cell Defects in a Transgenic Mouse Model of Human Deafness. *PLoS ONE* **2013**, *8*, e56520. [CrossRef]
55. Rance, G.; Starr, A. Pathophysiological Mechanisms and Functional Hearing Consequences of Auditory Neuropathy. *Brain* **2015**, *138*, 3141–3158. [CrossRef] [PubMed]
56. Surel, C.; Guillet, M.; Lenoir, M.; Bourien, J.; Sendin, G.; Joly, W.; Delprat, B.; Lesperance, M.M.; Puel, J.-L.; Nouvian, R. Remodeling of the Inner Hair Cell Microtubule Meshwork in a Mouse Model of Auditory Neuropathy AUNA1. *eNeuro* **2016**, *3*. [CrossRef]
57. Manchaiah, V.K.C.; Zhao, F.; Danesh, A.A.; Duprey, R. The Genetic Basis of Auditory Neuropathy Spectrum Disorder (ANSD). *Int. J. Pediatr. Otorhinolaryngol.* **2011**, *75*, 151–158. [CrossRef]
58. Rendtorff, N.D.; Lodahl, M.; Boulahbel, H.; Johansen, I.R.; Pandya, A.; Welch, K.O.; Norris, V.W.; Arnos, K.S.; Bitner-Glindzicz, M.; Emery, S.B.; et al. Identification of p.A684V Missense Mutation in the WFS1 Gene as a Frequent Cause of Autosomal Dominant Optic Atrophy and Hearing Impairment. *Am. J. Med. Genet. Part A* **2011**, *155*, 1298–1313. [CrossRef]
59. Morlet, T.; Nagao, K.; Bean, S.C.; Mora, S.E.; Hopkins, S.E.; Hobson, G.M. Auditory Function in Pelizaeus-Merzbacher Disease. *J. Neurol.* **2018**, *265*, 1580–1589. [CrossRef]
60. Han, K.-H.; Oh, D.-Y.; Lee, S.; Lee, C.; Han, J.H.; Kim, M.Y.; Park, H.-R.; Park, M.K.; Kim, N.K.D.; Lee, J.; et al. ATP1A3 Mutations Can Cause Progressive Auditory Neuropathy: A New Gene of Auditory Synaptopathy. *Sci. Rep.* **2017**, *7*, 16504. [CrossRef]

61. Lupski, J.R.; de Oca-Luna, R.M.; Slaugenhaupt, S.; Pentao, L.; Guzzetta, V.; Trask, B.J.; Saucedo-Cardenas, O.; Barker, D.F.; Killian, J.M.; Garcia, C.A.; et al. DNA Duplication Associated with Charcot-Marie-Tooth Disease Type 1A. *Cell* **1991**, *66*, 219–232. [CrossRef] [PubMed]
62. Rance, G.; Ryan, M.M.; Bayliss, K.; Gill, K.; O'Sullivan, C.; Whitechurch, M. Auditory Function in Children with Charcot-Marie-Tooth Disease. *Brain* **2012**, *135*, 1412–1422. [CrossRef] [PubMed]
63. Raglan, E.; Prasher, D.K.; Trinder, E.; Rudge, P. Auditory Function in Hereditary Motor and Sensory Neuropathy (Charcot-Marie-Tooth Disease). *Acta Oto-Laryngol.* **1987**, *103*, 50–55. [CrossRef]
64. Kovach, M.J.; Campbell, K.C.M.; Herman, K.; Waggoner, B.; Gelber, D.; Hughes, L.F.; Kimonis, V.E. Anticipation in a Unique Family with Charcot-Marie-Tooth Syndrome and Deafness: Delineation of the Clinical Features and Review of the Literature. *Am. J. Med. Genet.* **2002**, *108*, 295–303. [CrossRef]
65. Choi, J.E.; Seok, J.M.; Ahn, J.; Ji, Y.S.; Lee, K.M.; Hong, S.H.; Choi, B.-O.; Moon, I.J. Hidden Hearing Loss in Patients with Charcot-Marie-Tooth Disease Type 1A. *Sci. Rep.* **2018**, *8*, 10335. [CrossRef] [PubMed]
66. Johnston, P.B.; Gaster, R.N.; Smith, V.C.; Tripathi, R.C. A Clinicopathologic Study of Autosomal Dominant Optic Atrophy. *Am. J. Ophthalmol.* **1979**, *88*, 868–875. [CrossRef] [PubMed]
67. Alexander, C.; Votruba, M.; Pesch, U.E.; Thiselton, D.L.; Mayer, S.; Moore, A.; Rodriguez, M.; Kellner, U.; Leo-Kottler, B.; Auburger, G.; et al. OPA1, Encoding a Dynamin-Related GTPase, Is Mutated in Autosomal Dominant Optic Atrophy Linked to Chromosome 3q28. *Nat. Genet.* **2000**, *26*, 211–215. [CrossRef] [PubMed]
68. Delettre, C.; Lenaers, G.; Griffoin, J.M.; Gigarel, N.; Lorenzo, C.; Belenguer, P.; Pelloquin, L.; Grosgeorge, J.; Turc-Carel, C.; Perret, E.; et al. Nuclear Gene OPA1, Encoding a Mitochondrial Dynamin-Related Protein, Is Mutated in Dominant Optic Atrophy. *Nat. Genet.* **2000**, *26*, 207–210. [CrossRef]
69. Lenaers, G.; Neutzner, A.; Le Dantec, Y.; Jüschke, C.; Xiao, T.; Decembrini, S.; Swirski, S.; Kieninger, S.; Agca, C.; Kim, U.S.; et al. Dominant Optic Atrophy: Culprit Mitochondria in the Optic Nerve. *Prog. Retin. Eye Res.* **2021**, *83*, 100935. [CrossRef]
70. Amati-Bonneau, P.; Guichet, A.; Olichon, A.; Chevrollier, A.; Viala, F.; Miot, S.; Ayuso, C.; Odent, S.; Arrouet, C.; Verny, C.; et al. OPA1 R445H Mutation in Optic Atrophy Associated with Sensorineural Deafness. *Ann. Neurol.* **2005**, *58*, 958–963. [CrossRef]
71. Lodi, R.; Tonon, C.; Valentino, M.L.; Iotti, S.; Clementi, V.; Malucelli, E.; Barboni, P.; Longanesi, L.; Schimpf, S.; Wissinger, B.; et al. Deficit of in Vivo Mitochondrial ATP Production in OPA1-Related Dominant Optic Atrophy. *Ann. Neurol.* **2004**, *56*, 719–723. [CrossRef] [PubMed]
72. Olichon, A.; Baricault, L.; Gas, N.; Guillou, E.; Valette, A.; Belenguer, P.; Lenaers, G. Loss of OPA1 Perturbates the Mitochondrial Inner Membrane Structure and Integrity, Leading to Cytochrome c Release and Apoptosis. *J. Biol. Chem.* **2003**, *278*, 7743–7746. [CrossRef] [PubMed]
73. Frezza, C.; Cipolat, S.; Martins de Brito, O.; Micaroni, M.; Beznoussenko, G.V.; Rudka, T.; Bartoli, D.; Polishuck, R.S.; Danial, N.N.; De Strooper, B.; et al. OPA1 Controls Apoptotic Cristae Remodeling Independently from Mitochondrial Fusion. *Cell* **2006**, *126*, 177–189. [CrossRef] [PubMed]
74. Amati-Bonneau, P.; Valentino, M.L.; Reynier, P.; Gallardo, M.E.; Bornstein, B.; Boissière, A.; Campos, Y.; Rivera, H.; de la Aleja, J.G.; Carroccia, R.; et al. OPA1 Mutations Induce Mitochondrial DNA Instability and Optic Atrophy "plus" Phenotypes. *Brain* **2008**, *131*, 338–351. [CrossRef]
75. Belenguer, P.; Pellegrini, L. The Dynamin GTPase OPA1: More than Mitochondria? *Biochim. Et Biophys. Acta* **2013**, *1833*, 176–183. [CrossRef]
76. Elachouri, G.; Vidoni, S.; Zanna, C.; Pattyn, A.; Boukhaddaoui, H.; Gaget, K.; Yu-Wai-Man, P.; Gasparre, G.; Sarzi, E.; Delettre, C.; et al. OPA1 Links Human Mitochondrial Genome Maintenance to MtDNA Replication and Distribution. *Genome Res.* **2011**, *21*, 12–20. [CrossRef]
77. Carelli, V.; Ross-Cisneros, F.N.; Sadun, A.A. Mitochondrial Dysfunction as a Cause of Optic Neuropathies. *Prog. Retin. Eye Res.* **2004**, *23*, 53–89. [CrossRef]
78. Baker, M.R.; Fisher, K.M.; Whittaker, R.G.; Griffiths, P.G.; Yu-Wai-Man, P.; Chinnery, P.F. Subclinical Multisystem Neurologic Disease in "Pure" OPA1 Autosomal Dominant Optic Atrophy. *Neurology* **2011**, *77*, 1309–1312. [CrossRef]
79. Yu-Wai-Man, P.; Griffiths, P.G.; Gorman, G.S.; Lourenco, C.M.; Wright, A.F.; Auer-Grumbach, M.; Toscano, A.; Musumeci, O.; Valentino, M.L.; Caporali, L.; et al. Multi-System Neurological Disease Is Common in Patients with OPA1 Mutations. *Brain* **2010**, *133*, 771–786. [CrossRef]
80. Leruez, S.; Milea, D.; Defoort-Dhellemmes, S.; Colin, E.; Crochet, M.; Procaccio, V.; Ferré, M.; Lamblin, J.; Drouin, V.; Vincent-Delorme, C.; et al. Sensorineural Hearing Loss in OPA1-Linked Disorders. *Brain* **2013**, *136*, e236. [CrossRef]
81. Liskova, P.; Ulmanova, O.; Tesina, P.; Melsova, H.; Diblik, P.; Hansikova, H.; Tesarova, M.; Votruba, M. Novel OPA1 Missense Mutation in a Family with Optic Atrophy and Severe Widespread Neurological Disorder. *Acta Ophthalmol.* **2013**, *91*, e225–e231. [CrossRef] [PubMed]
82. Lenaers, G.; Hamel, C.; Delettre, C.; Amati-Bonneau, P.; Procaccio, V.; Bonneau, D.; Reynier, P.; Milea, D. Dominant Optic Atrophy. *Orphanet J. Rare Dis.* **2012**, *7*, 46. [CrossRef] [PubMed]
83. Huang, T.; Santarelli, R.; Starr, A. Mutation of OPA1 Gene Causes Deafness by Affecting Function of Auditory Nerve Terminals. *Brain Res.* **2009**, *1300*, 97–104. [CrossRef]
84. Santarelli, R. Information from Cochlear Potentials and Genetic Mutations Helps Localize the Lesion Site in Auditory Neuropathy. *Genome Med.* **2010**, *2*, 91. [CrossRef] [PubMed]

85. Adams, J.H.; Blackwood, W.; Wilson, J. Further Clinical and Pathological Observations on Leber's Optic Atrophy. *Brain* **1966**, *89*, 15–26. [CrossRef]
86. Ceranić, B.; Luxon, L.M. Progressive Auditory Neuropathy in Patients with Leber's Hereditary Optic Neuropathy. *J. Neurol. Neurosurg. Psychiatry* **2004**, *75*, 626–630. [CrossRef]
87. Meyer, E.; Michaelides, M.; Tee, L.J.; Robson, A.G.; Rahman, F.; Pasha, S.; Luxon, L.M.; Moore, A.T.; Maher, E.R. Nonsense Mutation in TMEM126A Causing Autosomal Recessive Optic Atrophy and Auditory Neuropathy. *Mol. Vis.* **2010**, *16*, 650–664.
88. Dürr, A.; Cossee, M.; Agid, Y.; Campuzano, V.; Mignard, C.; Penet, C.; Mandel, J.L.; Brice, A.; Koenig, M. Clinical and Genetic Abnormalities in Patients with Friedreich's Ataxia. *N. Engl. J. Med.* **1996**, *335*, 1169–1175. [CrossRef]
89. Harding, A.E. Friedreich's Ataxia: A Clinical and Genetic Study of 90 Families with an Analysis of Early Diagnostic Criteria and Intrafamilial Clustering of Clinical Features. *Brain* **1981**, *104*, 589–620. [CrossRef]
90. Lynch, D.R.; Farmer, J.M.; Balcer, L.J.; Wilson, R.B. Friedreich Ataxia: Effects of Genetic Understanding on Clinical Evaluation and Therapy. *Arch. Neurol.* **2002**, *59*, 743–747. [CrossRef]
91. Rance, G.; Barker, E.J. Speech Perception in Children with Auditory Neuropathy/Dyssynchrony Managed with Either Hearing AIDS or Cochlear Implants. *Otol. Neurotol.* **2008**, *29*, 179–182. [CrossRef] [PubMed]
92. Rance, G.; Corben, L.; Barker, E.; Carew, P.; Chisari, D.; Rogers, M.; Dowell, R.; Jamaluddin, S.; Bryson, R.; Delatycki, M.B. Auditory Perception in Individuals with Friedreich's Ataxia. *Audiol. Neurotol.* **2010**, *15*, 229–240. [CrossRef]
93. Jabbari, B.; Schwartz, D.M.; MacNeil, D.M.; Coker, S.B. Early Abnormalities of Brainstem Auditory Evoked Potentials in Friedreich's Ataxia: Evidence of Primary Brainstem Dysfunction. *Neurology* **1983**, *33*, 1071–1074. [CrossRef] [PubMed]
94. Santarelli, R.; Cama, E.; Pegoraro, E.; Scimemi, P. Abnormal Cochlear Potentials in Friedreich's Ataxia Point to Disordered Synchrony of Auditory Nerve Fiber Activity. *Neurodegener. Dis.* **2015**, *15*, 114–120. [CrossRef] [PubMed]
95. Koohi, N.; Thomas-Black, G.; Giunti, P.; Bamiou, D.-E. Auditory Phenotypic Variability in Friedreich's Ataxia Patients. *Cerebellum* **2021**, *20*, 497–508. [CrossRef] [PubMed]
96. Bahmad, F., Jr.; Merchant, S.N.; Nadol, J.B., Jr.; Tranebjærg, L. Otopathology in Mohr-Tranebjærg Syndrome. *Laryngoscope* **2007**, *117*, 1202–1208. [CrossRef]
97. Mulligan, R.C. The Basic Science of Gene Therapy. *Science* **1993**, *260*, 926–932. [CrossRef]
98. Sacheli, R.; Delacroix, L.; Vandenackerveken, P.; Nguyen, L.; Malgrange, B. Gene Transfer in Inner Ear Cells: A Challenging Race. *Gene Ther.* **2013**, *20*, 237–247. [CrossRef]
99. Wang, J.; Puel, J.-L. Toward Cochlear Therapies. *Physiol. Rev.* **2018**, *98*, 2477–2522. [CrossRef]
100. Reisinger, E.; Bresee, C.; Neef, J.; Nair, R.; Reuter, K.; Bulankina, A.; Nouvian, R.; Koch, M.; Bückers, J.; Kastrup, L.; et al. Probing the Functional Equivalence of Otoferlin and Synaptotagmin 1 in Exocytosis. *J. Neurosci.* **2011**, *31*, 4886–4895. [CrossRef]
101. Beurg, M.; Michalski, N.; Safieddine, S.; Bouleau, Y.; Schneggenburger, R.; Chapman, E.R.; Petit, C.; Dulon, D. Control of Exocytosis by Synaptotagmins and Otoferlin in Auditory Hair Cells. *J. Neurosci.* **2010**, *30*, 13281–13290. [CrossRef] [PubMed]
102. Safieddine, S.; Wenthold, R.J. SNARE Complex at the Ribbon Synapses of Cochlear Hair Cells: Analysis of Synaptic Vesicle- and Synaptic Membrane-Associated Proteins. *Eur. J. Neurosci.* **1999**, *11*, 803–812. [CrossRef] [PubMed]
103. Akil, O.; Dyka, F.; Calvet, C.; Emptoz, A.; Lahlou, G.; Nouaille, S.; Boutet de Monvel, J.; Hardelin, J.-P.; Hauswirth, W.W.; Avan, P.; et al. Dual AAV-Mediated Gene Therapy Restores Hearing in a DFNB9 Mouse Model. *Proc. Natl. Acad. Sci. USA* **2019**, *116*, 4496–4501. [CrossRef]
104. Ghosh, A.; Yue, Y.; Duan, D. Efficient Transgene Reconstitution with Hybrid Dual AAV Vectors Carrying the Minimized Bridging Sequences. *Hum. Gene Ther.* **2011**, *22*, 77–83. [CrossRef] [PubMed]
105. Rankovic, V.; Vogl, C.; Dörje, N.M.; Bahader, I.; Duque-Afonso, C.J.; Thirumalai, A.; Weber, T.; Kusch, K.; Strenzke, N.; Moser, T. Overloaded Adeno-Associated Virus as a Novel Gene Therapeutic Tool for Otoferlin-Related Deafness. *Front. Mol. Neurosci.* **2020**, *13*, 600051. [CrossRef]
106. Zhao, X.; Liu, H.; Liu, H.; Cai, R.; Wu, H. Gene Therapy Restores Auditory Functions in an Adult Vglut3 Knockout Mouse Model. *Hum. Gene Ther.* **2022**, *33*, 729–739. [CrossRef]
107. Valentijn, L.J.; Bolhuis, P.A.; Zorn, I.; Hoogendijk, J.E.; van den Bosch, N.; Hensels, G.W.; Stanton, V.P.; Housman, D.E.; Fischbeck, K.H.; Ross, D.A. The Peripheral Myelin Gene PMP-22/GAS-3 Is Duplicated in Charcot-Marie-Tooth Disease Type 1A. *Nat. Genet.* **1992**, *1*, 166–170. [CrossRef]
108. Timmerman, V.; Nelis, E.; Van Hul, W.; Nieuwenhuijsen, B.W.; Chen, K.L.; Wang, S.; Ben Othman, K.; Cullen, B.; Leach, R.J.; Hanemann, C.O. The Peripheral Myelin Protein Gene PMP-22 Is Contained within the Charcot-Marie-Tooth Disease Type 1A Duplication. *Nat. Genet.* **1992**, *1*, 171–175. [CrossRef]
109. Matsunami, N.; Smith, B.; Ballard, L.; Lensch, M.W.; Robertson, M.; Albertsen, H.; Hanemann, C.O.; Müller, H.W.; Bird, T.D.; White, R. Peripheral Myelin Protein-22 Gene Maps in the Duplication in Chromosome 17p11.2 Associated with Charcot-Marie-Tooth 1A. *Nat. Genet.* **1992**, *1*, 176–179. [CrossRef]
110. Lee, J.-S.; Chang, E.H.; Koo, O.J.; Jwa, D.H.; Mo, W.M.; Kwak, G.; Moon, H.W.; Park, H.T.; Hong, Y.B.; Choi, B.-O. Pmp22 Mutant Allele-Specific siRNA Alleviates Demyelinating Neuropathic Phenotype in Vivo. *Neurobiol. Dis.* **2017**, *100*, 99–107. [CrossRef]
111. Gautier, B.; Hajjar, H.; Soares, S.; Berthelot, J.; Deck, M.; Abbou, S.; Campbell, G.; Ceprian, M.; Gonzalez, S.; Fovet, C.-M.; et al. AAV2/9-Mediated Silencing of PMP22 Prevents the Development of Pathological Features in a Rat Model of Charcot-Marie-Tooth Disease 1 A. *Nat. Commun.* **2021**, *12*, 2356. [CrossRef] [PubMed]

112. Lee, J.-S.; Kwak, G.; Kim, H.J.; Park, H.-T.; Choi, B.-O.; Hong, Y.B. MiR-381 Attenuates Peripheral Neuropathic Phenotype Caused by Overexpression of PMP22. *Exp. Neurobiol.* **2019**, *28*, 279–288. [CrossRef] [PubMed]
113. Boutary, S.; Caillaud, M.; El Madani, M.; Vallat, J.-M.; Loisel-Duwattez, J.; Rouyer, A.; Richard, L.; Gracia, C.; Urbinati, G.; Desmaële, D.; et al. Squalenoyl SiRNA PMP22 Nanoparticles Are Effective in Treating Mouse Models of Charcot-Marie-Tooth Disease Type 1 A. *Commun. Biol.* **2021**, *4*, 317. [CrossRef]
114. Serfecz, J.; Bazick, H.; Al Salihi, M.O.; Turner, P.; Fields, C.; Cruz, P.; Renne, R.; Notterpek, L. Downregulation of the Human Peripheral Myelin Protein 22 Gene by MiR-29a in Cellular Models of Charcot-Marie-Tooth Disease. *Gene Ther.* **2019**, *26*, 455–464. [CrossRef]
115. Zhao, H.T.; Damle, S.; Ikeda-Lee, K.; Kuntz, S.; Li, J.; Mohan, A.; Kim, A.; Hung, G.; Scheideler, M.A.; Scherer, S.S.; et al. PMP22 Antisense Oligonucleotides Reverse Charcot-Marie-Tooth Disease Type 1A Features in Rodent Models. *J. Clin. Investig.* **2018**, *128*, 359–368. [CrossRef] [PubMed]
116. Lee, J.-S.; Lee, J.Y.; Song, D.W.; Bae, H.S.; Doo, H.M.; Yu, H.S.; Lee, K.J.; Kim, H.K.; Hwang, H.; Kwak, G.; et al. Targeted PMP22 TATA-Box Editing by CRISPR/Cas9 Reduces Demyelinating Neuropathy of Charcot-Marie-Tooth Disease Type 1A in Mice. *Nucleic Acids Res.* **2020**, *48*, 130–140. [CrossRef]
117. Berger, A.; Maire, S.; Gaillard, M.-C.; Sahel, J.-A.; Hantraye, P.; Bemelmans, A.-P. MRNA Trans-Splicing in Gene Therapy for Genetic Diseases. *Wiley Interdisc. Rev. RNA* **2016**, *7*, 487–498. [CrossRef]
118. Sahenk, Z.; Ozes, B. Gene Therapy to Promote Regeneration in Charcot-Marie-Tooth Disease. *Brain Res.* **2020**, *1727*, 146533. [CrossRef]
119. Sahenk, Z.; Nagaraja, H.N.; McCracken, B.S.; King, W.M.; Freimer, M.L.; Cedarbaum, J.M.; Mendell, J.R. NT-3 Promotes Nerve Regeneration and Sensory Improvement in CMT1A Mouse Models and in Patients. *Neurology* **2005**, *65*, 681–689. [CrossRef]
120. Sahenk, Z.; Galloway, G.; Clark, K.R.; Malik, V.; Rodino-Klapac, L.R.; Kaspar, B.K.; Chen, L.; Braganza, C.; Montgomery, C.; Mendell, J.R. AAV1.NT-3 Gene Therapy for Charcot-Marie-Tooth Neuropathy. *Mol. Ther.* **2014**, *22*, 511–521. [CrossRef]
121. Marchbank, N.J.; Craig, J.E.; Leek, J.P.; Toohey, M.; Churchill, A.J.; Markham, A.F.; Mackey, D.A.; Toomes, C.; Inglehearn, C.F. Deletion of the OPA1 Gene in a Dominant Optic Atrophy Family: Evidence That Haploinsufficiency Is the Cause of Disease. *J. Med. Genet.* **2002**, *39*, e47. [CrossRef] [PubMed]
122. Sarzi, E.; Seveno, M.; Piro-Mégy, C.; Elzière, L.; Quilès, M.; Péquignot, M.; Müller, A.; Hamel, C.P.; Lenaers, G.; Delettre, C. OPA1 Gene Therapy Prevents Retinal Ganglion Cell Loss in a Dominant Optic Atrophy Mouse Model. *Sci. Rep.* **2018**, *8*, 2468. [CrossRef] [PubMed]
123. Jüschke, C.; Klopstock, T.; Catarino, C.B.; Owczarek-Lipska, M.; Wissinger, B.; Neidhardt, J. Autosomal Dominant Optic Atrophy: A Novel Treatment for OPA1 Splice Defects Using U1 SnRNA Adaption. *Mol. Ther. Nucleic Acids* **2021**, *26*, 1186–1197. [CrossRef]
124. Sladen, P.E.; Perdigão, P.R.L.; Salsbury, G.; Novoselova, T.; van der Spuy, J.; Chapple, J.P.; Yu-Wai-Man, P.; Cheetham, M.E. CRISPR-Cas9 Correction of OPA1 c.1334G>A: P.R445H Restores Mitochondrial Homeostasis in Dominant Optic Atrophy Patient-Derived IPSCs. *Mol. Ther. Nucleic Acids* **2021**, *26*, 432–443. [CrossRef]
125. Sahel, J.-A.; Newman, N.J.; Yu-Wai-Man, P.; Vignal-Clermont, C.; Carelli, V.; Biousse, V.; Moster, M.L.; Sergott, R.; Klopstock, T.; Sadun, A.A.; et al. Gene Therapies for the Treatment of Leber Hereditary Optic Neuropathy. *Int. Ophthalmol. Clin.* **2021**, *61*, 195–208. [CrossRef]
126. Hage, R.; Vignal-Clermont, C. Leber Hereditary Optic Neuropathy: Review of Treatment and Management. *Front. Neurol.* **2021**, *12*, 651639. [CrossRef] [PubMed]
127. Ellouze, S.; Augustin, S.; Bouaita, A.; Bonnet, C.; Simonutti, M.; Forster, V.; Picaud, S.; Sahel, J.-A.; Corral-Debrinski, M. Optimized Allotopic Expression of the Human Mitochondrial ND4 Prevents Blindness in a Rat Model of Mitochondrial Dysfunction. *Am. J. Hum. Genet.* **2008**, *83*, 373–387. [CrossRef]
128. Marella, M.; Seo, B.B.; Thomas, B.B.; Matsuno-Yagi, A.; Yagi, T. Successful Amelioration of Mitochondrial Optic Neuropathy Using the Yeast NDI1 Gene in a Rat Animal Model. *PLoS ONE* **2010**, *5*, e11472. [CrossRef]
129. Shi, H.; Gao, J.; Pei, H.; Liu, R.; Hu, W.; Wan, X.; Li, T.; Li, B. Adeno-Associated Virus-Mediated Gene Delivery of the Human ND4 Complex I Subunit in Rabbit Eyes. *Clin. Exp. Ophthalmol.* **2012**, *40*, 888–894. [CrossRef]
130. Yu, H.; Koilkonda, R.D.; Chou, T.-H.; Porciatti, V.; Ozdemir, S.S.; Chiodo, V.; Boye, S.L.; Boye, S.E.; Hauswirth, W.W.; Lewin, A.S.; et al. Gene Delivery to Mitochondria by Targeting Modified Adenoassociated Virus Suppresses Leber's Hereditary Optic Neuropathy in a Mouse Model. *Proc. Natl. Acad. Sci. USA* **2012**, *109*, E1238–E1247. [CrossRef]
131. Chadderton, N.; Palfi, A.; Millington-Ward, S.; Gobbo, O.; Overlack, N.; Carrigan, M.; O'Reilly, M.; Campbell, M.; Ehrhardt, C.; Wolfrum, U.; et al. Intravitreal Delivery of AAV-NDI1 Provides Functional Benefit in a Murine Model of Leber Hereditary Optic Neuropathy. *Eur. J. Hum. Genet.* **2013**, *21*, 62–68. [CrossRef] [PubMed]
132. Koilkonda, R.D.; Yu, H.; Chou, T.-H.; Feuer, W.J.; Ruggeri, M.; Porciatti, V.; Tse, D.; Hauswirth, W.W.; Chiodo, V.; Boye, S.L.; et al. Safety and Effects of the Vector for the Leber Hereditary Optic Neuropathy Gene Therapy Clinical Trial. *JAMA Ophthalmol.* **2014**, *132*, 409–420. [CrossRef] [PubMed]
133. Koilkonda, R.; Yu, H.; Talla, V.; Porciatti, V.; Feuer, W.J.; Hauswirth, W.W.; Chiodo, V.; Erger, K.E.; Boye, S.L.; Lewin, A.S.; et al. LHON Gene Therapy Vector Prevents Visual Loss and Optic Neuropathy Induced by G11778A Mutant Mitochondrial DNA: Biodistribution and Toxicology Profile. *Investig. Ophthalmol. Vis. Sci.* **2014**, *55*, 7739–7753. [CrossRef] [PubMed]
134. Hsu, P.D.; Lander, E.S.; Zhang, F. Development and Applications of CRISPR-Cas9 for Genome Engineering. *Cell* **2014**, *157*, 1262–1278. [CrossRef]

135. Gao, X.; Tao, Y.; Lamas, V.; Huang, M.; Yeh, W.-H.; Pan, B.; Hu, Y.-J.; Hu, J.H.; Thompson, D.B.; Shu, Y.; et al. Treatment of Autosomal Dominant Hearing Loss by in Vivo Delivery of Genome Editing Agents. *Nature* **2018**, *553*, 217–221. [CrossRef]
136. Hauswirth, W.W.; Aleman, T.S.; Kaushal, S.; Cideciyan, A.V.; Schwartz, S.B.; Wang, L.; Conlon, T.J.; Boye, S.L.; Flotte, T.R.; Byrne, B.J.; et al. Treatment of Leber Congenital Amaurosis Due to RPE65 Mutations by Ocular Subretinal Injection of Adeno-Associated Virus Gene Vector: Short-Term Results of a Phase I Trial. *Hum. Gene Ther.* **2008**, *19*, 979–990. [CrossRef]
137. Bainbridge, J.W.B.; Smith, A.J.; Barker, S.S.; Robbie, S.; Henderson, R.; Balaggan, K.; Viswanathan, A.; Holder, G.E.; Stockman, A.; Tyler, N.; et al. Effect of Gene Therapy on Visual Function in Leber's Congenital Amaurosis. *N. Engl. J. Med.* **2008**, *358*, 2231–2239. [CrossRef]
138. Cideciyan, A.V.; Aleman, T.S.; Boye, S.L.; Schwartz, S.B.; Kaushal, S.; Roman, A.J.; Pang, J.-J.; Sumaroka, A.; Windsor, E.A.M.; Wilson, J.M.; et al. Human Gene Therapy for RPE65 Isomerase Deficiency Activates the Retinoid Cycle of Vision but with Slow Rod Kinetics. *Proc. Natl. Acad. Sci. USA* **2008**, *105*, 15112–15117. [CrossRef]
139. Wang, D.; Tai, P.W.L.; Gao, G. Adeno-Associated Virus Vector as a Platform for Gene Therapy Delivery. *Nat. Rev. Drug Discov.* **2019**, *18*, 358–378. [CrossRef]
140. HHTM. Decibel Therapeutics Announces Submission of Clinical Trial Applications for Lead Gene Therapy Candidate DB-OTO–HHTM. *Hearing News Watch*. Available online: https://hearinghealthmatters.org/hearingnewswatch/2022/decibel-therapeutics-clinical-trial-submission/ (accessed on 30 November 2022).
141. Sensorion Receives US FDA Rare Pediatric Disease Designation for Gene Therapy. Available online: https://www.biopharma-reporter.com/Article/2022/11/07/sensorion-receives-us-fda-rare-pediatric-disease-designation-for-gene-therapy (accessed on 30 November 2022).

Disclaimer/Publisher's Note: The statements, opinions and data contained in all publications are solely those of the individual author(s) and contributor(s) and not of MDPI and/or the editor(s). MDPI and/or the editor(s) disclaim responsibility for any injury to people or property resulting from any ideas, methods, instructions or products referred to in the content.

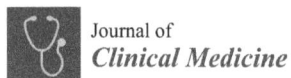

Review

Extracellular Vesicles in Inner Ear Therapies—Pathophysiological, Manufacturing, and Clinical Considerations

Athanasia Warnecke [1,2,*], Hinrich Staecker [3], Eva Rohde [4,5,6], Mario Gimona [4,5,7], Anja Giesemann [8], Agnieszka J. Szczepek [9,10], Arianna Di Stadio [11], Ingeborg Hochmair [12] and Thomas Lenarz [1,2]

[1] Department of Otolaryngology, Hannover Medical School, 30625 Hannover, Germany
[2] Cluster of Excellence of the German Research Foundation (DFG; "Deutsche Forschungsgemeinschaft") "Hearing4all", 30625 Hannover, Germany
[3] Department of Otolaryngology Head and Neck Surgery, University of Kansas School of Medicine, Rainbow Blvd., Kansas City, KS 66160, USA
[4] GMP Unit, Spinal Cord Injury & Tissue Regeneration Centre Salzburg (SCI-TReCS), Paracelsus Medical University, 5020 Salzburg, Austria
[5] Transfer Centre for Extracellular Vesicle Theralytic Technologies (EV-TT), 5020 Salzburg, Austria
[6] Department of Transfusion Medicine, University Hospital, Salzburger Landeskliniken GesmbH (SALK) Paracelsus Medical University, 5020 Salzburg, Austria
[7] Research Program "Nanovesicular Therapies", Paracelsus Medical University, 5020 Salzburg, Austria
[8] Department of Diagnostic and Interventional Neuroradiology, Hannover Medical School, Carl-Neuberg-Str. 1, 30625 Hannover, Germany
[9] Department of Otorhinolaryngology, Head and Neck Surgery, Charité-Universitätsmedizin Berlin, 10117 Berlin, Germany
[10] Faculty of Medicine and Health Sciences, University of Zielona Gora, 65-046 Zielona Gora, Poland
[11] Department GF Ingrassia, University of Catania, 95124 Catania, Italy
[12] MED-EL Medical Electronics, Fürstenweg 77a, 6020 Innsbruck, Austria
* Correspondence: warnecke.athanasia@mh-hannover.de

Abstract: (1) Background: Sensorineural hearing loss is a common and debilitating condition. To date, comprehensive pharmacologic interventions are not available. The complex and diverse molecular pathology that underlies hearing loss may limit our ability to intervene with small molecules. The current review focusses on the potential for the use of extracellular vesicles in neurotology. (2) Methods: Narrative literature review. (3) Results: Extracellular vesicles provide an opportunity to modulate a wide range of pathologic and physiologic pathways and can be manufactured under GMP conditions allowing for their application in the human inner ear. The role of inflammation in hearing loss with a focus on cochlear implantation is shown. How extracellular vesicles may provide a therapeutic option for complex inflammatory disorders of the inner ear is discussed. Additionally, manufacturing and regulatory issues that need to be addressed to develop EVs as advanced therapy medicinal product for use in the inner ear are outlined. (4) Conclusion: Given the complexities of inner ear injury, novel therapeutics such as extracellular vesicles could provide a means to modulate inflammation, stress pathways and apoptosis in the inner ear.

Keywords: extracellular vesicles; exosomes; multipotent mesenchymal stromal cells; umbilical cord; inflammation; oxidative stress; cochlea; hearing loss; cochlear implantation

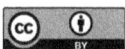

1. Introduction

More than 450 million people worldwide suffer from hearing loss [1]. According to the World Health Organization, one in twenty individuals is affected by hearing loss [2] and at risk of developing associated co-morbidities such as depression and dementia [3]. Although the importance of treating hearing loss to prevent these conditions has been demonstrated [4], pharmacological treatments are still unavailable, leaving most patients not adequately treated. Because some forms of hearing loss are age-related, the increase in the elderly population affects the prevalence of this symptom. For this reason, identifying effective treatments is fundamental also to reducing co-morbidities, i.e., cognitive decline [5].

A comprehensive understanding of the molecular pathophysiology of different inner ear diseases is lacking. Understanding the exact molecular mechanisms that lead to damage to the inner ear and induce hearing loss would accelerate the development of effective precision treatments. With innovations in molecular biology, some cellular and molecular changes related to hearing loss are elucidated and suggest the involvement of multiple diverse injury and stress pathways which are unlikely to be completely treated using standard pharmacological therapy. The current review focuses on the molecular changes associated with inner ear damage and hearing loss, which may be treatable using extracellular vesicles to directly target the molecular changes related to aging and inner ear damage. Finally, manufacturing and clinical considerations associated with introducing EV-related treatment strategies in the clinic will be discussed. This narrative review is based on searches performed in PubMed and ClinicalTrials.gov.

2. Hearing Loss

The causes for hearing loss are diverse and include genetic predisposition, ototoxic agents, and environmental factors such as noise and aging. Depending on the severity of the insult, different grades of damage are observed within the cochlea leading to different phenotypes of hearing loss and ranging from reversible to permanent: starting from molecular damage such as induced by excitotoxicity (e.g., loss of ribbon synapses) to more pronounced cellular and structural degeneration (loss of connectivity from neurons to hair cells, loss of hair cells, spiral ganglion neurons and cells of the stria vascularis). Ultimately, the neuroepithelium degenerates, leaving a flat non-functional epithelium in the organ of Corti [6,7]. Different prosthetic devices are available for hearing restoration depending on the severity of the hearing loss. Patients with moderate hearing loss can be treated with hearing aids (HA) (simple sound amplification). Unfortunately, many patients refuse daily use of their HA due to a lack of benefit in many everyday listening situations [8,9]. Cochlear implantation for direct electrical stimulation of the auditory neurons is performed in cases with severe hearing loss across all frequencies. In recent years, the use of cochlear implantation has been expanded to patients with residual hearing (high-frequency hearing loss but preserved hearing for lower frequencies). In these cases, hybrid stimulation is provided via a hearing aid (that amplifies low-frequency information acoustically) in combination with a cochlear implant (that electrically stimulates the high-frequency regions) [10,11]. With this strategy, patients develop a superior speech understanding even in challenging listening situations [12,13]. However, a significant portion of these patients loses their residual hearing after cochlear implantation [14] limiting the long-term efficacy of hybrid stimulation. There is an unmet clinical need for effective treatment strategies to protect residual hearing. In patients with residual hearing, the apical regions responsible for processing acoustic stimuli in lower frequency have intact inner ear cytoarchitecture and preserved electrolyte homeostasis and blood supply despite a damaged basal region (the area processing high-frequency sound).

3. Inflammation in Hearing Loss

Acute inflammation is an adaptive response to combat invading pathogens or to repair damaged tissues. An acute inflammatory reaction is a highly coordinated process [15]. Resolution of inflammation is critical to restore organ homeostasis and to prevent ongoing inflammatory responses leading to tissue damage [15–18].

The inflammation arises as a common hallmark underlying hearing loss [18]. Cellular stress leads to producing reactive oxygen species (ROS) [19–21], activating pro-survival pathways and increasing endogenous antioxidant molecules to maintain redox homeostasis [22]. Excessive ROS can cause either damage to the tissue directly by oxidation and reduction of cochlear blood flow [23] or indirectly by up-regulating pro-inflammatory cytokines, e.g., interleukin-6 (IL-6) and tumor necrosis factor-alpha (TNFα) [23]. These cytokines, in turn, induce apoptosis or necrosis [23]. Endogenous pathways that initiate the inflammation depend mainly on ROS [24]. Accumulation of ROS precedes any morphological sign of damage [25]. It spreads from the basal to the apical part of the cochlea [26], subsequently damaging initially unaffected parts as has been shown, e.g., for noise-exposure, ototoxicity, aging, Ménière's disease, and in cochlear implantation [22,23,25–31]. In fact, cochlear implantation can add additional damage to an already diseased organ through the surgical opening of the cochlea and insertion of a foreign body (the electrode). Specifically, foreign body insertion can lead to a phagocytic reflex in macrophages and activation of the NACHT-, leucine-rich repeat-and pyrin-domain-containing protein (NALP3 or NLRP3) inflammasome, which is a sensor of inflammation [24]. Thus, we create a wound not only at the opening site but also within the cochlea that elicits a trauma reaction with inflammation [32,33] leading to tissue remodeling and fibrosis [34,35]. Postmortem analyses of human temporal bones have confirmed that implantation trauma can result in severe damage of the cochlear structural and ultrastructural components [34–37] and loss of residual hearing [30,32,38].

The impact of the molecular changes associated with electrode insertion trauma has been recently reviewed in detail [39]. Injury to the stria vascularis in the lateral cochlear wall can be caused when inserting stiff straight electrode arrays, and this injury leads to an increase in ROS and induces inflammation. Consequently, the vascularization of the stria vascularis decreases [39], as has been shown in an animal model of cochlear implantation with residual hearing [40]. The fibrocytes that reside in the cochlear lateral wall are thought to mediate inflammation after noise exposure by the release of pro-inflammatory factors [41,42] such as interleukin (IL)-1β, TNF-α, inducible nitric oxide (NO), monocyte chemoattractant protein-1 (MCP-1), macrophage inflammatory protein (MIP), intercellular adhesion molecule-1 (ICAM-1), nuclear factor kappa B [43], and vascular endothelial growth factor (VEGF) [44]. Resident macrophages are activated and up-regulated by inner ear damage, as has been shown for noise exposure or aminoglycoside toxicity [44,45]. Indeed, the inhibition of macrophages resulted in protection against aminoglycoside toxicity [46].

Acute inflammation upon an insult may also be considered a necessary host reaction to restore cochlear homeostasis and glial-neuronal interactions. For example, neuroactive molecules such as TNFα and IL-1β are also released in patients with sudden sensorineural hearing loss, and increased levels can be measured in their peripheral blood [47,48]. The release of such cytokines might be essential to induce inflammation, followed by a timely resolution in order to prevent auditory dysfunction [18]. Indeed, maladaptive inflammation is acknowledged as a cause of neurodegenerative diseases, asthma, allergy, diabetes, fibrosis, cardiovascular disease, and metabolic disorders [17]. Four phases characterize inflammatory responses, starting with initiation, transition, resolution, and finally, restoration of homeostasis [15–18]. Others classify inflammation by the onset, resolution, and post-resolution phases [49]. Inflammation is initiated by recognizing pathogen- and/or damage-associated molecular patterns [17]. This phase is characterized by a coordinated delivery of blood components to the site of infection or injury [24] mediated by increased blood flow, capillary dilatation, leukocyte infiltration, as well as production of pro-inflammatory mediators, including cytokines, chemokines, vasoactive amines, and eicosanoids [49,50]. The release of pro-resolving chemical mediators characterizes the resolution phase, which aims to eliminate the inflammatory trigger, the clearance of immune cells from the inflamed sites, the reduction in extravasation of cells from the circulation, and the change from pro-inflammatory to pro-tissue repair signaling pathways [24].

On a molecular level, connexin43 channels and hemichannels have been demonstrated to amplify and perpetuate inflammation [50]. Inflammation can be initiated and maintained via adenosine triphosphate (ATP) released by connexin hemichannels [50]. In the cochlea, ATP release has also been shown to occur via connexin 26 and 30 hemichannels [51,52]. An increase in ATP concentration has been demonstrated in the cochlea, particularly after noise trauma, and may impair cochlear function [53]. Connexin hemichannels are located on the non-junctional cell surface and are not involved in forming gap junctions; they can open due to depolarization, hyperpolarization, or metabolic stress and release increased ATP [52]. The ribbon synapse protein CtBP can detect NAD+ and NADH levels and is therefore considered a metabolic biosensor [54,55]. Moreover, changes in the NAD(H) redox status can affect the formation of CtBP and, thus, that of the synapses [54,56]. Mitochondria are localized near the presynaptic ribbons in hair cells [54]. Mitochondria are the energy producers of the cell and the primary source of cellular ATP. As by-products, reactive oxygen species are also produced and released in the mitochondria while providing ATP. ATP is formed after the oxidation of carbohydrates, lipids, and proteins as energy storage. Other metabolites such as inositol 1,4,5 trisphosphate (IP3), glutamate, lactate, and D-serine are also released. ATP activates the NLRP3 inflammasome [50]. The exact mechanisms leading to a prolonged or dysregulated resolution of inflammation in the cochlea and other organ systems are unknown.

The late enhancement on magnetic resonance imaging is a potential sign of cochlear inflammation that can be visualized. Intralabyrinthine enhancement has been a diagnostic finding in T1-weighted magnetic resonance imaging (MRI) for many years. This enhancement usually refers to an enhancement a few minutes after intravenous (i.v.) contrast administration and is found in the acute stage of labyrinthitis ossificans and intracochlear schwannoma. Other causes are rarely encountered. In the last decade, the so-called "hydrops"-imaging has been performed to visualize an enlargement of the membranous spaces of the inner ear [57]. It is performed 4 to 6 h after i.v. contrast administration. A certain amount of contrast that gets into the perilymphatic space distinguishes the scala vestibuli and the scala tympani from the scala media on heavily T2-weighted 3D Flair images. At the same time, substantial enhancement was associated with several conditions. In patients with vestibular neuritis an enhancement can be seen regularly [58]. The same is true for about 20% of the patients with otosclerosis [59]. Single cases were attributed to a herpes infection. In many other cases, the causes remain unknown, but autoimmune diseases such as Cogan syndrome or accompanying inflammation in cases with known scleroderma or rheumatoid arthritis were discussed. Further studies have to evaluate the possible causes for the impaired blood–labyrinth barrier in detail—but late intralabyrinthine enhancement in MRI is a promising tool to detect infectious and inflammatory conditions of the cochlea and the vestibule.

4. Electrotoxicity

Damage of synaptic contacts due to electrical stimulation might be another reason for loss of residual hearing after cochlear implantation [60,61]. Indeed, chronic electrical stimulation leads to hearing loss, as has been demonstrated in animal models and the loss of hearing seems to be histologically attributed to the loss of synapses [40,60]. In the organ of Corti explants, a reduced density of ribbon synapses, an increase in free reactive oxygen species, and morphological changes in stereocilia bundles were observed under electrical stimulation [62,63]. The treatment with dexamethasone [64] could partially prevent the damage induced by experimental electrical stimulation. The exact molecular mechanisms and the conditions under which electrical stimulation may damage hair cells, and spiral ganglion neurons are unknown. In vitro experiments using charge-balanced biphasic electrical stimulation showed a reduced neurite outgrowth from the spiral ganglion and a reduced density in Schwann cells, possibly due to calcium influx through multiple types of voltage-gated calcium channels [65]. Although calcium overload and oxidative stress are assumed to be the leading cause of spiral ganglion neuron degeneration, decreased intracellular levels of calcium have been observed in neurons damaged by electrical stimulation [66]. Indeed, neuronal death has been observed under low and high calcium levels, and an imbalance in intracellular calcium homeostasis might increase the vulnerability of spiral ganglion neurons under electrical stimulation [66]. A retrospective analysis of patients enrolled in the multicenter Hybrid S8 trial who were treated with a Nucleus Contour Advance perimodiolar standard length electrode array or a Nucleus 422 Slim Straight electrode array showed an acceleration of hearing loss after activation of the device [61]. In addition, high charge exposure with the same devices also led to accelerated loss of residual hearing [61]. To our knowledge, this is the first and only report on humans showing a correlation between electrical activation and hearing loss. The authors also corroborated their results experimentally on the organ of Corti explants showing that high voltage ES damaged afferent nerve fibers [61]. Whether and under which stimulation parameter electrotoxicity can be mediated via all cochlear implants in humans is unknown hitherto.

5. Extracellular Vesicles

The term "extracellular vesicles" refers to a heterogeneous set of cell-derived membranous nano- and microvesicles that can be harvested for diagnostic and therapeutic purposes from the secretome of cells and any body fluid. Small EVs display a diameter ranging from 50–150 nm and are also called exosomes. Larger microvesicles up to 1000 nm and apoptotic bodies have also been identified. Potentially all pro- and eukaryotic cells release EVs into their secretome. There are two ways for the biogenesis of extracellular vesicles. By the inward budding of the plasma membrane or the trans-Golgi network, early endosomes are formed and mature into late endosomes to finally become multivesicular endosomal bodies (MVBs) [67,68]. After trafficking to the cell membrane, a fusion of MBV with the plasma membrane leads to the release of exosomes into the extracellular space. Another mechanism is the plasma membrane rearrangement leading to the budding of microvesicles from the cell membrane [67,68]. Through various isolation techniques, EVs can be enriched in a vesicular secretome fraction [69,70]. Depending on their source, EVs can be involved in physiological or pathophysiological processes. For example, exosomes derived from malignant cells can promote tumor growth, local invasion, and distant metastasis [71–74]. During pregnancy, placental exosomes are involved in the regulation and progression of a normal pregnancy and pathological conditions that can arise during pregnancy [75]. Depending on their source, EVs exert differential effects. For example, anti-apoptotic [76,77], anti-fibrotic [78–80], pro-angiogenic [81,82], and immunomodulatory [83–90] effects are mediated by EVs derived from naïve umbilical cord mesenchymal stromal cells (UC-MSC).

6. Extracellular Vesicles as Anti-Inflammatory and Anti-Oxidative Treatment

Growth factors such as the neurotrophins brain-derived neurotrophic factor (BDNF) and neurotrophin-3 (NT-3) are essential regulators in embryonic development [91,92] and in the maintenance of the adult auditory system [93–95]. In addition, individual neurotrophins have also been shown to exert immunomodulatory effects [96,97]. However, in terms of potency, a cocktail of various growth factors was more effective in the protection of neuronal survival than single factors [98–100]. For the delivery of human neuroprotective factor cocktails to the inner ear, we have investigated cell-based approaches such as platelet-rich plasma [101] or autologous mononuclear cells derived from human bone marrow [102] as potent regulators of inflammation and oxidative stress and as a source of a balanced composition of endogenous neuroprotective factors. We assume that extracellular vesicles (EVs) are the main contributors to neuroprotection and regulation of inflammation when using cell-based approaches.

Extracellular vesicles mainly target immune-competent cells such as T cells, B cells, and natural killer cells. Like their parental cells, MSC-EVs can impede the maturation of dendritic cells and modify their function, thereby suppressing antigen uptake [103]. In addition, the cytokine production profile of dendritic cells was changed from pro-inflammatory to immunoregulatory after exposure to MSC-EVs [103]. A phenotype change from pro-inflammatory to immunoregulatory was also observed in macrophages after exposure to EVs [104]. Specific microRNAs involved in the development and maturation of dendritic cells are highly enriched in MSC-EVs and might account for the anti-inflammatory and immunomodulating effects [103]. Chronic unresolved inflammation with an accumulation of pro-inflammatory macrophages is the hallmark of metabolic diseases, including diabetes.

The release of pro-inflammatory cytokines such as tumor necrosis factor-alpha (TNF-α) and interleukin-1-beta (IL-1β) are critical drivers for the maintenance of inflammation and the induction of insulin resistance. Indeed, macrophages exposed to high glucose levels and oxidative stress release EVs with an altered microRNA profile that can induce atherosclerosis [105]. Th2 cytokines such as IL-4 and IL-13 polarize macrophages towards an anti-inflammatory phenotype [106–108] with associated changes in their EV-cargo [105,109] and protective effects against cardiometabolic disease [109].

Excessive release of pro-inflammatory cytokines leading to an overwhelming systemic inflammation is the main cause of severe organ damage and failure in sepsis developed after infectious diseases [110,111]. Mesenchymal stromal cells have an immunomodulatory effect and could be ideal candidates for modulating the deregulated immune response in sepsis [112–114]. When primed with IL-1β the immunomodulatory efficacy of MSC could be increased [87]. A significant upregulation of miR-146a expression and packaging within exosomes seems to be the mechanism by which priming with IL-1β increases the potency of MSC to ameliorate the symptoms associated with sepsis and prevent organ injury [87]. Additionally, MSC and MSC-EVs mediate a transition of macrophages from a pro-inflammatory to an immunomodulatory phenotype that is beneficial for recovery from sepsis [87]. Derived from macrophages with an anti-inflammatory phenotype, EVs have been shown efficient in reducing excessive cytokine release and oxidative stress leading to multiple organ damage in mice challenged with bacterial endotoxins [115]. Specifically, the release of pro-inflammatory cytokines TNF-α and IL-6 is reduced [115]. That is important since TNF-α is the primary activator of the pro-inflammatory NF-κB pathway amplifying the inflammatory cascade leading to lethal toxic shock [115–117].

The cytokines TNF-α and IL-6 are also involved in severe steroid-resistant asthma and exacerbate airway inflammation and lung tissue damage [118,119]. Indeed, MSC-EVs were able to ameliorate inflammation via the NF-κB and PI3K/AKT signaling pathways by reducing the expression of the TNF-receptor-associated factor 1 (TRAF1) [83]. TRAF1 is involved in regulating inflammation and apoptosis and is known to activate NF-κB [83]. Thus, MSC-EVs may present an ideal targeted therapeutic for severe steroid-resistant asthma.

Suppression of lymphocyte proliferation [86], specifically B cells and natural killer cells, was mediated by anti-inflammatory factors such as indoleamine 2 3-dioxygenase (IDO) [86]. In inflammatory skin diseases such as psoriasis, IL-17A, and its upstream regulator IL-23 are two critical molecules involved in the pathogenesis and thus present key targets for targeted treatment [120]. Extracellular vesicles derived from UC-MSC promote a shift from a Th1 or Th17 into a Treg phenotype, thus, exhibiting the ability to silence Th17 signaling in patients with psoriasis [85]. Multiple sclerosis (MS) is characterized by the proliferation of conventional T cells and their differentiation into an autoreactive phenotype in response to self-antigens [121]. Treatment with EVs reduced IFN-γ and IL-17 release from lymphocytes derived from patients with MS [84].

The emerging role of EVs in promoting intracellular defense against oxidative stress by inhibiting the formation of excess ROS, thereby improving mitochondrial performance, has been discussed in a recent review article [122]. Thus, EVs may be effective therapeutics to treat oxidative stress. For example, EVs derived from patients' blood after myocardial infarction have an antioxidative effect on the endothelium [123]. In response to heat shock, EVs can protect cultured neurons from oxidative stress [124]. Derived from hypoxia preconditioned MSC, EVs have been shown to protect cardiomyocytes from apoptosis by targeting a protein [125] (thioredoxin-interacting protein) involved in oxidative stress responses [126]. In diabetic cardiomyopathy, the platelet inhibitor ticagrelor modulates the cargo of EVs to enhance the suppression of cellular stress and ROS production [127]. Several heat shock proteins are involved in oxidative stress, either protective or damaging. The heat shock protein B8 (HSPB8) is involved in removing cytotoxic proteins, thereby facilitating autophagy and reducing oxidative stress. Endogenous HSPB8 mRNA expression is increased by the uptake of EVs derived from oligodendrocytes [128]. However, the protective effect of EVs from oxidative stress is not inherent and depends on the source and the content of EVs. The transcription factor nuclear factor (erythroid-derived 2)-like 2 (Nrf2) regulates the expression of antioxidant and anti-inflammatory proteins in response to oxidative stress [129]. However, the effects of EVs are not inherent and depend on the source and the content of EVs. As a result, EVs can contribute to the healing process but also induce inflammation and disease. The transcription factor nuclear factor (erythroid-derived 2)-like 2 (Nrf2) regulates the expression of antioxidant and anti-inflammatory proteins in response to oxidative stress [129]. Cardiac-derived EVs isolated from the circulation of rats and patients suffering from chronic heart failure have a miRNA profile associated with inhibition of the Nrf2/anti-oxidant signaling pathway, thereby contributing not only to the heart disease but also to the neuroinflammation and redox imbalance at distant sites such as the brain [129]. Altering the cargo of EVs or inhibiting the responsible miRNA may present a therapeutic strategy for treating chronic heart failure.

7. Extracellular Vesicles as a Novel Therapeutic in Neurotology

There is a lack of specific inner ear therapeutics for the protection and regeneration of cochlear cells alongside an antioxidative and anti-inflammatory/immunomodulatory treatment.

The first report about the release of EVs from rats' primary cultured inner ear cells was published by Wong et al. in 2018 [130]. The authors also showed that exosomes could potentially be used as a biomarker reflecting the state of the inner ear [130]. For example, there was a change in concentration and proteomic cargo upon induction of ototoxic stress by exposure to cisplatin or gentamycin [130]. The authors state that the isolated exosomes may be derived from the organ of Corti [130]. Furthermore, EVs isolated from a murine auditory cell line (HEI-OC1) showed a distinct protein and surface marker profile of HEI-OC1-EVs [131] when compared to the EVs content listed in ExoCarta, a manually curated database of exosomal proteins, RNA, and lipids. Moreover, the authors stated that HEI-OC1-EVs could be loaded with anti-inflammatory drugs and pro-resolving mediators and used as drug nanocarriers [131,132].

For the first time, using human perilymph, we could isolate EVs carrying hair cell-specific proteins [133], demonstrating not only the presence of EVs in the perilymph but also suggesting hair cells as a potential source of the exosomes. Cochlear tissues derived from different postnatal developmental stages were analyzed for EVs' presence and content. Indeed, EVs had a specific miRNA and proteome profile related to the development of the inner ear and auditory nervous system [134]. Although that study suggests that EVs may be involved in inner ear development, the presence and role of exosomes in the adult inner ear are still unclear. As in other organ systems, EVs might contribute to physiological and pathophysiological processes in the adult inner ear. For example, it has been shown that EVs derived from human vestibular schwannoma (VS) cell culture can exert differential effects on hair cells and auditory neurons [135]. Exosomes derived from patients diagnosed with VS and hearing impairment were more likely to damage hair cells and auditory neurons than exosomes derived from patients with VS and good hearing [135].

The protective role of exosomes in otology has been demonstrated in several preclinical studies [136–143]. Breglio et al. were the first to demonstrate in 2020 that utricle-derived exosomes are mediators of heat stress response in the inner ear and can protect hair cells against aminoglycoside-induced death [142]. We were the first to also demonstrate in 2020 that umbilical cord-derived MSC-EVs exerted immunomodulatory activity on T cells and microglial cells and significantly improved spiral ganglion neurons' survival in vitro [143]. We furthermore could show that MSC-EVs contain BDNF and that local post-traumatic application of MSC-EVs to the cochlea attenuated hearing loss and protected auditory hair cells from noise-induced trauma in vivo [143]. Our results were corroborated by Tsai et al., who also showed later that post-traumatic administration of UC-MSC-EVs significantly improved hearing loss and rescued the loss of cochlear hair cells in mice receiving chronic cisplatin injection [140]. Preconditioning of MSC may increase the therapeutic efficacy of thereof derived EVs. For example, hypoxia-preconditioned MSC-EVs have an up-regulated expression of HIF-1α, leading to increased potency in the treatment of cisplatin-induced ototoxicity [139]. Heat shock-preconditioned MSCs release EVs with an increased HSP70 content and an increased efficacy against cisplatin-induced hair cell loss [136]. HSP70 might be one of the mediators of EV-related protective effects. Interestingly, the co-culture of MSC and cochlear explants led to an increase in HSP70 content in EVs and was able to protect explants from cisplatin-induced toxicity [139]. Also, exosomal HSP70 treatment decreased the concentration of pro-inflammatory cytokines IL-1β, IL-6, and TNF-α and increased the concentrations of anti-inflammatory cytokine IL-10 in cisplatin-exposed mice inner ears [136]. Neural progenitor cells also release EVs. Specifically, EVs derived from miRNA-21-overexpressing progenitors, showed increased anti-inflammatory activity and prevented hearing loss after ischemia-reperfusion injury [137]. Interestingly, the effects were also mediated by a decrease of IL-1β, IL-6, TNF-α, and an increase of IL-10 [137]. Exosomes derived from spiral ganglion progenitor cells isolated from neonatal mice cochlear explants were able to protect the hearing threshold in mice exposed to ischemia-reperfusion injury [141].

The feasibility of applying allogeneic human MSC-EVs into the inner ear was recently demonstrated in the first report of EV application into the scala tympani during cochlear implantation [144]. The goal of cochlear implantation would be to limit the potential damage induced in the inner ear by a foreign body reaction, inflammation caused by the surgical opening of the cochlea, and insertion of the electrode array, and to protect residual hearing for improved implant performance. Other application fields for EVs in neurotology are the increase of efficacy of viral vector gene therapy approaches. It has been shown that exosomes applied in conjunction with AAV could rescue hearing in a mouse model of hereditary deafness [145]. Indeed, robust transduction with AAV was also observed in other organ systems, such as the eye or the nervous systems, by combining gene therapy with exosome treatment [146].

For a better overview on the studies demonstrating inner ear protection by EVs, Table 1 summarizes all to our knowledge currently published reports. Based on the potent anti-inflammatory efficacy of EVs and to the lack of specific treatment alternatives, treatment of autoimmune-mediated hearing loss, Meniere's disease, and insertion of trauma-mediated immune responses could present potential clinical applications. To our knowledge, there are no clinical trials investigating the effect of EVs in the inner ear.

Table 1. Summary of the studies demonstrating inner ear protection by EVs.

Authors	Title	Origin of EVs	Species	Journal and Year
Breglio, A.M. et al. [142]	Exosomes mediate sensory hair cells protection in the inner ear	Heat shocked utricles from mice	Mice	*J. Clin. Invest.* 2020
Lai, S.-W. et al. [97]	Exosomes derived from mouse inner ear stem cells attenuate gentamicin-induced ototoxicity in vitro through the miR-182-5p/FOXO3 axis	Inner ear stem cells from mice	Mice	*Mol. Neurobiol.* 2018
Warnecke, A. et al. [143]	Extracellular vesicles from human multipotent stromal cells protect against hearing loss after noise trauma in vivo	Human umbilical mesenchymal stromal cells	Mice	*Clin. Trans. Med.* 2020
Warnecke, A. et al. [144]	First-in-human intracochlear application of human stromal cell-derived extracellular vesicles	Human umbilical mesenchymal stromal cells	Human	*J. Extracell. Vesicles* 2021
Tsai, S.C.-S. et al. [140]	Umbilical Cord Mesenchymal Stromal Cell-Derived Exosomes Rescue the Loss of Outer Hair Cells and Repair Cochlear Damage in Cisplatin-Injected Mice	Umbilical mesenchymal stromal cells (presumably human; but not specified in publication)	Mice	*Int. J. Mol. Sci.* 2021
Yang, T. et al. [141]	Exosomes derived from cochlear spiral ganglion progenitor cells prevent cochlea damage from ischemia-reperfusion injury via inhibiting the inflammatory process	Spiral ganglion progenitor cells from mice	Mice	*Cell Tissue Res.* 2021

Table 1. Cont.

Authors	Title	Origin of EVs	Species	Journal and Year
Jiang, P. et al. [134]	Characterization of the microRNA transcriptomes and proteomics of cochlear tissue-derived small extracellular vesicles from mice of different ages after birth	Cochlear tissue from mice	-	Cell Mol. Life Sci. 2022
Hao, F. et al. [137]	Exosomes Derived from microRNA-21 Overexpressing Neural Progenitor Cells Prevent Hearing Loss from Ischemia-Reperfusion Injury in Mice via Inhibiting the Inflammatory Process in the Cochlea	Neural progenitor cells from mice transfected with miR-21	Mice	ACS Chem. Neurosci. 2022

8. Manufacturing Considerations

EV-based therapeutics derived from genetically unmodified mesenchymal stromal cells are considered to belong to the pharmaceutical category of biological medicinal products in Europe, the United States of Amerika, Australia, and Japan [147]. A "biological medicine is a medicine that contains one or more active substances made by or derived from a biological cell" [147]. According to the European Medicines Agency (EMA, Amsterdam), medicines for human use that are based on genes, tissues, or cells are classified as advanced therapy medicinal products (ATMPs) [148]. "They offer ground breaking new opportunities for the treatment of disease and injury" [148]. The inherent heterogeneity and biological or technological complexity hamper the identification of the therapeutically active component or components in EV formulations and the mode of action. The latter depends on the parental cell type, handling and culture conditions, and materials or medical devices used for EV isolation and administration [149]. When considering translating the use of EVs towards clinical application, several considerations concerning their manufacturing are mandatory.

Harmonized guidelines are available, and the International Council for Harmonisation of Technical Requirements for Pharmaceuticals for Human Use connects regulatory authorities with researchers and biotechnology companies to discuss and regulate scientific and technical aspects of drug registration globally [149]. The goal is to ensure safety, effectiveness, and high quality for the manufacturing of ATMPs.

Product specifications related to purity, identity, quantity, potency, and sterility need to be defined according to pharmaceutical manufacturing regulations. Since EVs include a wide variety of membrane-bounded vesicles, exosomes are restricted by size and surface markers. Since part of the EV-based secretome includes soluble molecules such as proteins, lipids, and extracellular RNA species either from tissue or from in vitro expanded cell cultures, several factors may influence the composition of EVs. Electron microscopy data show that even highly purified EV preparations for analytical purposes contain co-purifying components [150]. Segregation of EVs from co-purifying components during large-scale clinical manufacturing will not be possible entirely, so an increasing fraction of secretome components will be present in the final preparation [149]. Thus, there is heterogeneity and complexity of secretome-based preparations, and an attempt to find a terminology that embraces all biological components and therapeutic aspects without eliminating the central claim is problematic. From a cell biology standpoint and not limiting the definition to a purely proteomic view, the secretome can be seen as the totality of organic molecules and inorganic elements secreted by cells into the extracellular space, either in a soluble or packaged form. Although the EVs' manufacturing and enrichment process eliminates a large portion of soluble proteome components, the co-purifying fraction is still challenging to determine. Thus, the manufacturing strategy aims to enrich (and not necessarily purify) membrane-bounded vesicular structures [149]. The product may then be considered as a vesicular secretome fraction. This terminology can also accommodate fractions containing co-purifying soluble serum components in those cases where the manufacturing process requires the use of (vesicle-depleted) serum. Nevertheless, and fully considering the above, we will adhere to the EV terminology for simplicity. The product is a biological containing cell-derived EVs. The cell source for the production of EVs is manifold. Multipotent mesenchymal stromal cells-derived EVs might be favorable for a rapid clinical translation. From 2015–2021, 416 clinical trials comprising MSCs were registered [151]. In mid-2021, 1014 MSC-based clinical trials were registered in the ClinicalTrials.gov database either as completed or in progress [152]. A recent search in ClinicalTrials.gov (using the terms 'application' and 'human umbilical cord-derived MSC') showed that by October 2022, a total of 135 trials investigated the application of human umbilical cord-derived MSC in many diseases affecting adults and infants. Thus, abundant clinical data are available on the safety and efficacy of MSCs, specifically of UC-MSC.

The allogeneic human UC-MSCs grown in a fibrinogen-depleted growth medium containing pooled human platelet lysate (pHPL) serve as an alternative source for xenogeneic growth factors. The tissue of human origin must be collected following the Helsinki Declaration after the written informed consent of adult donors. A Master Cell Bank needs to be generated to provide a pool of producer cells for EVs. Since the final product should be a ready-to-inject solution, the sterilized product needs to be dissolved, e.g., in Ringer's lactate, and filled at a defined dose in aseptic glass vials. The use of EV-based therapeutics instead of the cells themselves has several advantages: the possibility of filter sterilization of the final product immediately prior to aseptic filling and the stability after freeze–thaw cycles, as well as flexibility in the choice of storage buffers. However, compared to the cells as a product, EV manufacturing includes additional steps such as isolation, enrichment, and characterization of vesicles [149,153].

9. Regulatory Affairs

National competent authorities are responsible for approving clinical trials in the respective country and providing scientific and regulatory advice on drug development and the planning and conduct of clinical trials. Regulatory advice and authorization for drugs and ATMPs for human use are granted in Germany by the Paul Ehrlich Institute (PEI) or the Federal Institute for Drugs and Medical Devices (BfArM). When granted, European marketing authorizations are coordinated by the EMA and are valid for the entire European Union (EU).

The biological medicinal product must be manufactured under GMP-compliant conditions, and the guidelines apply to the whole manufacturing chain. Pharmaceutical production includes harvesting the tissue, isolation of the parental cells, culture environment, cultivation system, culture medium, isolation and purification of EVs, fill and finish as well as storage of the final product. According to the requirements of a state-of-the-art pharmaceutical quality management system, the quality and therapeutic activity of the EV-based novel product have to be confirmed by defined release testing. Biodistribution, bioavailability, cytotoxicity, and pharmacokinetics are cornerstones in the non-clinical development of a biological therapy toward an investigational medicinal product. Overall low toxicity of EVs has been demonstrated in several phase I clinical trials [154–157]. Labeling of EVs is mandatory for biodistribution studies if in vivo tracking of unlabeled EVs is not feasible in the relevant disease-specific animal models. Besides clinically approved radioisotopes, superparamagnetic particle loading is an alternative to investigating the distribution of EVs after application [149].

Validated in vitro and in vivo potency assays are necessary to systematically evaluate the expected biological activity and/or therapeutic potency in adequate models [149]. Depending on the disease and envisaged clinical application, potency assays, proof-of-concept, and application modes need thorough consideration and investigation. Of course, information about the therapeutically active substance of such complex novel biological therapies and the mode of action would help to accelerate translation to the clinic. Unfortunately, the molecules responsible for efficacy in the inner ear and EV mode of action are incompletely understood. Before the completion of the phase 2 clinical trial, there is no necessity to fully characterize and identify the active substance or to provide a detailed concept about the mode of action of an investigational medicinal product [147,158]. Outcome measures need not only be defined for planned clinical trials but also included as endpoints in preclinical experiments for an improved transfer and comparability. To this aim, an early and repeatedly seeking of advice from the responsible national and international authorities is highly recommended.

Partnerships between approving authorities, academia, and industry should be considered to pave and accelerate the road to the clinic for vesicle-based therapeutics. The International Society for Extracellular Vesicles ISEV has therefore built a "Task Force on Regulatory Affairs and Clinical Use of EV-based Therapeutics" to identify existing or develop novel applicable regulatory guidance [159]. The aim is to provide a safe and efficient evaluation of EVs in clinical trials for an evidence-based application of EV therapeutics for various pathological conditions.

10. Conclusions

The development of EV-based therapeutics in all fields, especially in neurotology, is on the rise and offers vast unexploited potential. Scalable and reproducible purification protocols are already available based on robust data and qualified potency assays in disease-specific in vitro and in vivo models. Following regulatory requirements and GMP compliance, high-quality clinical trials are rising in other medical fields. As such, EV products will be available for clinical use in the near future (Figure 1). Following the philosophy that "the developmental process is indeed the product", each manufacturing step of EV-therapeutics needs to be standardized as much as possible. Thus, with the patient's benefit in mind, joined efforts of regulatory authorities, academic experts, and biotechnological manufacturing teams can address the unmet clinical needs and will hopefully lead to a new era for treating acute and chronic diseases, especially in neurotology.

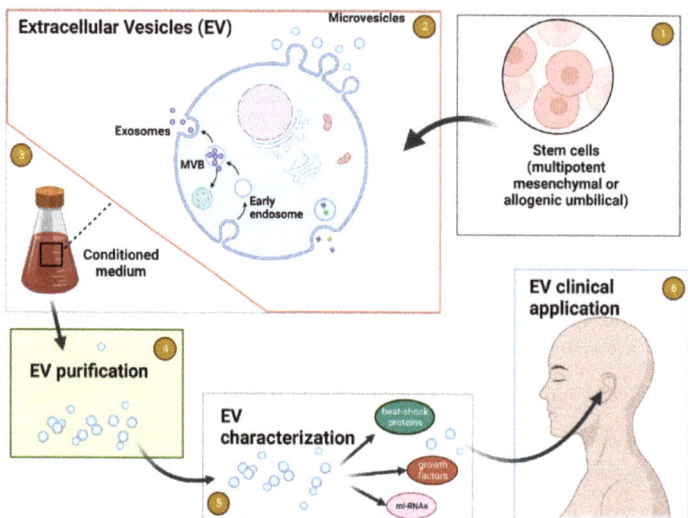

Figure 1. Schematic flow of EV production for medicinal use in Neurotology. (1) Establishing the cell source for EV. (2) Cells release the EV 3 to the tissue culture media. (3) Collection of the conditioned medium. (4) EVs purification. (5) EVs characterization. (6) Clinical application of purified and characterized EVs for the inner ear conditions. Created with BioRender.com.

Author Contributions: Conceptualization, A.W. and H.S.; methodology, A.W.; data curation, A.W., H.S., A.G., E.R., M.G., T.L., A.J.S., A.D.S. and I.H.; writing—original draft preparation, A.W.; writing—review and editing, H.S., A.G., E.R., M.G., T.L., A.J.S., A.D.S. and I.H.; visualization, A.J.S.; supervision, T.L. All authors have read and agreed to the published version of the manuscript.

Funding: This research received no external funding.

Institutional Review Board Statement: Not applicable.

Informed Consent Statement: Not applicable.

Data Availability Statement: The data are available upon request from the corresponding author.

Conflicts of Interest: The authors declare no conflict of interest.

References

1. WHO. 10 Facts about Deafness. Available online: http://www.who.int/features/factfiles/deafness/en/ (accessed on 5 October 2022).
2. WHO. Deafness and Hearing Loss Fact Sheet. 2018. Available online: https://www.who.int/news-room/fact-sheets/detail/deafness-and-hearing-loss (accessed on 5 October 2022).
3. Livingston, G.; Sommerlad, A.; Orgeta, V.; Costafreda, S.G.; Huntley, J.; Ames, D.; Ballard, C.; Banerjee, S.; Burns, A.; Cohen-Mansfield, J.; et al. Dementia prevention, intervention, and care. *Lancet* **2017**, *390*, 2673–2734. [CrossRef] [PubMed]
4. Di Stadio, A.; Ralli, M.; Roccamatisi, D.; Scarpa, A.; Della Volpe, A.; Cassandro, C.; Ricci, G.; Greco, A.; Bernitsas, E. Hearing loss and dementia: Radiologic and biomolecular basis of their shared characteristics. A systematic review. *Neurol. Sci.* **2021**, *42*, 579–588. [CrossRef]
5. Bisogno, A.; Scarpa, A.; Di Girolamo, S.; De Luca, P.; Cassandro, C.; Viola, P.; Ricciardiello, F.; Greco, A.; De Vincentiis, M.; Ralli, M.; et al. Hearing Loss and Cognitive Impairment: Epidemiology, Common Pathophysiological Findings, and Treatment Considerations. *Life* **2021**, *11*, 1102. [CrossRef]
6. Izumikawa, M.; Batts, S.A.; Miyazawa, T.; Swiderski, D.L.; Raphael, Y. Response of the flat cochlear epithelium to forced expression of Atoh1. *Hear. Res.* **2008**, *240*, 52–56. [CrossRef]
7. He, L.; Guo, J.-Y.; Liu, K.; Wang, G.-P.; Gong, S.-S. Research Progress on Flat Epithelium of the Inner Ear. *Physiol. Res.* **2020**, *69*, 775. [CrossRef] [PubMed]
8. Korkmaz, M.H.; Bayır, Ö.; Er, S.; Işık, E.; Saylam, G.; Tatar, E.; Özdek, A. Satisfaction and compliance of adult patients using hearing aid and evaluation of factors affecting them. *Eur. Arch. Oto-Rhino-Laryngology* **2016**, *273*, 3723–3732. [CrossRef] [PubMed]
9. Salonen, J.; Johansson, R.; Karjalainen, S.; Vahlberg, T.; Jero, J.P.; Isoaho, R. Hearing aid compliance in the elderly. *B-ENT* **2013**, *9*, 23–28.
10. von Ilberg, C.A.; Baumann, U.; Kiefer, J.; Tillein, J.; Adunka, O.F. Electric-Acoustic Stimulation of the Auditory System: A Review of the First Decade. *Audiol. Neurotol.* **2011**, *16*, 1–30. [CrossRef]
11. Vonilberg, C.; Kiefer, J.; Tillein, J.; Pfenningdorff, T.; Hartmann, R.; Stürzebecher, E.; Klinke, R. Electric-Acoustic Stimulation of the Auditory System: New technology for severe hearing loss. *ORL* **1999**, *61*, 334–340. [CrossRef]
12. Büchner, A.; Illg, A.; Majdani, O.; Lenarz, T. Investigation of the effect of cochlear implant electrode length on speech comprehension in quiet and noise compared with the results with users of electro-acoustic-stimulation, a retrospective analysis. *PLoS ONE* **2017**, *12*, e0174900. [CrossRef]
13. Hochmair, I.; Nopp, P.; Jolly, C.; Schmidt, M.; Schösser, H.; Garnham, C.; Anderson, I. MED-EL Cochlear Implants: State of the Art and a Glimpse into the Future. *Trends Amplif.* **2006**, *10*, 201–219. [CrossRef] [PubMed]
14. Maria, P.L.S.; Gluth, M.B.; Yuan, Y.; Atlas, M.D.; Blevins, N.H. Hearing Preservation Surgery for Cochlear Implantation. *Otol. Neurotol.* **2014**, *35*, e256–e269. [CrossRef] [PubMed]
15. Sansbury, B.E.; Spite, M. Resolution of Acute Inflammation and the Role of Resolvins in Immunity, Thrombosis, and Vascular Biology. *Circ. Res.* **2016**, *119*, 113–130. [CrossRef] [PubMed]
16. Sugimoto, M.A.; Sousa, L.P.; Pinho, V.; Perretti, M.; Teixeira, M.M. Resolution of Inflammation: What Controls Its Onset? *Front. Immunol.* **2016**, *7*, 160. [CrossRef] [PubMed]
17. Serhan, C.N.; Gupta, S.K.; Perretti, M.; Godson, C.; Brennan, E.; Li, Y.; Soehnlein, O.; Shimizu, T.; Werz, O.; Chiurchiù, V.; et al. The Atlas of Inflammation Resolution (AIR). *Mol. Asp. Med.* **2020**, *74*, 100894. [CrossRef]
18. Kalinec, G.M.; Lomberk, G.; Urrutia, R.A.; Kalinec, F. Resolution of Cochlear Inflammation: Novel Target for Preventing or Ameliorating Drug-, Noise- and Age-related Hearing Loss. *Front. Cell. Neurosci.* **2017**, *11*, 192. [CrossRef]
19. Furness, D.N. Molecular basis of hair cell loss. *Cell Tissue Res.* **2015**, *361*, 387–399. [CrossRef]
20. Böttger, E.C.; Schacht, J. The mitochondrion: A perpetrator of acquired hearing loss. *Hear. Res.* **2013**, *303*, 12–19. [CrossRef]
21. Yang, C.-H.; Schrepfer, T.; Schacht, J. Age-related hearing impairment and the triad of acquired hearing loss. *Front. Cell. Neurosci.* **2015**, *9*, 276. [CrossRef]
22. Calabrese, V.; Cornelius, C.; Maiolino, L.; Luca, M.; Chiaramonte, R.; A Toscano, M.; Serra, A. Oxidative Stress, Redox Homeostasis and Cellular Stress Response in Ménière's Disease: Role of Vitagenes. *Neurochem. Res.* **2010**, *35*, 2208–2217. [CrossRef]

23. Kurabi, A.; Keithley, E.M.; Housley, G.D.; Ryan, A.F.; Wong, A.C.-Y. Cellular mechanisms of noise-induced hearing loss. *Hear. Res.* **2017**, *349*, 129–137. [CrossRef] [PubMed]
24. Medzhitov, R. Origin and physiological roles of inflammation. *Nature* **2008**, *454*, 428–435. [CrossRef] [PubMed]
25. Choung, Y.; Taura, A.; Pak, K.; Choi, S.; Masuda, M.; Ryan, A. Generation of highly-reactive oxygen species is closely related to hair cell damage in rat organ of corti treated with gentamicin. *Neuroscience* **2009**, *161*, 214–226. [CrossRef]
26. Yamane, H.; Nakai, Y.; Takayama, M.; Iguchi, H.; Nakagawa, T.; Kojima, A. Appearance of free radicals in the guinea pig inner ear after noise-induced acoustic trauma. *Eur. Arch. Oto-Rhino-Laryngol.* **1995**, *252*, 504–508. [CrossRef] [PubMed]
27. Kamogashira, T.; Fujimoto, C.; Yamasoba, T. Reactive Oxygen Species, Apoptosis, and Mitochondrial Dysfunction in Hearing Loss. *BioMed Res. Int.* **2015**, *2015*, 1–7. [CrossRef] [PubMed]
28. Wong, A.C.; Ryan, A.F. Mechanisms of sensorineural cell damage, death and survival in the cochlea. *Front. Aging Neurosci.* **2015**, *7*, 58. [CrossRef] [PubMed]
29. Eshraghi, A.A.; Van De Water, T.R. Cochlear implantation trauma and noise-induced hearing loss: Apoptosis and therapeutic strategies. *Anat. Rec. Part A Discov. Mol. Cell. Evol. Biol.* **2006**, *288*, 473–481. [CrossRef]
30. Bas, E.; Gupta, C.; Van De Water, T.R. A Novel Organ of Corti Explant Model for the Study of Cochlear Implantation Trauma. *Anat. Rec.* **2012**, *295*, 1944–1956. [CrossRef]
31. de Beeck, K.O.; Schacht, J.; Van Camp, G. Apoptosis in acquired and genetic hearing impairment: The programmed death of the hair cell. *Hear. Res.* **2011**, *281*, 18–27. [CrossRef]
32. Bas, E.; Goncalves, S.; Adams, M.; Dinh, C.T.; Bas, J.M.; Van De Water, T.R.; Eshraghi, A.A. Spiral ganglion cells and macrophages initiate neuro-inflammation and scarring following cochlear implantation. *Front. Cell. Neurosci.* **2015**, *9*, 303. [CrossRef]
33. Seyyedi, M.; Nadol, J.B. Intracochlear Inflammatory Response to Cochlear Implant Electrodes in Humans. *Otol. Neurotol.* **2014**, *35*, 1545–1551. [CrossRef] [PubMed]
34. Quesnel, A.M.; Nakajima, H.H.; Rosowski, J.J.; Hansen, M.R.; Gantz, B.J.; Nadol, J.B. Delayed loss of hearing after hearing preservation cochlear implantation: Human temporal bone pathology and implications for etiology. *Hear. Res.* **2015**, *333*, 225–234. [CrossRef] [PubMed]
35. Ishai, R.; Herrmann, B.S.; Nadol, J.B.; Quesnel, A.M. The pattern and degree of capsular fibrous sheaths surrounding cochlear electrode arrays. *Hear. Res.* **2017**, *348*, 44–53. [CrossRef]
36. Clark, G.M.; Clark, J.; Cardamone, T.; Clarke, M.; Nielsen, P.; Jones, R.; Arhatari, B.; Birbilis, N.; Curtain, R.; Xu, J.; et al. Biomedical studies on temporal bones of the first multi-channel cochlear implant patient at the University of Melbourne. *Cochlea- Implant. Int.* **2014**, *15*, S1–S15. [CrossRef] [PubMed]
37. Somdas, M.A.; Li, P.M.; Whiten, D.M.; Eddington, D.K.; Nadol, J.J.B. Quantitative Evaluation of New Bone and Fibrous Tissue in the Cochlea following Cochlear Implantation in the Human. *Audiol. Neurotol.* **2007**, *12*, 277–284. [CrossRef]
38. Astolfi, L.; Simoni, E.; Giarbini, N.; Giordano, P.; Pannella, M.; Hatzopoulos, S.; Martini, A. Cochlear implant and inflammation reaction: Safety study of a new steroid-eluting electrode. *Hear. Res.* **2016**, *336*, 44–52. [CrossRef]
39. Gao, J.; Yi, H. Molecular mechanisms and roles of inflammatory responses on low-frequency residual hearing after cochlear implantation. *J. Otol.* **2021**, *17*, 54–58. [CrossRef]
40. Tanaka, C.; Nguyen-Huynh, A.; Loera, K.; Stark, G.; Reiss, L. Factors associated with hearing loss in a normal-hearing guinea pig model of hybrid cochlear implants. *Hear. Res.* **2014**, *316*, 82–93. [CrossRef]
41. Okano, T. Immune system of the inner ear as a novel therapeutic target for sensorineural hearing loss. *Front. Pharmacol.* **2014**, *5*, 205. [CrossRef]
42. Tan, W.J.T.; Thorne, P.R.; Vlajkovic, S.M. Characterisation of cochlear inflammation in mice following acute and chronic noise exposure. *Histochem. Cell Biol.* **2016**, *146*, 219–230. [CrossRef]
43. Merchant, S.N.; Adams, J.C.; Nadol, J.B. Pathology and Pathophysiology of Idiopathic Sudden Sensorineural Hearing Loss. *Otol. Neurotol.* **2005**, *26*, 151–160. [CrossRef] [PubMed]
44. Fuentes-Santamaría, V.; Alvarado, J.C.; Melgar-Rojas, P.; Gabaldón-Ull, M.C.; Miller, J.M.; Juiz, J.M. The Role of Glia in the Peripheral and Central Auditory System Following Noise Overexposure: Contribution of TNF-α and IL-1β to the Pathogenesis of Hearing Loss. *Front. Neuroanat.* **2017**, *11*, 9. [CrossRef] [PubMed]
45. Ladrech, S.; Wang, J.; Simonneau, L.; Puel, J.-L.; Lenoir, M. Macrophage contribution to the response of the rat organ of Corti to amikacin. *J. Neurosci. Res.* **2007**, *85*, 1970–1979. [CrossRef]
46. Sun, S.; Yu, H.; Yu, H.; Honglin, M.; Ni, W.; Zhang, Y.; Guo, L.; He, Y.; Xue, Z.; Ni, Y.; et al. Inhibition of the Activation and Recruitment of Microglia-Like Cells Protects Against Neomycin-Induced Ototoxicity. *Mol. Neurobiol.* **2014**, *51*, 252–267. [CrossRef]
47. Tsinaslanidou, Z.; Tsaligopoulos, M.; Angouridakis, N.; Vital, V.; Kekes, G.; Constantinidis, J. The Expression of TNFα, IL-6, IL-2 and IL-8 in the Serum of Patients with Idiopathic Sudden Sensorineural Hearing Loss: Possible Prognostic Factors of Response to Corticosteroid Treatment. *Audiol. Neurotol. Extra* **2016**, *6*, 9–19. [CrossRef]
48. Yoon, S.H.; E Kim, M.; Kim, H.Y.; Lee, J.S.; Jang, C.H. Inflammatory cytokines and mononuclear cells in sudden sensorineural hearing loss. *J. Laryngol. Otol.* **2019**, *133*, 95–101. [CrossRef] [PubMed]
49. Fullerton, J.N.; Gilroy, D.W. Resolution of inflammation: A new therapeutic frontier. *Nat. Rev. Drug Discov.* **2016**, *15*, 551–567. [CrossRef] [PubMed]

50. Mugisho, O.O.; Green, C.R.; Kho, D.T.; Zhang, J.; Graham, E.S.; Acosta, M.L.; Rupenthal, I.D. The inflammasome pathway is amplified and perpetuated in an autocrine manner through connexin43 hemichannel mediated ATP release. *Biochim. Biophys. Acta Gen. Subj.* **2018**, *1862*, 385–393. [CrossRef]
51. Anselmi, F.; Hernandez, V.H.; Crispino, G.; Seydel, A.; Ortolano, S.; Roper, S.D.; Kessaris, N.; Richardson, W.; Rickheit, G.; Filippov, M.A.; et al. ATP release through connexin hemichannels and gap junction transfer of second messengers propagate Ca^{2+} signals across the inner ear. *Proc. Natl. Acad. Sci. USA* **2008**, *105*, 18770–18775. [CrossRef]
52. Zhao, H.-B.; Yu, N.; Fleming, C.R. Gap junctional hemichannel-mediated ATP release and hearing controls in the inner ear. *Proc. Natl. Acad. Sci. USA* **2005**, *102*, 18724–18729. [CrossRef]
53. Muñoz, D.J.; Thorne, P.R.; Housley, G.D.; Billett, T.E.; Battersby, J.M. Extracellular adenosine 5′-triphosphate (ATP) in the endolymphatic compartment influences cochlear function. *Hear. Res.* **1995**, *90*, 106–118. [CrossRef] [PubMed]
54. Wong, H.-T.C.; Zhang, Q.; Beirl, A.J.; Petralia, R.S.; Wang, Y.-X.; Kindt, K. Synaptic mitochondria regulate hair-cell synapse size and function. *eLife* **2019**, *8*, e48914. [CrossRef] [PubMed]
55. Stankiewicz, T.R.; Gray, J.J.; Winter, A.N.; Linseman, D.A. C-terminal binding proteins: Central players in development and disease. *Biomol. Concepts* **2014**, *5*, 489–511. [CrossRef]
56. Thio, S.S.C. The CtBP2 co-repressor is regulated by NADH-dependent dimerization and possesses a novel N-terminal repression domain. *Nucleic Acids Res.* **2004**, *32*, 1836–1847. [CrossRef]
57. Naganawa, S.; Yamazaki, M.; Kawai, H.; Bokura, K.; Sone, M.; Nakashima, T. Imaging of Ménière's Disease after Intravenous Administration of Single-dose Gadodiamide: Utility of Multiplication of MR Cisternography and HYDROPS Image. *Magn. Reson. Med Sci.* **2013**, *12*, 63–68. [CrossRef] [PubMed]
58. Eliezer, M.; Maquet, C.; Horion, J.; Gillibert, A.; Toupet, M.; Bolognini, B.; Magne, N.; Kahn, L.; Hautefort, C.; Attyé, A. Detection of intralabyrinthine abnormalities using post-contrast delayed 3D-FLAIR MRI sequences in patients with acute vestibular syndrome. *Eur. Radiol.* **2018**, *29*, 2760–2769. [CrossRef]
59. Laine, J.; Hautefort, C.; Attye, A.; Guichard, J.-P.; Herman, P.; Houdart, E.; Fraysse, M.-J.; Fraysse, B.; Gillibert, A.; Kania, R.; et al. MRI evaluation of the endolymphatic space in otosclerosis and correlation with clinical findings. *Diagn. Interv. Imaging* **2020**, *101*, 537–545. [CrossRef]
60. Reiss, L.A.; Stark, G.; Nguyen-Huynh, A.T.; Spear, K.A.; Zhang, H.; Tanaka, C.; Li, H. Morphological correlates of hearing loss after cochlear implantation and electro-acoustic stimulation in a hearing-impaired Guinea pig model. *Hear. Res.* **2015**, *327*, 163–174. [CrossRef]
61. Kopelovich, J.C.; Reiss, L.; Etler, C.P.; Xu, L.; Bertroche, J.T.; Gantz, B.; Hansen, M.R. Hearing Loss After Activation of Hearing Preservation Cochlear Implants Might Be Related to Afferent Cochlear Innervation Injury. *Otol. Neurotol.* **2015**, *36*, 1035–1044. [CrossRef]
62. Peter, M.N.; Paasche, G.; Reich, U.; Lenarz, T.; Warnecke, A. Reaktionen im Corti-Organ auf elektrische Stimulation: StED technology for detecting changes. *HNO* **2019**, *67*, 251–257. [CrossRef]
63. Peter, M.N.; Warnecke, A.; Reich, U.; Olze, H.; Szczepek, A.J.; Lenarz, T.; Paasche, G. Influence of In Vitro Electrical Stimulation on Survival of Spiral Ganglion Neurons. *Neurotox. Res.* **2019**, *36*, 204–216. [CrossRef] [PubMed]
64. Peter, M.N.; Paasche, G.; Reich, U.; Lenarz, T.; Warnecke, A. Differential Effects of Low- and High-Dose Dexamethasone on Electrically Induced Damage of the Cultured Organ of Corti. *Neurotox. Res.* **2020**, *38*, 487–497. [CrossRef] [PubMed]
65. Shen, N.; Liang, Q.; Liu, Y.; Lai, B.; Li, W.; Wang, Z.; Li, S. Charge-balanced biphasic electrical stimulation inhibits neurite extension of spiral ganglion neurons. *Neurosci. Lett.* **2016**, *624*, 92–99. [CrossRef] [PubMed]
66. Shen, N.; Zhou, L.; Lai, B.; Li, S. The Influence of Cochlear Implant-Based Electric Stimulation on the Electrophysiological Characteristics of Cultured Spiral Ganglion Neurons. *Neural Plast.* **2020**, *2020*, e3108490. [CrossRef]
67. Teng, F.; Fussenegger, M. Shedding Light on Extracellular Vesicle Biogenesis and Bioengineering. *Adv. Sci.* **2020**, *8*, e202003505. [CrossRef]
68. Abels, E.R.; Breakefield, X.O. Introduction to Extracellular Vesicles: Biogenesis, RNA Cargo Selection, Content, Release, and Uptake. *Cell. Mol. Neurobiol.* **2016**, *36*, 301–312. [CrossRef]
69. Brennan, K.; Martin, K.; Fitzgerald, S.P.; O'Sullivan, J.; Wu, Y.; Blanco, A.; Richardson, C.; Mc Gee, M.M. A comparison of methods for the isolation and separation of extracellular vesicles from protein and lipid particles in human serum. *Sci. Rep.* **2020**, *10*, 1039. [CrossRef]
70. Crescitelli, R.; Lässer, C.; Lötvall, J. Isolation and characterization of extracellular vesicle subpopulations from tissues. *Nat. Protoc.* **2021**, *16*, 1548–1580. [CrossRef]
71. Dai, J.; Su, Y.; Zhong, S.; Cong, L.; Liu, B.; Yang, J.; Tao, Y.; He, Z.; Chen, C.; Jiang, Y. Exosomes: Key players in cancer and potential therapeutic strategy. *Signal Transduct. Target. Ther.* **2020**, *5*, 145. [CrossRef]
72. Lan, J.; Sun, L.; Xu, F.; Liu, L.; Hu, F.; Song, D.; Hou, Z.; Wu, W.; Luo, X.; Wang, J.; et al. M2 Macrophage-Derived Exosomes Promote Cell Migration and Invasion in Colon Cancer. *Cancer Res* **2019**, *79*, 146–158. [CrossRef]
73. Chen, W.; Jiang, J.; Xia, W.; Huang, J. Tumor-Related Exosomes Contribute to Tumor-Promoting Microenvironment: An Immunological Perspective. *J. Immunol. Res.* **2017**, *2017*, e1073947. [CrossRef] [PubMed]
74. Hosseinikhah, S.M.; Gheybi, F.; Moosavian, S.A.; Shahbazi, M.-A.; Jaafari, M.R.; Sillanpää, M.; Kesharwani, P.; Alavizadeh, S.H.; Sahebkar, A. Role of exosomes in tumour growth, chemoresistance and immunity: State-of-the-art. *J. Drug Target.* **2022**, *21*, e2114000. [CrossRef] [PubMed]

75. Maligianni, I.; Yapijakis, C.; Nousia, K.; Bacopoulou, F.; Chrousos, G.P. Exosomes and exosomal non-coding RNAs throughout human gestation (Review). *Exp. Ther. Med.* **2022**, *24*, e11518. [CrossRef] [PubMed]
76. Sun, L.; Li, D.; Song, K.; Wei, J.; Yao, S.; Li, Z.; Su, X.; Ju, X.; Chao, L.; Deng, X.; et al. Exosomes derived from human umbilical cord mesenchymal stem cells protect against cisplatin-induced ovarian granulosa cell stress and apoptosis in vitro. *Sci. Rep.* **2017**, *7*, 2552. [CrossRef]
77. Joerger-Messerli, M.S.; Oppliger, B.; Spinelli, M.; Thomi, G.; Di Salvo, I.; Schneider, P.; Schoeberlein, A. Extracellular Vesicles Derived from Wharton's Jelly Mesenchymal Stem Cells Prevent and Resolve Programmed Cell Death Mediated by Perinatal Hypoxia-Ischemia in Neuronal Cells. *Cell Transplant.* **2018**, *27*, 168–180. [CrossRef]
78. Huang, Y.-J.; Cao, J.; Lee, C.-Y.; Wu, Y.-M. Umbilical cord blood plasma-derived exosomes as a novel therapy to reverse liver fibrosis. *Stem Cell Res. Ther.* **2021**, *12*, 1–13. [CrossRef]
79. Kolios, G.; Paspaliaris, V. Mesenchyme Stem Cell-Derived Conditioned Medium as a Potential Therapeutic Tool in Idiopathic Pulmonary Fibrosis. *Biomedicines* **2022**, *10*, 2298. [CrossRef]
80. Li, T.; Yan, Y.; Wang, B.; Qian, H.; Zhang, X.; Shen, L.; Wang, M.; Zhou, Y.; Zhu, W.; Li, W.; et al. Exosomes Derived from Human Umbilical Cord Mesenchymal Stem Cells Alleviate Liver Fibrosis. *Stem Cells Dev.* **2013**, *22*, 845–854. [CrossRef]
81. Burger, D.; Viñas, J.L.; Akbari, S.; Dehak, H.; Knoll, W.; Gutsol, A.; Carter, A.; Touyz, R.M.; Allan, D.S.; Burns, K.D. Human endothelial colony-forming cells protect against acute kidney injury: Role of exosomes. *Am. J. Pathol.* **2015**, *185*, 2309–2323. [CrossRef]
82. Li, L.; Mu, J.; Zhang, Y.; Zhang, C.; Ma, T.; Chen, L.; Huang, T.; Wu, J.; Cao, J.; Feng, S.; et al. Stimulation by Exosomes from Hypoxia Preconditioned Human Umbilical Vein Endothelial Cells Facilitates Mesenchymal Stem Cells Angiogenic Function for Spinal Cord Repair. *ACS Nano* **2022**, *16*, 10811–10823. [CrossRef]
83. Dong, B.; Wang, C.; Zhang, J.; Zhang, J.; Gu, Y.; Guo, X.; Zuo, X.; Pan, H.; Hsu, A.C.-Y.; Wang, G.; et al. Exosomes from human umbilical cord mesenchymal stem cells attenuate the inflammation of severe steroid-resistant asthma by reshaping macrophage polarization. *Stem Cell Res. Ther.* **2021**, *12*, 1–17. [CrossRef] [PubMed]
84. Baharlooi, H.; Salehi, Z.; Moeini, M.M.; Rezaei, N.; Azimi, M. Immunomodulatory Potential of Human Mesenchymal Stem Cells and their Exosomes on Multiple Sclerosis. *Adv. Pharm. Bull.* **2021**, *12*, 389–397. [CrossRef] [PubMed]
85. Rodrigues, S.C.; Cardoso, R.M.S.; Freire, P.C.; Gomes, C.F.; Duarte, F.V.; das Neves, R.P.; Simões-Correia, J. Immunomodulatory Properties of Umbilical Cord Blood-Derived Small Extracellular Vesicles and Their Therapeutic Potential for Inflammatory Skin Disorders. *Int. J. Mol. Sci.* **2021**, *22*, 9797. [CrossRef] [PubMed]
86. Baharlooi, H.; Nouraei, Z.; Azimi, M.; Moghadasi, A.N.; Tavassolifar, M.J.; Moradi, B.; Sahraian, M.A.; Izad, M. Umbilical cord mesenchymal stem cells as well as their released exosomes suppress proliferation of activated PBMCs in multiple sclerosis. *Scand. J. Immunol.* **2020**, *93*, e13013. [CrossRef]
87. Song, Y.; Dou, H.; Li, X.; Zhao, X.; Li, Y.; Liu, D.; Ji, J.; Liu, F.; Ding, L.; Ni, Y.; et al. Exosomal miR-146a Contributes to the Enhanced Therapeutic Efficacy of Interleukin-1β-Primed Mesenchymal Stem Cells Against Sepsis. *STEM CELLS* **2017**, *35*, 1208–1221. [CrossRef]
88. Taghavi-Farahabadi, M.; Mahmoudi, M.; Rezaei, N.; Hashemi, S.M. Wharton's Jelly Mesenchymal Stem Cells Exosomes and Conditioned Media Increased Neutrophil Lifespan and Phagocytosis Capacity. *Immunol. Investig.* **2020**, *50*, 1042–1057. [CrossRef]
89. Sun, W.; Yan, S.; Yang, C.; Yang, J.; Wang, H.; Li, C.; Zhang, L.; Zhao, L.; Zhang, J.; Cheng, M.; et al. Mesenchymal Stem Cells-derived Exosomes Ameliorate Lupus by Inducing M2 Macrophage Polarization and Regulatory T Cell Expansion in MRL/lpr Mice. *Immunol. Investig.* **2022**, *51*, 1785–1803. [CrossRef]
90. Heidari, N.; Abbasi-Kenarsari, H.; Namaki, S.; Baghaei, K.; Zali, M.R.; Mirsanei, Z.; Hashemi, S.M. Regulation of the Th17/Treg balance by human umbilical cord mesenchymal stem cell-derived exosomes protects against acute experimental colitis. *Exp. Cell Res.* **2022**, *419*, e113296. [CrossRef]
91. Fritzsch, B.; Pirvola, U.; Ylikoski, J. Making and breaking the innervation of the ear: Neurotrophic support during ear development and its clinical implications. *Cell Tissue Res.* **1999**, *295*, 369–382. [CrossRef]
92. Pirvola, U.; Ylikoski, J.; Palgi, J.; Lehtonen, E.; Arumäe, U.; Saarma, M. Brain-derived neurotrophic factor and neurotrophin 3 mRNAs in the peripheral target fields of developing inner ear ganglia. *Proc. Natl. Acad. Sci. USA* **1992**, *89*, 9915–9919. [CrossRef]
93. Bailey, E.M.; Green, S.H. Postnatal Expression of Neurotrophic Factors Accessible to Spiral Ganglion Neurons in the Auditory System of Adult Hearing and Deafened Rats. *J. Neurosci.* **2014**, *34*, 13110–13126. [CrossRef] [PubMed]
94. Lagarde, M.M.M.; Cox, B.C.; Fang, J.; Taylor, R.; Forge, A.; Zuo, J. Selective Ablation of Pillar and Deiters' Cells Severely Affects Cochlear Postnatal Development and Hearing in Mice. *J. Neurosci.* **2013**, *33*, 1564–1576. [CrossRef] [PubMed]
95. May, L.A.; Kramarenko, I.I.; Brandon, C.S.; Voelkel-Johnson, C.; Roy, S.; Truong, K.; Francis, S.P.; Monzack, E.L.; Lee, F.-S.; Cunningham, L.L. Inner ear supporting cells protect hair cells by secreting HSP70. *J. Clin. Investig.* **2013**, *123*, 3577–3587. [CrossRef] [PubMed]
96. Asami, T.; Ito, T.; Fukumitsu, H.; Nomoto, H.; Furukawa, Y.; Furukawa, S. Autocrine activation of cultured macrophages by brain-derived neurotrophic factor. *Biochem. Biophys. Res. Commun.* **2006**, *344*, 941–947. [CrossRef] [PubMed]
97. Lai, S.-W.; Chen, J.-H.; Lin, H.-Y.; Liu, Y.-S.; Tsai, C.-F.; Chang, P.-C.; Lu, D.-Y.; Lin, C. Regulatory Effects of Neuroinflammatory Responses through Brain-Derived Neurotrophic Factor Signaling in Microglial Cells. *Mol. Neurobiol.* **2018**, *55*, 7487–7499. [CrossRef] [PubMed]

98. Kaiser, O.; Paasche, G.; Stöver, T.; Ernst, S.; Lenarz, T.; Kral, A.; Warnecke, A. TGF-beta superfamily member activin A acts with BDNF and erythropoietin to improve survival of spiral ganglion neurons in vitro. *Neuropharmacology* **2013**, *75*, 416–425. [CrossRef]
99. Kranz, K.; Warnecke, A.; Lenarz, T.; Durisin, M.; Scheper, V. Phosphodiesterase Type 4 Inhibitor Rolipram Improves Survival of Spiral Ganglion Neurons In Vitro. *PLoS ONE* **2014**, *9*, e92157. [CrossRef]
100. Schwieger, J.; Warnecke, A.; Lenarz, T.; Esser, K.-H.; Scheper, V. Neuronal Survival, Morphology and Outgrowth of Spiral Ganglion Neurons Using a Defined Growth Factor Combination. *PLoS ONE* **2015**, *10*, e0133680. [CrossRef]
101. Stolle, M.; Schulze, J.; Roemer, A.; Lenarz, T.; Durisin, M.; Warnecke, A. Human Plasma Rich in Growth Factors Improves Survival and Neurite Outgrowth of Spiral Ganglion Neurons In Vitro. *Tissue Eng. Part A* **2018**, *24*, 493–501. [CrossRef]
102. Roemer, A.; Köhl, U.; Majdani, O.; Klöß, S.; Falk, C.; Haumann, S.; Lenarz, T.; Kral, A.; Warnecke, A. Biohybrid cochlear implants in human neurosensory restoration. *Stem Cell Res. Ther.* **2016**, *7*, 1–14. [CrossRef]
103. Reis, M.; Mavin, E.; Nicholson, L.; Green, K.; Dickinson, A.M.; Wang, X.-N. Mesenchymal Stromal Cell-Derived Extracellular Vesicles Attenuate Dendritic Cell Maturation and Function. *Front. Immunol.* **2018**, *9*, 2538. [CrossRef] [PubMed]
104. Malvicini, R.; Santa-Cruz, D.; De Lazzari, G.; Tolomeo, A.M.; Sanmartin, C.; Muraca, M.; Yannarelli, G.; Pacienza, N. Macrophage bioassay standardization to assess the anti-inflammatory activity of mesenchymal stromal cell-derived small extracellular vesicles. *Cytotherapy* **2022**, *24*, 999–1012. [CrossRef] [PubMed]
105. Bouchareychas, L.; Duong, P.; Phu, T.A.; Alsop, E.; Meechoovet, B.; Reiman, R.; Ng, M.; Yamamoto, R.; Nakauchi, H.; Gasper, W.J.; et al. High glucose macrophage exosomes enhance atherosclerosis by driving cellular proliferation & hematopoiesis. *iScience* **2021**, *24*, e102847. [CrossRef]
106. Orecchioni, M.; Ghosheh, Y.; Pramod, A.B.; Ley, K. Macrophage Polarization: Different Gene Signatures in M1(LPS+) vs. Classically and M2(LPS−) vs. Alternatively Activated Macrophages. *Front. Immunol.* **2019**, *10*, 1084. [CrossRef]
107. Gerrick, K.Y.; Gerrick, E.R.; Gupta, A.; Wheelan, S.J.; Yegnasubramanian, S.; Jaffee, E.M. Transcriptional profiling identifies novel regulators of macrophage polarization. *PLoS ONE* **2018**, *13*, e0208602. [CrossRef]
108. Celik, M.; Labuz, D.; Keye, J.; Glauben, R.; Machelska, H. IL-4 induces M2 macrophages to produce sustained analgesia via opioids. *JCI Insight* **2020**, *5*, e133093. [CrossRef]
109. Phu, T.A.; Ng, M.; Vu, N.K.; Bouchareychas, L.; Raffai, R.L. IL-4 polarized human macrophage exosomes control cardiometabolic inflammation and diabetes in obesity. *Mol. Ther.* **2022**, *30*, 2274–2297. [CrossRef]
110. Huang, C.; Wang, Y.; Li, X.; Ren, L.; Zhao, J.; Hu, Y.; Zhang, L.; Fan, G.; Xu, J.; Gu, X.; et al. Clinical features of patients infected with 2019 novel coronavirus in Wuhan, China. *Lancet* **2020**, *395*, 497–506. [CrossRef]
111. Coperchini, F.; Chiovato, L.; Croce, L.; Magri, F.; Rotondi, M. The cytokine storm in COVID-19: An overview of the involvement of the chemokine/chemokine-receptor system. *Cytokine Growth Factor Rev.* **2020**, *53*, 25–32. [CrossRef]
112. Chen, J.; Li, C.; Liang, Z.; Li, C.; Li, Y.; Zhao, Z.; Qiu, T.; Hao, H.; Niu, R.; Chen, L. Human mesenchymal stromal cells small extracellular vesicles attenuate sepsis-induced acute lung injury in a mouse model: The role of oxidative stress and the mitogen-activated protein kinase/nuclear factor kappa B pathway. *Cytotherapy* **2021**, *23*, 918–930. [CrossRef]
113. Xu, Z.; Huang, Y.; Zhou, J.; Deng, X.; He, W.; Liu, X.; Li, Y.; Zhong, N.; Sang, L. Current Status of Cell-Based Therapies for COVID-19: Evidence from Mesenchymal Stromal Cells in Sepsis and ARDS. *Front. Immunol.* **2021**, *12*, e738697. [CrossRef] [PubMed]
114. Alp, E.; Gonen, Z.B.; Gundogan, K.; Esmaoglu, A.; Kaynar, L.; Cetin, A.; Karakukcu, M.; Cetin, M.; Kalin, G.; Doganay, M. The Effect of Mesenchymal Stromal Cells on the Mortality of Patients with Sepsis and Septic Shock: A Promising Therapy. *Emerg. Med. Int.* **2022**, *2022*, e9222379. [CrossRef] [PubMed]
115. Wang, Y.; Liu, S.; Li, L.; Li, L.; Zhou, X.; Wan, M.; Lou, P.; Zhao, M.; Lv, K.; Yuan, Y.; et al. Peritoneal M2 macrophage-derived extracellular vesicles as natural multitarget nanotherapeutics to attenuate cytokine storms after severe infections. *J. Control. Release* **2022**, *349*, 118–132. [CrossRef] [PubMed]
116. Karki, R.; Kanneganti, T.-D. The 'cytokine storm': Molecular mechanisms and therapeutic prospects. *Trends Immunol.* **2021**, *42*, 681–705. [CrossRef]
117. Faulkner, L.; Cooper, A.; Fantino, C.; Altmann, D.; Sriskandan, S. The Mechanism of Superantigen-Mediated Toxic Shock: Not a Simple Th1 Cytokine Storm. *J. Immunol.* **2005**, *175*, 6870–6877. [CrossRef]
118. Chung, K.F. Cytokines in chronic obstructive pulmonary disease. *Eur. Respir. J. Suppl.* **2001**, *34*, 50s–59s. [CrossRef]
119. Hansbro, P.M.; Kaiko, G.E.; Foster, P.S. Cytokine/anti-cytokine therapy—Novel treatments for asthma? *Br. J. Pharmacol.* **2011**, *163*, 81–95. [CrossRef]
120. Karimkhani, C.; Dellavalle, R.P.; Coffeng, L.E.; Flohr, C.; Hay, R.J.; Langan, S.; Nsoesie, E.O.; Ferrari, A.; Erskine, H.E.; Silverberg, J.I.; et al. Global Skin Disease Morbidity and Mortality: An Update from the Global Burden of Disease Study 2013. *JAMA Dermatol.* **2017**, *153*, 406–412. [CrossRef]
121. Nylander, A.; Hafler, D.A. Multiple sclerosis. *J. Clin. Investig.* **2012**, *122*, 1180–1188. [CrossRef]
122. Xia, C.; Dai, Z.; Jin, Y.; Chen, P. Emerging Antioxidant Paradigm of Mesenchymal Stem Cell-Derived Exosome Therapy. *Front. Endocrinol.* **2021**, *12*, e727272. [CrossRef]
123. Žėkas, V.; Kurg, R.; Kurg, K.; Bironaitė, D.; Radzevičius, M.; Karčiauskaitė, D.; Matuzevičienė, R.; Kučinskienė, Z.A. Oxidative Properties of Blood-Derived Extracellular Vesicles in 15 Patients After Myocardial Infarction. *J. Pharmacol. Exp. Ther.* **2022**, *28*, e935291. [CrossRef] [PubMed]

124. Huber, C.C.; Callegari, E.A.; Paez, M.D.; Romanova, S.; Wang, H. Heat Shock-Induced Extracellular Vesicles Derived from Neural Stem Cells Confer Marked Neuroprotection Against Oxidative Stress and Amyloid-β-Caused Neurotoxicity. *Mol. Neurobiol.* **2022**, *59*, 7404–7412. [CrossRef] [PubMed]
125. Mao, C.-Y.; Zhang, T.-T.; Li, D.-J.; Zhou, E.; Fan, Y.-Q.; He, Q.; Wang, C.-Q.; Zhang, J.-F. Extracellular vesicles from hypoxia-preconditioned mesenchymal stem cells alleviates myocardial injury by targeting thioredoxin-interacting protein-mediated hypoxia-inducible factor-1α pathway. *World J. Stem Cells* **2022**, *14*, 183–199. [CrossRef] [PubMed]
126. Domingues, A.; Jolibois, J.; de Rougé, P.M.; Nivet-Antoine, V. The Emerging Role of TXNIP in Ischemic and Cardiovascular Diseases; A Novel Marker and Therapeutic Target. *Int. J. Mol. Sci.* **2021**, *22*, 1693. [CrossRef]
127. Bitirim, C.V.; Ozer, Z.B.; Aydos, D.; Genc, K.; Demirsoy, S.; Akcali, K.C.; Turan, B. Cardioprotective effect of extracellular vesicles derived from ticagrelor-pretreated cardiomyocyte on hyperglycemic cardiomyocytes through alleviation of oxidative and endoplasmic reticulum stress. *Sci. Rep.* **2022**, *12*, 1–15. [CrossRef]
128. Broek, B.V.D.; Wuyts, C.; Sisto, A.; Pintelon, I.; Timmermans, J.-P.; Somers, V.; Timmerman, V.; Hellings, N.; Irobi, J. Oligodendroglia-derived extracellular vesicles activate autophagy via LC3B/BAG3 to protect against oxidative stress with an enhanced effect for HSPB8 enriched vesicles. *Cell Commun. Signal.* **2022**, *20*, 1–19. [CrossRef]
129. Tian, C.; Gao, L.; Rudebush, T.L.; Yu, L.; Zucker, I.H. Extracellular Vesicles Regulate Sympatho-Excitation by Nrf2 in Heart Failure. *Circ. Res.* **2022**, *31*, 687–700. [CrossRef]
130. Wong, E.H.C.; Dong, Y.Y.; Coray, M.; Cortada, M.; Levano, S.; Schmidt, A.; Brand, Y.; Bodmer, D.; Muller, L. Inner ear exosomes and their potential use as biomarkers. *PLoS ONE* **2018**, *13*, e0198029. [CrossRef]
131. Kalinec, G.M.; Cohn, W.; Whitelegge, J.P.; Faull, K.F.; Kalinec, F.; Cohn, B.W. Preliminary Characterization of Extracellular Vesicles from Auditory HEI-OC1 Cells. *Ann. Otol. Rhinol. Laryngol.* **2019**, *128*, 52S–60S. [CrossRef]
132. Kalinec, G.M.; Gao, L.; Cohn, W.; Whitelegge, J.P.; Faull, K.F.; Kalinec, F. Extracellular Vesicles from Auditory Cells as Nanocarriers for Anti-inflammatory Drugs and Pro-resolving Mediators. *Front. Cell. Neurosci.* **2019**, *13*, 530. [CrossRef]
133. Zhuang, P.; Phung, S.; Warnecke, A.; Arambula, A.; Peter, M.S.; He, M.; Staecker, H. Isolation of sensory hair cell specific exosomes in human perilymph. *Neurosci. Lett.* **2021**, *764*, 136282. [CrossRef] [PubMed]
134. Jiang, P.; Ma, X.; Han, S.; Ma, L.; Ai, J.; Wu, L.; Zhang, Y.; Xiao, H.; Tian, M.; Tao, W.A.; et al. Characterization of the microRNA transcriptomes and proteomics of cochlear tissue-derived small extracellular vesicles from mice of different ages after birth. *Cell. Mol. Life Sci.* **2022**, *79*, 154. [CrossRef] [PubMed]
135. Soares, V.Y.R.; Atai, N.A.; Fujita, T.; Dilwali, S.; Sivaraman, S.; Landegger, L.D.; Hochberg, F.H.; Oliveira, C.A.P.C.; Bahmad, F.; Breakefield, X.O.; et al. Extracellular vesicles derived from human vestibular schwannomas associated with poor hearing damage cochlear cells. *Neuro-Oncology* **2016**, *18*, 1498–1507. [CrossRef] [PubMed]
136. Yang, T.; Li, W.; Peng, A.; Wang, Q. Exosomes derived from heat shock preconditioned bone marrow mesenchymal stem cells alleviate cisplatin-induced ototoxicity in mice. *J. Biol. Eng.* **2022**, *16*, 1–9. [CrossRef]
137. Hao, F.; Shan, C.; Zhang, Y.; Zhang, Y.; Jia, Z. Exosomes Derived from microRNA-21 Overexpressing Neural Progenitor Cells Prevent Hearing Loss from Ischemia-Reperfusion Injury in Mice via Inhibiting the Inflammatory Process in the Cochlea. *ACS Chem. Neurosci.* **2022**, *13*, 2464–2472. [CrossRef]
138. Yang, T.; Li, W.; Peng, A.; Liu, J.; Wang, Q. Exosomes Derived from Bone Marrow-Mesenchymal Stem Cells Attenuates Cisplatin-Induced Ototoxicity in a Mouse Model. *J. Clin. Med.* **2022**, *11*, 4743. [CrossRef]
139. Park, D.J.; Park, J.-E.; Lee, S.H.; Eliceiri, B.P.; Choi, J.S.; Seo, Y.J. Protective effect of MSC-derived exosomes against cisplatin-induced apoptosis via heat shock protein 70 in auditory explant model. *Nanomedicine Nanotechnol. Biol. Med.* **2021**, *38*, 102447. [CrossRef]
140. Tsai, S.C.-S.; Yang, K.D.; Chang, K.-H.; Lin, F.C.-F.; Chou, R.-H.; Li, M.-C.; Cheng, C.-C.; Kao, C.-Y.; Chen, C.-P.; Lin, H.-C.; et al. Umbilical Cord Mesenchymal Stromal Cell-Derived Exosomes Rescue the Loss of Outer Hair Cells and Repair Cochlear Damage in Cisplatin-Injected Mice. *Int. J. Mol. Sci.* **2021**, *22*, 6664. [CrossRef]
141. Yang, T.; Cai, C.; Peng, A.; Liu, J.; Wang, Q. Exosomes derived from cochlear spiral ganglion progenitor cells prevent cochlea damage from ischemia-reperfusion injury via inhibiting the inflammatory process. *Cell Tissue Res.* **2021**, *386*, 239–247. [CrossRef]
142. Breglio, A.M.; May, L.A.; Barzik, M.; Welsh, N.C.; Francis, S.P.; Costain, T.Q.; Wang, L.; Anderson, D.E.; Petralia, R.S.; Wang, Y.-X.; et al. Exosomes mediate sensory hair cell protection in the inner ear. *J. Clin. Investig.* **2020**, *130*, 2657–2672. [CrossRef]
143. Warnecke, A.; Harre, J.; Staecker, H.; Prenzler, N.; Strunk, D.; Couillard-Despres, S.; Romanelli, P.; Hollerweger, J.; Lassacher, T.; Auer, D.; et al. Extracellular vesicles from human multipotent stromal cells protect against hearing loss after noise trauma in vivo. *Clin. Transl. Med.* **2020**, *10*, e262. [CrossRef] [PubMed]
144. Warnecke, A.; Prenzler, N.; Harre, J.; Köhl, U.; Gärtner, L.; Lenarz, T.; Laner-Plamberger, S.; Wietzorrek, G.; Staecker, H.; Lassacher, T.; et al. First-in-human intracochlear application of human stromal cell-derived extracellular vesicles. *J. Extracell. Vesicles* **2021**, *10*, e12094. [CrossRef] [PubMed]
145. György, B.; Sage, C.; Indzhykulian, A.A.; Scheffer, D.I.; Brisson, A.R.; Tan, S.; Wu, X.; Volak, A.; Mu, D.; Tamvakologos, P.I.; et al. Rescue of Hearing by Gene Delivery to Inner-Ear Hair Cells Using Exosome-Associated AAV. *Mol. Ther.* **2016**, *25*, 379–391. [CrossRef]
146. György, B.; Maguire, C.A. Extracellular vesicles: Nature's nanoparticles for improving gene transfer with adeno-associated virus vectors. *WIREs Nanomed. Nanobiotechnol.* **2017**, *10*, e1488. [CrossRef] [PubMed]

147. Lener, T.; Gimona, M.; Aigner, L.; Börger, V.; Buzas, E.; Camussi, G.; Chaput, N.; Chatterjee, D.; Court, F.A.; Del Portillo, H.A.; et al. Applying extracellular vesicles based therapeutics in clinical trials—An ISEV position paper. *J. Extracell. Vesicles* **2015**, *4*, 30087. [CrossRef]
148. European Medicines Agency. Advanced Therapy Medicinal Products: Overview. Available online: https://www.ema.europa.eu/en/human-regulatory/overview/advanced-therapy-medicinal-products-overview (accessed on 5 October 2022).
149. Gimona, M.; Pachler, K.; Laner-Plamberger, S.; Schallmoser, K.; Rohde, E. Manufacturing of Human Extracellular Vesicle-Based Therapeutics for Clinical Use. *Int. J. Mol. Sci.* **2017**, *18*, 1190. [CrossRef]
150. Marquez-Curtis, L.A.; Janowska-Wieczorek, A.; McGann, L.E.; Elliott, J.A. Mesenchymal stromal cells derived from various tissues: Biological, clinical and cryopreservation aspects. *Cryobiology* **2015**, *71*, 181–197. [CrossRef]
151. Galderisi, U.; Peluso, G.; Di Bernardo, G. Clinical Trials Based on Mesenchymal Stromal Cells are Exponentially Increasing: Where are We in Recent Years? *Stem Cell Rev. Rep.* **2021**, *18*, 23–36. [CrossRef]
152. Jovic, D.; Yu, Y.; Wang, D.; Wang, K.; Li, H.; Xu, F.; Liu, C.; Liu, J.; Luo, Y. A Brief Overview of Global Trends in MSC-Based Cell Therapy. *Stem Cell Rev. Rep.* **2022**, *18*, 1525–1545. [CrossRef]
153. Rohde, E.; Pachler, K.; Gimona, M. Manufacturing and characterization of extracellular vesicles from umbilical cord–derived mesenchymal stromal cells for clinical testing. *Cytotherapy* **2019**, *21*, 581–592. [CrossRef]
154. Besse, B.; Charrier, M.; Lapierre, V.; Dansin, E.; Lantz, O.; Planchard, D.; Le Chevalier, T.; Livartoski, A.; Barlesi, F.; Laplanche, A.; et al. Dendritic cell-derived exosomes as maintenance immunotherapy after first line chemotherapy in NSCLC. *OncoImmunology* **2016**, *5*, e1071008. [CrossRef] [PubMed]
155. Morse, M.A.; Garst, J.; Osada, T.; Khan, S.; Hobeika, A.; Clay, T.M.; Valente, N.; Shreeniwas, R.; Sutton, M.A.; Delcayre, A.; et al. A phase I study of dexosome immunotherapy in patients with advanced non-small cell lung cancer. *J. Transl. Med.* **2005**, *3*, 9. [CrossRef] [PubMed]
156. Escudier, B.; Dorval, T.; Chaput, N.; André, F.; Caby, M.-P.; Novault, S.; Flament, C.; Leboulaire, C.; Borg, C.; Amigorena, S.; et al. Vaccination of metastatic melanoma patients with autologous dendritic cell (DC) derived-exosomes: Results of thefirst phase I clinical trial. *J. Transl. Med.* **2005**, *3*, 1–13. [CrossRef] [PubMed]
157. Dai, S.; Wei, D.; Wu, Z.; Zhou, X.; Wei, X.; Huang, H.; Li, G. Phase I Clinical Trial of Autologous Ascites-derived Exosomes Combined With GM-CSF for Colorectal Cancer. *Mol. Ther.* **2008**, *16*, 782–790. [CrossRef]
158. Bailey, A.M.; Mendicino, M.; Au, P. An FDA perspective on preclinical development of cell-based regenerative medicine products. *Nat. Biotechnol.* **2014**, *32*, 721–723. [CrossRef]
159. International Society for Extracellular Vesicles. Regulatory Affairs Task Force. Available online: https://www.isev.org/regulatory-affairs-task-force (accessed on 5 October 2022).

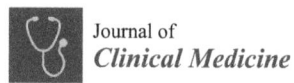

Review

Inner Ear Diagnostics and Drug Delivery via Microneedles

Stephen Leong [1], Aykut Aksit [2], Sharon J. Feng [1], Jeffrey W. Kysar [2,3] and Anil K. Lalwani [1,2,3,*]

1. Vagelos College of Physicians & Surgeons, Columbia University Irving Medical Center, New York, NY 10032, USA
2. Department of Mechanical Engineering, Columbia University, New York, NY 10027, USA
3. Department of Otolaryngology—Head & Neck Surgery, New-York Presbyterian/Columbia University Irving Medical Center, New York, NY 10032, USA
* Correspondence: akl2144@cumc.columbia.edu; Tel.: +1-212-305-3319

Abstract: Objectives: Precision medicine for inner ear disorders has seen significant advances in recent years. However, unreliable access to the inner ear has impeded diagnostics and therapeutic delivery. The purpose of this review is to describe the development, production, and utility of novel microneedles for intracochlear access. Methods: We summarize the current work on microneedles developed using two-photon polymerization (2PP) lithography for perforation of the round window membrane (RWM). We contextualize our findings with the existing literature in intracochlear diagnostics and delivery. Results: Two-photon polymerization lithography produces microneedles capable of perforating human and guinea pig RWMs without structural or functional damage. Solid microneedles may be used to perforate guinea pig RWMs in vivo with full reconstitution of the membrane in 48–72 h, and hollow microneedles may be used to aspirate perilymph or inject therapeutics into the inner ear. Microneedles produced with two-photon templated electrodeposition (2PTE) have greater strength and biocompatibility and may be used to perforate human RWMs. Conclusions: Microneedles produced with 2PP lithography and 2PTE can safely and reliably perforate the RWM for intracochlear access. This technology is groundbreaking and enabling in the field of inner ear precision medicine.

Keywords: microneedle; round window membrane; intracochlear delivery; precision medicine; gene therapy

Citation: Leong, S.; Aksit, A.; Feng, S.J.; Kysar, J.W.; Lalwani, A.K. Inner Ear Diagnostics and Drug Delivery via Microneedles. *J. Clin. Med.* **2022**, *11*, 5474. https://doi.org/10.3390/jcm11185474

Academic Editor: Giuseppe Magliulo

Received: 14 August 2022
Accepted: 13 September 2022
Published: 17 September 2022

Publisher's Note: MDPI stays neutral with regard to jurisdictional claims in published maps and institutional affiliations.

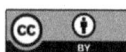

Copyright: © 2022 by the authors. Licensee MDPI, Basel, Switzerland. This article is an open access article distributed under the terms and conditions of the Creative Commons Attribution (CC BY) license (https://creativecommons.org/licenses/by/4.0/).

1. Introduction

The ears are vital to one's perception of and interaction with the world, providing constant information to the brain to allow for both effective hearing and balance. Inner ear dysfunction—resulting from a combination of genetic and environmental factors, and characterized by hearing loss, tinnitus, and vertigo—is quite prevalent in the general population (Table 1) [1]. Untreated, auditory and vestibular disturbance can significantly impact function and can have debilitating effects on one's quality of life. With the identification of over a hundred deafness genes and the recent demonstration of mammalian hair cell regeneration, stem cell therapy, and gene editing technology, we are on the cusp of precision therapy for inner ear disorders [2].

A significant impediment to implementing precision medicine for inner ear disorders is safe and reliable access to the inner ear for diagnostics and therapeutic delivery. Without a means to sample inner ear fluid for electrochemical, RNA, or proteomic analysis, precise intervention is not possible. Furthermore, current options for intracochlear delivery, including systemic administration, intratympanic (IT) injection, and direct injection into the cochlea, are imprecise. Although systemic administration may achieve high drug levels in the cochlea, it is more frequently associated with systemic toxicity. IT injection is a more precise delivery method, but is hampered by variable efficacy, as it must rely on simple diffusion across the round window membrane (RWM). Additionally, the injected medication can leak down the Eustachian tube, be impeded by debris in the round window niche, or escape out of the external canal, thus resulting in highly variable medication levels between patients [3]. Direct placement of therapeutic agents on the RWM in a biodegradable carrier substance, such as gelatin, hydrogel, or nanoparticles, may overcome some of these limitations [4–6]; however, the rate of drug delivery to the inner ear is inevitably limited by molecular diffusion across the RWM. These limitations may have been responsible for the recent failures of two promising large clinical trials: AM-111 in the treatment of sudden sensorineural hearing loss, and sustained release dexamethasone in Poloxamer 407 gel for Meniere's Disease [7,8].

Table 1. Hearing loss data based on National Health Statistics Reports 2020 [1].

	All Ages 18+	Ages 18–44	Ages 45–64	Ages 65–74	Age 75+
Severe hearing loss	2.4% (2.0–2.8)	0.4% (0.2–0.6)	1.9% (1.5–2.5)	6.0% (4.2–8.3)	13.4% (10.2–17.2)
Mild–moderate hearing loss	13.6% (12.7–14.4)	5.3% (4.6–6.1)	16.7% (15.3–18.2)	31.2% (28.0–34.6)	36.4% (31.2–41.9)
Balance issues	18.7% (17.7–19.7)	14.2% (12.9–15.6)	21.1% (19.5–22.7)	27.1% (24.0–30.4)	30.1% (25.3–35.2)

Direct intracochlear drug administration results in significantly higher and less variable drug levels compared to IT injection, with a much smaller concentration gradient from base to apex [9]. Various methods of intracochlear delivery have been developed, including osmotic mini-pump infusion into the scala tympani via the round window [10–13], infusion or microinjection into the scala tympani through a cochleostomy [13–17], and intracochlear injection through the RWM [18–21]. Though these methods are a step toward precise inner ear delivery, all of them breach the inner ear and consequently risk hearing impairment. A safe and reliable method for intracochlear delivery thus remains to be developed.

The RWM is the only soft tissue portal from the middle ear into the cochlea and, therefore, is an ideal candidate for intracochlear access. Microneedle-mediated perforation of the RWM is a novel means of achieving intracochlear access and can facilitate reliable and predictable perforation of the RWM, with minimal anatomic and functional damage [22,23]. Using microneedles, drug concentrations within the inner ear may be controlled with a precision that IT injections cannot provide. The application of microneedles is not a departure from current clinical practices, but rather a natural progression from the current practice. Microneedle technology promises increased safety and efficacy over the current techniques for inner ear therapy, and may potentially be applied in an office setting.

2. Properties of the Round Window Membrane

A significant challenge to intracochlear delivery is perforation of the RWM without inducing tearing or ripping. As will be discussed in a later section, the size of such a perforation must necessarily be at least an order of magnitude smaller than the RWM itself, which means that the perforations should be no wider than about 200 µm through the 2 mm wide and 70–80 µm thick RWM. Designing microneedles for this purpose requires knowledge of the RWM microanatomy and mechanical properties. The RWM has a connective tissue core containing fibroblasts, collagen, and elastic fibers, providing mechanical strength to the RWM to bear the perilymphatic pressure [24,25]. Over the last several years, the microanatomy and mechanical properties of the RWM have been extensively studied, and a detailed finite element model (FEM) simulation that has directly impacted microneedle design has been developed [26–29].

Using micro-CT (µ-CT) with 1 µm resolution and white laser interferometry, we demonstrated in a guinea pig model that much of the surface of the RWM can be approximated as a hyperbolic paraboloid (HP)—like a saddle or a Pringle potato chip—that sits in a bony sulcus reminiscent of the tympanic annulus and the tympanic membrane. Using immunostaining and sectioning, confocal and multi-photon microscopy, and scanning electron microscopy (SEM), we showed that RWM fibers are highly organized and share directionality and dispersion characteristics. In large portions of the RWM, fibers are primarily oriented in the direction of zero curvature which allows them to remain as straight as possible in their physiologically natural configuration. There is a strong correlation between elastic and collagen fiber directionality and the distance along the axis of the cochlea. The fibers also follow a direction that improves the behavior of the RWM when it is subjected to increased perilymphatic pressure from the inner ear side, which is consistent with the fact that the perilymph of a guinea pig (GP) is usually at a nominal physiological internal pressure of 0.2 kPa.

3. Microneedle Design and Testing

Since they were first demonstrated in 1998, microneedles have been extensively researched for sampling of biological fluids and therapeutic delivery [30]. While early research focused on transdermal sampling and delivery, microneedles have subsequently been used in many different tissues, including the oral cavity, genitourinary tract, gastrointestinal tract, vascular wall, eye, and skin [31–34]. Our group has specifically focused on the development of microneedle technology for inner ear access [35–38].

3.1. Design for RWM Perforation

A prototypical solid microneedle design from our group is shown in Figure 1a. It starts from a tip of radius R_t and tapers at an angle α to a constant shaft diameter D_n, with a taper-plus-shaft length of L and a base with maximum diameter D_b designed to fit into the lumen of a blunt stainless-steel needle. A Luer lock is affixed to the other end of the stainless-steel needle.

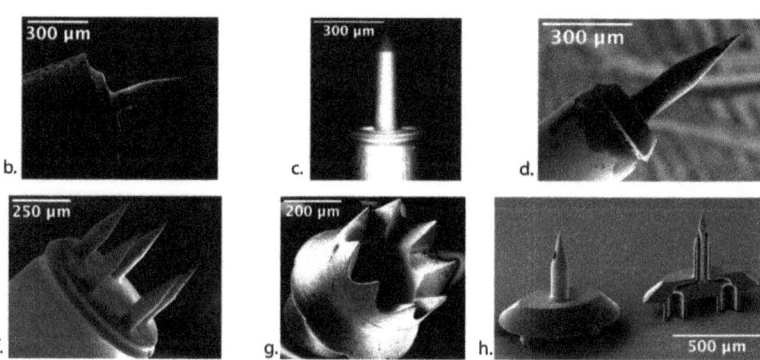

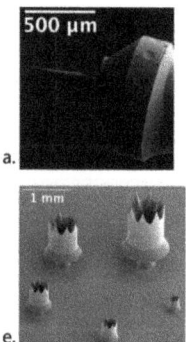

Figure 1. Suite of microneedles developed for the inner ear. (**a**) Solid polymeric microneedle. (**b**) Solid metallic microneedle. (**c**) Solid polymeric microneedle for human RWM use. (**d**) Hollow microneedle for perilymph aspiration and direct intracochlear injection. (**e**) Five differently sized "crown" needles to facilitate cochlear implantation. (**f**) Microneedle array for opening simultaneous microperforations on the RWM. (**g**) A 410 μm sized "crown" needle for cochlear implantation, fabricated via 2PTE. (**h**) Dual-lumen microneedle for simultaneous aspiration and injection of fluids across the RWM. (Adapted with permission from Ref. [35], 2018, Ref. [37], 2020, Ref. [38], 2020, Ref. [39], 2021, Jeffrey W. Kysar, PhD and Anil K. Lalwani, MD).

The human RWM is about 2 mm in diameter and 70–80 μm thick, with collagen and elastic fibers that endow the RWM with stiffness, strength and toughness; furthermore, the RWM is under a tensile prestrain [40]. Microneedles are designed to create perforations through the RWM to deliver drugs and aspirate fluids for diagnosis. The perforation must be minimally traumatic to promote rapid healing and avoid anatomic and functional consequences. Thus, the tip radius R_t should be sufficiently small to penetrate the RWM, while cutting as few collagen and elastic fibers as possible. Fortuitously, such a process minimizes the peak perforation force F_p that the microneedle exerts on the RWM and also minimizes the pressure increase in the cochlea during perforation.

Our group has found that the two most important design criteria are: (1) an ultra-sharp tip R_t to minimize both trauma and perforation force; (2) high strength and ductility to ensure the microneedle has a safe "bend not break" failure mode. Once these two criteria are fulfilled, the low perforation force F_p, coupled with a strong and ductile material, allow length L, shaft diameter D_n, and angle α to span large ranges while still maintaining microneedle structural integrity with a large factor of safety. We can then specify L, D_n, and α based on medical needs, rather than compromising these values for the sake of structural integrity.

Nonetheless, fabrication of strong, ductile, ultra-sharp microneedles is very challenging, and even more so for microneedles that are hollow or have complex geometries. To overcome this challenge, our group has developed a new paradigm for fabrication of microneedles.

3.2. Microneedle Fabrication

Methods to manufacture microneedles to perforate the RWM require three attributes: (1) accuracy and precision leading to ultra-sharp needles; (2) strong and ductile material; and (3) high design freedom to fabricate complex needle geometries for middle and inner ear anatomy. Figure 2 depicts these in a Venn diagram.

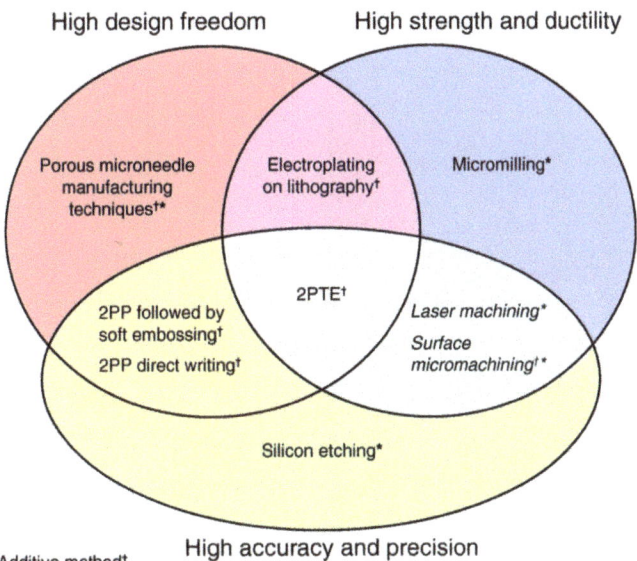

Figure 2. Attributes of different microneedle manufacturing techniques. [†] Additive method. [*] Subtractive method. [†*] Combination method. Italics: 2D method. (Reprinted with permission from Ref. [38], 2020, Jeffrey W. Kysar, PhD and Anil K. Lalwani, MD).

Existing microneedle manufacturing methods include: micromachining, direct writing techniques, laser machining, micromilling, electric discharge machining, laser sintering, electroplating and various combinations of lithography, molding, and hot/soft embossing techniques [30,41,42]. Materials used include: silicon, polysilicon, steel, nickel, gold, titanium, and a variety of different polymers. None of these methods and materials encompass all three attributes in Figure 2.

Our group has therefore employed a new, enabling manufacturing technology called two-photon polymerization (2PP) lithography that has become commercially available in the past few years [43]. The 2PP lithography method is an additive manufacturing (i.e., 3D printing) process that can produce highly complex geometries out of hard polymers with voxel spatial resolution approaching 100 nm. The sub-micrometer precision and accuracy, combined with the design freedom of 3D printing, enable the direct 3D writing of polymeric microneedles. Figure 1a shows a polymeric needle from our group with tip radius $R_t = 0.5$ µm and a shaft diameter $D_n = 100$ µm printed with 2PP lithography and mounted on the end of a 23-gauge blunt hollow stainless-steel needle [35].

To assess the effectiveness of the polymeric microneedles, our group designed—based on the RWM anatomic and mechanical characteristics described above—microneedles with $D_n = 100$ µm, $\alpha = 18°$, and $L_n = 200$ µm, and performed in vitro studies of GP RWM perforation [35]. Figure 3a shows a confocal microscopy image of the perforation introduced at the center of a GP RWM with a mean $F_p = 1.2$ mN; Figure 3b shows collagen and connective fiber separation, and demonstrates that the length of the lens-shaped perforation is approximately the same as the microneedle diameter.

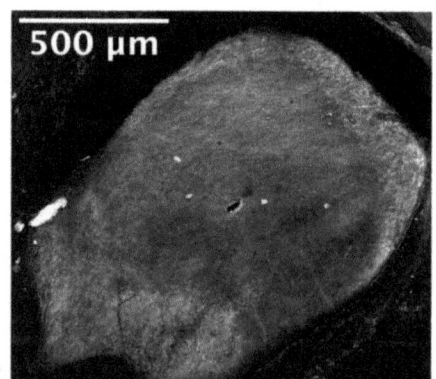
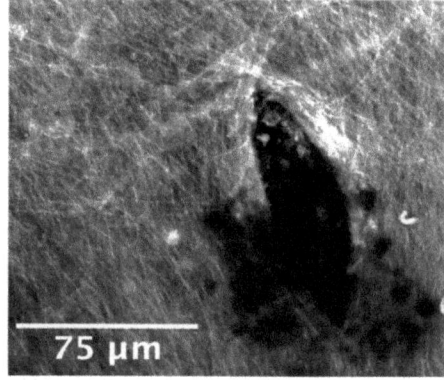

a.   b.

Figure 3. Confocal image of a guinea pig RWM around a perforation with (**a**) low magnification and (**b**) high magnification showing connective fibers of the membrane. (Reprinted with permission from Ref. [35], 2018, Jeffrey W. Kysar, PhD and Anil K. Lalwani, MD).

3.3. Anatomical and Functional Consequences of Perforation

To assess anatomic and functional consequences of microneedles on the RWM, our group used the same microneedles to perforate the GP RWM in vivo [36]. The ultra-sharp microneedles created precise, accurate, and stable perforations with separation of connective fibers (Figure 4). Confocal microscopy showed that the RWM perforation began to heal by 24 h and completely healed by 1 week; subsequently, we showed that complete closure of the RWM occurred between 48 and 72 h. Perforations could not be detected histologically at 1 week. From audiometric measurements, including compound action potential (CAP) and distortion product otoacoustic emissions (DPOAE) at 0–2 h, 24 h, 48 h, and 1-week post-perforation, there were no measurable audiologic consequences, although covert hearing loss cannot be ruled out. Of note, these experiments were performed in healthy GPs; models of auditory pathology, especially those producing pressure abnormalities in the inner ear, may result in different RWM healing properties.

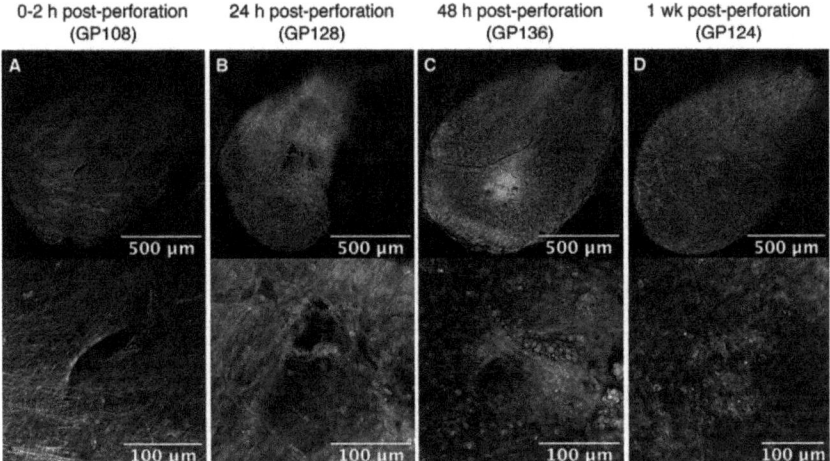

Figure 4. Guinea pig RWM healing after perforation with 100µm-diameter microneedle perforations under low magnification (**top**) and high magnification (**bottom**) at (**A**) 0–2 h, (**B**) 24 h, (**C**) 48 h, and (**D**) 1-week post-perforation. (Reprinted with permission from Ref. [36], 2020, Jeffrey W. Kysar, PhD and Anil K. Lalwani, MD).

Based on the mechanical properties of the human RWM, the human microneedle design was modified from the GP microneedle design to account for the stronger and thicker human RWM, with $\alpha = 60°$, $D_n = 150$ µm, and $L = 480$ µm; this microneedle is shown in Figure 1c. The polymeric microneedles designed for human use created precise and stable perforations that were slit-shaped via fiber separation, with a distinct major axis equal to the microneedle diameter, and aligned with the predominant fiber direction; the microneedles maintained their integrity during perforation [37]. Approximately $F_p = 60$ mN was required to perforate the RWM and microneedles needed to be displaced inward approximately 300 µm, which is sufficiently small so that the microneedles do not touch the closest structures behind the RWM during perforation, thus avoiding cochlear trauma. In summary, these microneedles designed for perforating the human RWM were durable, created precise perforations, and avoided cochlear trauma.

Thus, a microneedle with an ultra-sharp tip radius $R_t \approx 1$ µm is an achievable design specification with 2PP lithography. Furthermore, stable perforations of 100 µm in a GP model and 150 µm in human tissue can be introduced safely. Perforations of this size scale are known to significantly enhance the rate of diffusion of molecules across the GP RWM [44].

3.4. Design Freedom in Microneedle Synthesis

The 2PP method provides impressive flexibility to create polymeric microneedles with complex geometries. Figure 1f shows an array of five microneedles—each 100 µm in diameter—secured to a common base that is mounted on a stainless-steel blunt needle. Figure 1e shows five "crown" needles with different diameters for creating large perforations on the RWM, through which a cochlear implant can be inserted.

While the polymeric material from 2PP has good strength and ductility, it is not as strong and ductile as a metal, nor is the specific polymeric material biocompatible. Therefore, our group developed a new method to fabricate ultra-sharp metallic microneedles using a technique known as two-photon templated electrodeposition (2PTE). First, 2PP lithography is used to "print" polymeric mold structures containing cavities in the shape of the desired needle. The cavities are then filled with copper via electrochemical deposition. The polymeric molds are then dissolved, and the needles are recovered and mounted on a blunt stainless-steel needle, as shown in Figure 1b [38]. A biocompatible metallic coating is also applied onto the microneedles, consisting of a 1.5 µm conformal film of nickel followed by a 30–100 nm conformal film of gold. The final microneedle has a tip radius of 1.5 µm and shaft diameter of 100 µm, and has been tested in vitro in a GP RWM. The mean peak perforation was 4 mN and the ultra-sharp tip successfully separated RWM fibers.

The 2PTE process provides sub-micrometer resolution to create precise, ultra-sharp, high-ductility, high-strength, and biocompatible metallic microneedles that have significant design freedom [38]. Figure 1g illustrates one of the complex geometries that can be fabricated via 2PTE; specifically, a 410 µm crown needle to facilitate cochlear implantation across the RWM is shown. The combination of design freedom, precision, and material choice of the 2PTE process is unique in microneedle manufacturing, is ideal for microneedle development for inner ear precision medicine, and encompasses all three attributes outlined in Figure 2.

4. Clinical Applications of Microneedles

Our microneedle technology is critical for the field of otology because it allows for direct access into the cochlea without lasting effects on hearing. Thus, our microneedle technology makes precision medicine of the inner ear possible, in both diagnostic and therapeutic realms. We have developed hollow microneedles that are capable of both aspiration and injection of fluid; in this section, the diagnostic utility of perilymph aspiration and the therapeutic utility of direct intracochlear injection is discussed.

4.1. Hollow Microneedles for Aspiration

To assess the potential of aspiration for the diagnosis of cochlear disorders, our group designed and 2PP printed hollow microneedles with $D_n = 100$ µm, $L = 435$ µm, $\alpha = 24°$, and 35 µm diameter lumen and mounted them atop a 30-gauge blunt hollow stainless-steel needle, as shown in Figure 1d [39]. We then aspirated 1 µL of GP perilymph across the RWM in vivo for proteomic analysis. Over 400 proteins were identified; the inner ear protein cochlin, widely recognized as a perilymph marker, as well as proteins from the heat shock protein family, including heat shock protein 70, were detected in all samples tested. Results are shown in Figure 5. There were no measurable shifts in hearing thresholds, and perforations healed completely within 72 h. The ability to collect perilymph will overcome the methodological limitation of prior studies that required dissecting the whole cochlea from animals for adequate tissue samples.

Our group further tested the clinical utility of cochlear aspiration by determining if proteomic differences in systemic versus IT delivery of steroids could be detected in perilymph. Previous studies have demonstrated that local administration results in greater perilymph concentrations and favors the base, whereas systemic administration favors the apex [45,46]. Additionally, intratympanically delivered glucocorticoids have been found to affect thousands more inner ear genes compared to systemically delivered glucocorticoids in mice [47]. Through aspiration of 1 µL of GP perilymph using hollow microneedles, we demonstrated that systemically administered dexamethasone results in greater modulation of perilymph proteins compared to IT dexamethasone, with 14 modulated proteins in the systemic group and 3 modulated proteins in the IT group [48]. In both groups, the growth factor VGF was significantly upregulated and the regulatory protein 14-3-3γ was down-regulated; in particular, upregulation of VGF suggests an otoprotective role for steroids administered both systemically and via IT injection. Increased modulation of protein expression with systemically administered steroids conflicts with previous studies [47], but may suggest greater off-target effects for systemic therapy. In summary, our ability to distinguish between systemically and locally administered glucocorticoids via microneedle aspiration of perilymph further supports the efficacy of our technology.

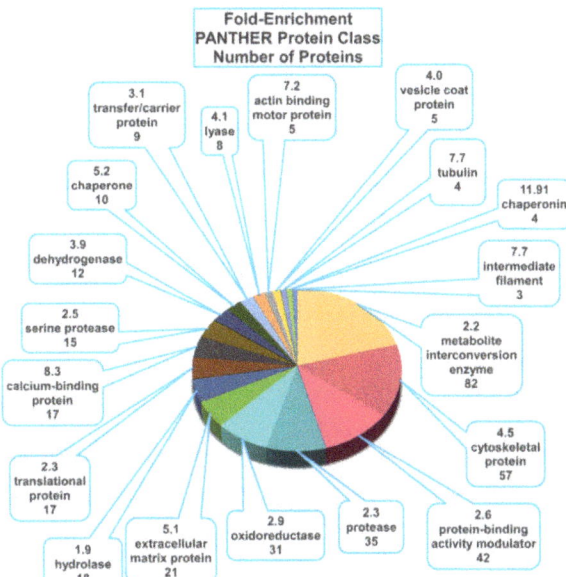

Figure 5. Composition of guinea pig perilymph proteome, by functional categories. The 620 gene names were searched against the mouse gene list in PANTHER (http://www/pantherdb.org (accessed on 1 September 2020)) to determine the distribution of proteins across functional classes. The fold-enrichment, PANTHER protein class, and the number of proteins within each class are presented. (Reprinted with permission from Ref. [39], 2021, Jeffrey W. Kysar, PhD and Anil K. Lalwani, MD).

4.2. Microneedles for Diffusion and Injection

Microperforations across the RWM can enhance diffusion of therapeutics across the RWM. Our group has shown that a single perforation occupying 0.22% of RWM leads to a 35-fold increase in diffusion of Rhodamine B (chosen because of its similarity to dexamethasone and gentamicin)—consistent with our predictions based on mathematical modeling [44]. Interestingly, the use of Poloxamer-407 gel as a reservoir for the Rhodamine B results in a slower diffusion rate than PBS solution, but with a smaller standard deviation. One concern when creating perforations within the RWM is the potential leakage of perilymph from the scala tympani into the middle ear due to perilymph pressure [19,49]. As the fluidic resistance to flow is inversely proportional to the diameter of the perforation to the fourth power, the risk of leakage can be further reduced by using multiple smaller microperforations in place of a single larger perforation to mediate drug diffusion [50]. We tested diffusion across multiple smaller holes using a filter paper model of the RWM in a horizontal Valia–Chien diffusion cell and a phosphate buffered saline (PBS) fluid in the reservoir donor chamber [51]. Our group demonstrated that the diffusion rate across the membrane from a liquid reservoir was directly correlated to aggregate area of perforation; thus, multiple smaller holes—potentially introduced by an array of microneedles—are equivalent to a single larger perforation in enhancing diffusion but have lower risk of perilymph leakage.

While solid needles have been found extremely successful in enhancing diffusion across the RWM, direct injection of the therapeutic into the cochlea is attractive as a more precise method of delivery. Direct injection has been proposed by several companies, including Akouos and Decibel. Since our 2PTE fabrication technology can create hollow microneedles that can be attached on top of common syringe needles, it is possible to directly inject precise amounts of therapeutics directly across the RWM. In guinea pigs, patency of the cochlear aqueduct allows for direct injection of agents without significant efflux of fluid through the perforation created by the microneedle. However, pressure relief through the cochlear aqueduct likely requires some level of pressure buildup within the cochlea; our group has demonstrated that injection of large volumes of fluid into the GP cochlea through a single-lumen hollow microneedle results in high-frequency hearing loss, which can be entirely avoided with injection of smaller volumes. In humans, the cochlear aqueduct is closed and direct injection will likely result in immediate efflux through the very perforation created. Solutions such as perforation of the stapes, semicircular canal, or apex of cochlea have been proposed to overcome this issue by providing a vent release for escape of cochlear fluid—but are invasive and damaging. As one possible solution, our group has designed a microneedle system with a second lumen that can act as a vent, so that cochlear fluid volume remains constant during injection of a large therapeutic volume (Figure 1h). Our group will continue developing microneedle technology to enable safe injection of therapeutics directly across the RWM.

4.3. Office-Based Diagnostic and Therapeutic Intervention

Our group has additionally been developing an endoscopic approach for microneedle-mediated perforation of the RWM and injection of agents. By mounting a hollow microneedle at the tip of a middle ear micro-endoscope, we have successfully perforated human cadaveric RWMs. Further development of this technology will allow our microneedle technology to be translated into the office setting, where otolaryngologists may use microneedles to deliver therapeutics as part of routine outpatient care.

5. Conclusions

Many current technologies used to access the inner ear are inherently traumatic and result in significant hearing loss. Microneedles offer a solution to this problem, for both diagnostic and therapeutic purposes. Our microneedle technology allows for direct sampling of perilymph and makes the clinical translation of a variety of intracochlear therapies possible. With our technology, we believe that precision therapeutics such as gene therapy will take hold in the field and revolutionize treatment for hearing loss.

Author Contributions: Conceptualization, S.L., A.A., S.J.F., J.W.K. and A.K.L.; methodology, S.L., A.A., S.J.F., J.W.K. and A.K.L.; software, S.L. and A.A.; validation, S.L. and A.A.; formal analysis, S.L. and A.A.; investigation, S.L. and A.A.; resources, S.L. and A.A.; data curation, S.L. and A.A.; writing—original draft preparation, S.L., A.A. and S.J.F.; writing—review and editing, S.L., A.A., S.J.F., J.W.K. and A.K.L.; visualization, S.L. and A.A.; supervision, J.W.K. and A.K.L.; project administration, J.W.K. and A.K.L.; funding acquisition, S.L., A.A., S.J.F., J.W.K. and A.K.L. All authors have read and agreed to the published version of the manuscript.

Funding: This research was supported by National Institutes of Health (NIH) National Institute on Deafness and Other Communication Disorders (NIDCD) with award number R01DC014547, and by the American Otological Society Fellowship Grant.

Institutional Review Board Statement: The animal study protocols were approved by the Institutional Review Board (or Ethics Committee) of Columbia University Irving Medical Center (protocol code AABA5450, date of approval 30 December 2021).

Informed Consent Statement: Not applicable.

Data Availability Statement: Not applicable.

Acknowledgments: We would like to acknowledge the veterinarians and veterinarian technicians at the Institute of Comparative Medicine at Columbia University Irving Medical Center for their assistance and expertise in animal handling.

Conflicts of Interest: Stephen Leong, BA: None. Aykut Aksit, MS: None. Sharon J. Feng, BA, BS: None. Elizabeth S. Olson, PhD: None. Jeffrey W. Kysar, PhD: None. Anil K. Lalwani, MD: Medical Advisory Board, Spiral Therapeutics. Anil K. Lalwani, MD, Jeffrey W. Kysar, PhD, and Aykut Aksit, PhD are the co-founders of Haystack Medical, Inc., that will commercialize microneedles and associated technologies to facilitate medical access to the middle and inner ear.

References

1. Lucas, J.W.; Zelaya, C.E. Hearing difficulty, vision trouble, and balance problems among male veterans and nonveterans. *Natl. Health Stat. Rep.* **2020**, *142*, 1–8.
2. Ahmed, H.; Shubina-Oleinik, O.; Holt, J.R. Emerging Gene Therapies for Genetic Hearing Loss. *JARO* **2017**, *18*, 649–670. [CrossRef] [PubMed]
3. Hoffer, M.E.; Allen, K.; Kopke, R.D.; Weisskopf, P.; Gottshall, K.; Wester, D. Transtympanic versus sustained-release administration of gentamicin: Kinetics, morphology, and function. *Laryngoscope* **2001**, *111*, 1343–1357. [CrossRef] [PubMed]
4. Zhang, L.; Xu, Y.; Cao, W.; Xie, S.; Wen, L.; Chen, G. Understanding the translocation mechanism of PLGA nanoparticles across round window membrane into the inner ear: A guideline for inner ear drug delivery based on nanomedicine. *Int. J. Nanomed.* **2018**, *13*, 479–492. [CrossRef] [PubMed]
5. Paulson, D.P.; Abuzeid, W.; Jiang, H.; Oe, T.; O'Malley, B.W.; Li, D. A novel controlled local drug delivery system for inner ear disease. *Laryngoscope* **2008**, *118*, 706–711. [CrossRef] [PubMed]
6. Li, L.; Ren, J.; Yin, T.; Liu, W. Intratympanic dexamethasone perfusion versus injection for treatment of refractory sudden sensorineural hearing loss. *Eur. Arch. Otorhinolaryngol.* **2012**, *270*, 861–867. [CrossRef] [PubMed]
7. Lambert, P.R.; Carey, J.; Mikulec, A.A.; LeBel, C.; on behalf of the Otonomy Ménière's Study Group. Intratympanic Sustained-Exposure Dexamethasone Thermosensitive Gel for Symptoms of Ménière's Disease: Randomized Phase 2b Safety and Efficacy Trial. *Otol. Neurotol.* **2016**, *37*, 1669–1676. [CrossRef]
8. Staecker, H.; Jokovic, G.; Karpishchenko, S.; Kienle-Gogolok, A.; Krzyzaniak, A.; Lin, C.-D.; Navratil, P.; Tzvetkov, V.; Wright, N.; Meyer, T. Efficacy and Safety of AM-111 in the Treatment of Acute Unilateral Sudden Deafness-A Double-blind, Randomized, Placebo-controlled Phase 3 Study. *Otol. Neurotol.* **2019**, *40*, 584–594. [CrossRef]
9. Hahn, H.; Salt, A.N.; Biegner, T.; Kammerer, B.; Delabar, U.; Hartsock, J.; Plontke, K.K. Dexamethasone levels and base to apex concentration gradients in scala tympani perilymph following intracochlear delivery in the guinea pig. *Otol. Neurotol.* **2012**, *33*, 660–665. [CrossRef]
10. Liu, H.; Hao, J.; Li, K.S. Current strategies for drug delivery to the inner ear. *Acta Pharm. Sin. B* **2013**, *3*, 86–96. [CrossRef]
11. Derby, M.L.; Sena-Esteves, M.; Breakefield, X.O.; Corey, D.P. Gene transfer into the mammalian inner ear using HSV-1 and vaccinia virus vectors. *Hear. Res.* **1999**, *134*, 1–8. [CrossRef]
12. Komeda, M.; Roessler, B.J.; Raphael, Y. The influence of interleukin-1 receptor antagonist transgene on spiral ganglion neurons. *Hear. Res.* **1999**, *131*, 1–8. [CrossRef]
13. Zhang, Y.; Zhang, W.; Johnston, A.H.; Newman, T.A.; Pyykk, I.; Zou, J. Comparison of the distribution pattern of PEG-b-PCL polymersomes delivered into the rat inner ear via different methods. *Acta Otolaryngol.* **2011**, *131*, 1249–1256. [CrossRef]
14. Wareing, M.; Mhatre, A.N.; Pettis, R.; Han, J.J.; Haut, T.; Pfister, M.H.; Hong, K.; Zheng, W.W.; Lalwani, A.K. Cationic liposome mediated transgene expression in the guinea pig cochlea. *Hear. Res.* **1999**, *128*, 61–69. [CrossRef]
15. Han, J.J.; Mhatre, A.N.; Wareing, M.; Pettis, R.; Gao, W.Q.; Zufferey, R.N.; Trono, D.; Lalwani, A.K. Transgene expression in the guinea pig cochlea mediated by a lentivirus-derived gene transfer vector. *Hum. Gene Ther.* **1999**, *10*, 1867–1873. [CrossRef]
16. Carvalho, G.J.; Lalwani, A.K. The effect of cochleostomy and intracochlear infusion on auditory brain stem response threshold in the guinea pig. *Am. J. Otol.* **1999**, *20*, 87–90.
17. Jero, J.; Tseng, C.J.; Mhatre, A.N.; Lalwani, A.K. A surgical approach appropriate for targeted cochlear gene therapy in the mouse. *Hear. Res.* **2001**, *151*, 106–114. [CrossRef]
18. Horváth, M.; Ribári, O.; Répássy, G.; Tóth, I.E.; Boldogkői, Z.; Palkovits, M. Intracochlear injection of pseudorabies virus labels descending auditory and monoaminerg projections to olivocochlear cells in guinea pig. *Eur. J. Neurosci.* **2003**, *18*, 1439–1447. [CrossRef]
19. Plontke, S.K.; Hartsock, J.J.; Gill, R.M.; Salt, A.N. Intracochlear Drug Injections through the Round Window Membrane: Measures to Improve Drug Retention. *Audiol. Neurotol.* **2016**, *21*, 72–79. [CrossRef]
20. Plontke, S.K.; Götze, G.; Rahne, T.; Liebau, A. Intracochlear drug delivery in combination with cochlear implants. *HNO* **2017**, *65*, 19–28. [CrossRef]
21. Prenzler, N.K.; Salcher, R.; Lenarz, T.; Gaertner, L.; Warnecke, A. Dose-Dependent Transient Decrease of Impedances by Deep Intracochlear Injection of Triamcinolone with a Cochlear Catheter Prior to Cochlear Implantation–1 Year Data. *Front. Neurol.* **2020**, *11*, 258. [CrossRef]
22. Szeto, B.; Chiang, H.; Valentini, C.; Yu, M.; Kysar, J.W.; Lalwani, A.K. Inner ear delivery: Challenges and opportunities. *Laryngoscope Investig. Otolaryngol.* **2020**, *5*, 122–131. [CrossRef] [PubMed]
23. Valentini, C.; Szeto, B.; Kysar, J.W.; Lalwani, A.K. Inner ear gene delivery: Vectors and routes. *Hear. Balance Commun.* **2020**, *18*, 278–285. [CrossRef]
24. Cheng, T.; Gan, R.Z. Experimental measurement and modeling analysis on mechanical properties of tensor tympani tendon. *Med. Eng. Phys.* **2008**, *30*, 358–366. [CrossRef]
25. Watanabe, H.; Kysar, J.W.; Lalwani, A.K. Round Window Membrane as a Portal for Inner Ear Therapy. *Recent Adv. Otolaryngol. Head Neck Surg.* **2017**, *6*, 39.
26. Goycoolea, M.V. Clinical aspects of round window membrane permeability under normal and pathological conditions. *Acta Oto-Laryngol.* **2001**, *121*, 437–447. [CrossRef]

27. Nordang, L.; Anniko, M. Hearing loss in relation to round window membrane morphology in experimental otitis media. *ORL* **2001**, *63*, 333–340. [CrossRef]
28. Sahni, R.S.; Paparella, M.M.; Schachern, P.A.; Goycoolea, M.V.; Le, C.T. Thickness of the human round window membrane in different forms of otitis media. *Arch Otolaryngol. Head Neck Surg.* **1987**, *113*, 630–634. [CrossRef]
29. Arriaga, M.; Arteaga, D.N.; Fafalis, D.; Yu, M.; Wang, X.; Kasza, K.E.; Lalwani, A.K.; Kysar, J.W. Membrane curvature and connective fiber alignment in guinea pig round window membrane. *Acta Biomater.* **2021**, *136*, 343–362. [CrossRef]
30. Henry, S.; McAllister, D.V.; Allen, M.G.; Prausnitz, M.R. Microfabricated microneedles: A novel approach to transdermal drug delivery. *J. Pharm. Sci.* **1999**, *88*, 948. [CrossRef]
31. Donnelly, R.F.; Raj Singh, T.R.; Woolfson, A.D. Microneedle-based drug delivery systems: Microfabrication, drug delivery, and safety. *Drug Deliv.* **2010**, *17*, 187–207. [CrossRef] [PubMed]
32. Donnelly, R.F.; Singh, T.R.R.; Tunney, M.M.; Morrow, D.I.J.; McCarron, P.A.; O'Mahony, C.; Woolfson, A.D. Microneedle arrays allow lower microbial penetration than hypodermic needles in vitro. *Pharm. Res.* **2009**, *26*, 2513–2522. [CrossRef] [PubMed]
33. Kim, Y.-C.; Park, J.-H.; Prausnitz, M.R. Microneedles for drug and vaccine delivery. *Adv. Drug Deliv. Rev.* **2012**, *64*, 1547–1568. [CrossRef] [PubMed]
34. Lee, J.; Prausnitz, M. Drug delivery using microneedle patches: Not just for skin. *Expert Opin. Drug Deliv.* **2018**, *15*, 541–543. [CrossRef]
35. Aksit, A.; Arteaga, D.; Arriaga, M.; Wang, X.; Watanabe, H.; Kasza, K.; Lalwani, A.; Kysar, J. In-vitro perforation of the round window membrane via direct 3-D printed microneedles. *Biomed. Microdevices* **2018**, *20*, 1–12. [CrossRef]
36. Yu, M.; Arteaga, D.N.; Aksit, A.; Chiang, H.; Olson, E.S.; Kysar, J.W.; Lalwani, A.K. Anatomical and Functional Consequences of Microneedle Perforation of Round Window Membrane. *Otol. Neurotol.* **2020**, *41*, e280–e287. [CrossRef]
37. Chiang, H.; Yu, M.; Aksit, A.; Wang, W.; Stern-Shavit, S.; Kysar, J.W.; Lalwani, A.K. 3D-printed Microneedles Create Precise Perforations in Human Round Window Membrane in situ. *Otol. Neurotol.* **2020**, *41*, 277–284. [CrossRef]
38. Aksit, A.; Rastogi, S.; Nadal, M.; Parker, A.; Lalwani, A.; West, A.; Kysar, J.W. Drug delivery device for the inner ear: Ultra-sharp fully metallic microneedles. *Drug Deliv. Transl. Res.* **2020**, *11*, 214–226. [CrossRef]
39. Szeto, B.; Aksit, A.; Valentini, C.; Yu, M.; Werth, E.G.; Goeta, S.; Tang, C.; Brown, L.M.; Olson, E.S.; Kysar, J.W.; et al. Novel 3D-printed hollow microneedles facilitate safe, reliable, and informative sampling of perilymph from guinea pigs. *Hear. Res.* **2021**, *400*, 108141. [CrossRef]
40. Watanabe, H.; Cardoso, L.; Lalwani, A.K.; Kysar, J.W. A dual wedge microneedle for sampling of perilymph solution via round window membrane. *Biomed. Microdevices* **2016**, *18*, 24. [CrossRef]
41. Park, J.-H.; Allen, M.G.; Prausnitz, M.R. Polymer Microneedles for Controlled-Release Drug Delivery. *Pharm. Res.* **2006**, *23*, 1008–1019. [CrossRef]
42. Larrañeta, E.; McCrudden, M.T.C.; Courtenay, A.J.; Donnelly, R.F. Microneedles: A New Frontier in Nanomedicine Delivery. *Pharm. Res.* **2016**, *33*, 1055–1073. [CrossRef]
43. Serbin, J.; Egbert, A.; Ostendorf, A.; Chichkov, B.N.; Houbertz, R.; Domann, G.; Schulz, J.; Cronauer, C.; Fröhlich, L.; Popall, M. Femtosecond laser-induced two-photon polymerization of inorganic–organic hybrid materials for applications in photonics. *Opt. Lett.* **2003**, *28*, 301–303. [CrossRef]
44. Kelso, C.M.; Watanabe, H.; Wazen, J.M.; Bucher, T.; Qian, Z.J.; Olson, E.S.; Kysar, J.W.; Lalwani, A.K. Microperforations Significantly Enhance Diffusion Across Round Window Membrane. *Otol. Neurotol.* **2015**, *36*, 694–700. [CrossRef]
45. Creber, N.J.; Eastwood, H.T.; Hampson, A.J.; Tan, J.; O'Leary, S.J. A comparison of cochlear distribution and glucocorticoid receptor activation in local and systemic dexamethasone drug delivery regimes. *Hear. Res.* **2018**, *368*, 75–85. [CrossRef]
46. Wang, Y.; Han, L.; Diao, T.; Jing, Y.; Wang, L.; Zheng, H.; Ma, X.; Qi, J.; Yu, L. A comparison of systemic and local dexamethasone administration: From perilymph/cochlear concentration to cochlear distribution. *Hear. Res.* **2018**, *370*, 1–10. [CrossRef]
47. Trune, D.R.; Shives, K.D.; Hausman, F.; Kempton, J.B.; MacArthur, C.J.; Choi, D. Intratympanically delivered steroids impact thousands more inner ear genes than systemic delivery. *Ann. Otol. Rhinol. Laryngol.* **2019**, *128* (Suppl. S6), 134S–138S. [CrossRef]
48. Szeto, B.; Valentini, C.; Aksit, A.; Werth, E.G.; Goeta, S.; Brown, L.M.; Olson, E.S.; Kysar, J.W.; Lalwani, A.K. Impact of Systemic versus Intratympanic Dexamethasone Administration on the Perilymph Proteome. *J. Proteom. Res.* **2021**, *20*, 4001–4009. [CrossRef]
49. Salt, A.N.; Sirjani, D.B.; Hartsock, J.J.; Gill, R.M.; Plontke, S.K. Marker retention in the cochlea following injections through the round window membrane. *Hear. Res.* **2007**, *232*, 78–86. [CrossRef]
50. Poiseuille, J. Ecoulement des Liquides: Societe Philomatique de Paris. *Extraits des Proces-Verbaux des Seances Pendant I'Annee* **1838**, *3*, 77–81.
51. Santimetaneedol, A.; Wang, Z.; Arteaga, D.N.; Aksit, A.; Prevoteau, C.; Yu, M.; Chiang, H.; Fafalis, D.; Lalwani, A.K.; Kysar, J.W. Small molecule delivery across a perforated artificial membrane by thermoreversible hydrogel poloxamer 407. *Colloids Surf. B Biointerfaces* **2019**, *182*, 110300. [CrossRef]

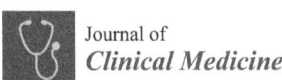

Review

A Window of Opportunity: Perilymph Sampling from the Round Window Membrane Can Advance Inner Ear Diagnostics and Therapeutics

Madeleine St. Peter [1], Athanasia Warnecke [2] and Hinrich Staecker [1,*]

1. Department of Otolaryngology-Head & Neck Surgery, University of Kansas Medical Center, Kansas City, KS 66160, USA; mstpeter@kumc.edu
2. Department of Otolaryngology Head and Neck Surgery, Hannover Medical School, D-30625 Hanover, Germany; warnecke.athanasia@mh-hannover.de
* Correspondence: hstaecker@kumc.edu

Abstract: In the clinical setting, the pathophysiology of sensorineural hearing loss is poorly defined and there are currently no diagnostic tests available to differentiate between subtypes. This often leaves patients with generalized treatment options such as steroids, hearing aids, or cochlear implantation. The gold standard for localizing disease is direct biopsy or imaging of the affected tissue; however, the inaccessibility and fragility of the cochlea make these techniques difficult. Thus, the establishment of an indirect biopsy, a sampling of inner fluids, is needed to advance inner ear diagnostics and allow for the development of novel therapeutics for inner ear disease. A promising source is perilymph, an inner ear liquid that bathes multiple structures critical to sound transduction. Intraoperative perilymph sampling via the round window membrane of the cochlea has been successfully used to profile the proteome, metabolome, and transcriptome of the inner ear and is a potential source of biomarker discovery. Despite its potential to provide insight into inner ear pathologies, human perilymph sampling continues to be controversial and is currently performed only in conjunction with a planned procedure where the inner ear is opened. Here, we review the safety of procedures in which the inner ear is opened, highlight studies where perilymph analysis has advanced our knowledge of inner ear diseases, and finally propose that perilymph sampling could be done as a stand-alone procedure, thereby advancing our ability to accurately classify sensorineural hearing loss.

Keywords: perilymph; round window; stapedectomy; cochlear implantation; sensorineural hearing loss

1. Introduction

Permanent hearing loss affects more than 5% of the world's population and is the most common sensory deficit in developed countries [1]. It can be divided into two categories: conductive hearing loss (CHL) and sensorineural hearing loss (SNHL). SNHL makes up 90% of the cases and can be caused by damage to any of the more than 20 inner ear cell types responsible for hearing [2–4]. As with all other tissues in the body, damage to the inner ear can be caused by genetic, infectious, inflammatory, toxic, or degenerative mechanisms. At present, SNHL is defined by the hearing threshold (i.e., mild, moderate, severe, severe to profound, and profound) combined with clinical features (progressive, sudden, fluctuating, etc.). The degree of hearing loss is determined by pure tone audiometry, which is a subjective patient response-based test. Objective auditory diagnostic testing such as otoacoustic emissions can localize hearing loss to a decline in outer hair cell function but is ineffective in more severe hearing losses [5]. Without accurate localization of disease and disease mechanisms, only rehabilitative treatment options such as hearing aids or cochlear implants can be offered. Those with severe or profound SNHL who identify 50%

or fewer words on key word testing can be offered cochlear implantation (CI), which can have variable outcomes.

The location and fragility of the cochlea poses a significant diagnostic challenge. The cochlea is buried deep within the temporal bone and is surrounded by a thick bony otic capsule, making it difficult to access for diagnostic profiling [6]. Violation of the tight junction system that separates the scala media (endolymph compartment) from the remainder of the inner ear results in complete loss of residual hearing, making it impossible to biopsy the inner ear. While postmortem and animal studies of the cochlea have offered invaluable insights, we still have a limited understanding of what is occurring on a molecular level in patients with active inner ear disease [7]. The successful development of hearing preservation cochlear implantation raises the possibility that perilymph in the scala tympani of the inner ear can be accessed without loss of residual hearing [8,9].

Perilymph is found in the scalae tympani, scala vestibuli, and in the balance portions of the inner ear and is similar in composition to cerebral spinal fluid (CSF). It bathes multiple structures necessary for signal transduction including spiral ganglion cell bodies, the auditory nerve, the hair cells, as well as portions of the lateral wall of the cochlea and is critical to sound transmission within the cochlea [10,11]. Perilymph can potentially be sampled during inner ear surgery such as stapedectomy, labyrinthectomy, and cochlear implantation, which allows for comparison between patient subpopulations with SNHL and CHL [12,13]. Since the advent of the sampling technique in the mid-1900s, human and animal studies have revealed proteins, metabolites, and microRNAs (miRNAs) specific to subtypes of SNHL in perilymph. In addition, perilymph profiles have been correlated to surgical outcomes and prognosis, specifically patient response to cochlear implantation (CI). We propose that perilymph sampling via the round window membrane (RWM) can be developed as a safe outpatient procedure and can serve as a "liquid biopsy" to guide diagnosis and treatment of SNHL.

2. History of Human Perilymph Sampling

2.1. Postmortem Profiling

Many perilymph profiling studies in humans have been performed using postmortem samples. These studies largely form the backbone of our current understanding of the chemical and protein makeup of human perilymph. In fact, postmortem studies were the first to accurately describe ionic concentrations of human perilymph [14,15] and investigate changes in ionic and protein compositions associated with inner ear diseases such as otosclerosis [16–18].

Postmortem perilymph sampling has also allowed for comparisons between CSF, serum, and perilymph, furthering our understanding of inner ear anatomy and the role of each fluid in hearing. Arrer et al. used proteome analysis to compare the levels of α1-antitrypsin and pre-albumin in the CSF, perilymph, and serum. Each fluid demonstrated a different pattern, suggesting that they are distinct fluids with different roles in the inner ear [19]. Later, Palva et al. used postmortem samples to compare the esterase composition of endolymph, perilymph, serum, and CSF. This study revealed distinct patterns of esterase concentration of endolymph and perilymph compared to serum and CSF, further suggesting that these are all separate fluids [17]. More recently, postmortem analysis of perilymph has been used to catalog the presence of miRNA in the cochlea. For example, over 500 miRNAs have been detected in the endolymph and perilymph of postmortem samples, with 481 differentially expressed in patients with a vestibular disorder called benign paroxysmal positional vertigo [20].

2.2. Intraoperative Sampling in Humans

Although many advances have been made using postmortem sampling, molecular analysis in these studies is limited because of rapid autolysis and degradation of DNA, RNA, and proteins [21]. To overcome this, human perilymph can be sampled from living subjects intraoperatively. Sampling during open ear surgeries dates back as far as 1950, when Waltner et al. extracted perilymph from the semicircular canal of patients with Meniere's disease (SNHL) during labyrinthectomy to compare perilymph and endolymph compositions [11]. Stapedectomy was the first surgical procedure in which the inner ear was routinely opened and, until the advent of cochlear implantation, yielded the bulk of data on perilymph composition.

Intraoperative perilymph sampling can also be used to assess direct and systemic drug delivery to the inner ear. Molecules perfused into a perilymph compartment (ideally the scala tympani) have direct access to the cells of the inner ear; therefore, optimal drug delivery to the inner ear depends on high concentrations in perilymph. Most studies have focused on quantifying steroid delivery specifically, given that intratympanic and intravenous steroids are commonly used as first line for certain subtypes of SNHL. Using intraoperative sampling during CI, it was found that inner ear levels are dependent on the systemic intravenous steroid dose received [22], and that intratympanic injections result in much higher drug delivery when compared to intravenous infusion [23].

3. Animal Models of Sensorineural Hearing Loss and Perilymph Sampling

3.1. Noise-Induced Hearing Loss

Noise-induced hearing loss (NIHL) accounts for one-third of all acquired cases of SNHL. Exposure to noises greater than 90 decibels for prolonged periods can cause mitochondrial pathology, excessive excitatory neurotransmitter release, and reduced blood flow to the cochlea, all of which result in the production of reactive oxygen species (ROS). ROS then inflict oxidative damage to the cochlear structures necessary for hearing [24].

Perilymph sampling in animal models has been used to measure changes in ROS, cytokines, and other metabolites in the cochlea before and after noise exposure. In mice, one hour of exposure to 110 dB causes a fourfold increase in hydroxy radical concentration in perilymph [25]. In guinea pigs, impulse noise exposure with subsequent perilymph analysis resulted in the discovery of seven altered metabolites following noise exposure [26]. Furthermore, inhalation of hydrogen gas was protective from ROS-mediated NIHL, and metabolic changes associated with hydrogen gas administration were reflected in perilymph [26]. Changes in cytokines such as tumor necrosis factor and interleukin 6 have also been detected after noise exposure using perilymph sampling in mice [20]. Although not currently relevant for understanding human disease, these findings suggest that profiling of ROS species and cytokines in human perilymph may lead to a further understanding of the mechanisms of NIHL as well as other subtypes of SNHL that may involve the ROS or inflammatory pathway.

3.2. Age-Related Hearing Loss

Age-related hearing loss (ARHL), also called presbycusis, is the most common subtype of SNHL and has a multifactorial etiology. It was hypothesized by Harman in 1956 that environmental exposures such as noise, ototoxic substances, and age-related cochlear hypoperfusion increase oxidative stress and contribute to the development of ARHL in those with genetic predisposition [27,28]. Though there are multiple animal models of ARHL and several lines of evidence supporting Harman's free radical theory in animals, there is currently a paucity of literature regarding animal models of perilymph profiles in ARHL.

3.3. Perilymph Expression Patterns across Species

Intraoperative perilymph sampling allows for direct comparison of human and animal tissues. It can therefore be used to identify feasible drug targets and guide animal model development. Although there is limited literature comparing animal and human perilymph, there are some studies that compare protein profiles. In 2011, Lysaght et al. found that perilymph from patients undergoing CI for SNHL had 31 orthologs in common with the mouse perilymph profile collected by Swan et al. in 2009 [29–31]. Comparison of human perilymph to guinea pigs has revealed a 64% overlap in protein profile, with apolipoproteins, enzymes, and immunoglobulins among the highly conserved classes [32]. This suggests that although useful, animal models are not a complete substitute for human data.

4. Human Perilymph Proteomics

4.1. Perilymph Proteins Specific to Subtypes of SNHL

Protein analysis of perilymph has elucidated the pathways involved in SNHL and has allowed for comparisons between subtypes of SNHL. Mass spectrometry has been used to create and compare comprehensive libraries of perilymph proteins in CI and vestibular schwannoma (VS) patients [31]. Although both patient groups have SNHL, comparison of their perilymph revealed differentially expressed proteins in VS samples including m-crystallin and LDL receptor related protein 2, which serve as the first potential markers of VS. Later studies by Rasmussen et al. discovered a protein that correlates with degree of tumor-associated hearing loss in VS perilymph: alpha-2-HS-glycoprotein [33]. In a large-scale analysis of perilymph from CI patients, proteins specific to infectious and congenital causes of SNHL were identified. In this same study, 97 proteins were found to be present only in adults with idiopathic SNHL when compared to children with idiopathic SNHL, revealing proteins potentially implicated in presbycusis [13,33].

Proteins specific to Meniere's disease (SNHL) have also been identified in human perilymph using liquid chromatography with tandem mass spectrometry. In 2019, Lin et al. compared the perilymph of Meniere's disease patients to the perilymph of normal hearing patients with skull-base meningiomas and discovered 38 proteins with differential abundance [29], four of which have known roles in the pathogenesis of Meniere's disease. Additional groups have used protein analysis to investigate entire pathways and protein families altered in patients with subtypes of SNHL, including inflammatory pathways, heat shock proteins, and neurotrophin pathways.

4.2. Inflammatory Pathways

Some patients with progressive or sudden SNHL are responsive to intratympanic injection of anti-inflammatory medications such as steroids. Therefore, identifying inflammatory protein mediators in the inner ear is of interest to researchers [34]. Warnecke et al. used perilymph from CI patients to perform protein multiplex analysis, which resulted in the discovery of key inflammatory mediators and potential drug targets for SNHL. In addition, protein patterns were correlated with residual hearing pre-CI [35]. Some of the proteins discovered in this study were also the targets of drugs with demonstrated efficacy in animal models. For instance, insulin-like growth factor binding protein 1 (IGFBP1), a known regulator of insulin-like growth factor 1 (IGF-1), was highly expressed in the perilymph of patients with complete loss of auditory function when compared to patients with residual hearing. Animal studies have shown that applying recombinant IGF-1 to the RWM protects against noise-induced hearing loss in guinea pigs and rats [35,36]. Furthermore, in a human trial, treating patients with sudden SNHL refractory to systemic steroids with middle ear IGF-1 was superior to intratympanic steroid injections [37]. This demonstrates that perilymph analysis and animal studies can be linked to potentially develop novel diagnostic and therapeutic interventions.

4.3. Neurotrophin Pathway

Studies of the mouse cochlea in vivo have demonstrated that neurotrophic factors such as brain-derived neurotrophic factor (BDNF) and neurotrophin 3 (NT-3) are essential to neuron survival, and application of these factors can rescue and protect spiral ganglia neurons, which are critical for signal transduction and hearing [38–40]. Consistent with these findings, human perilymph protein analysis revealed that higher levels of BDNF-regulated proteins are correlated to the presence of residual hearing prior to implantation and to better cochlear implant performance. Conversely, decreased levels of BDNF-regulated proteins were associated with profoundly deaf patients versus those with residual hearing [41].

4.4. Heat Shock Proteins

Heat shock proteins (HSPs) are thought to protect tissues by refolding denatured or misfolded proteins. They have been implicated in many disease processes, and recently in the pathogenesis of sudden SNHL, Meniere's disease, and idiopathic SNHL. Serum values of HSPs are significantly higher in those with sudden SNHL compared to normal hearing controls [42]. Additionally, antibodies to HSPs are present in patients with Meniere's disease and levels correlate with disease activity [43]. In human perilymph, 10 subgroups of HSPs have been identified, with higher levels present in patients with residual hearing before undergoing CI and VS removal [44].

5. Human Perilymph Metabolome and Transcriptome

5.1. Perilymph Metabolome

Characterizing the metabolic composition of perilymph fluid is critical for understanding the pathophysiology of deafness and predicting surgical outcomes. This is especially critical for CI patients, as the metabolites in perilymph interact directly with the electrode placed in the cochlea. Perilymph proteome analysis has revealed a relationship between the levels of metabolites such as N-acetylneuraminate, glutaric acid, cystine, 2-methylpropanoate, butanoate, and xanthine and the duration of SNHL [45]. Although there have been mixed results, there is some evidence that those with a longer duration of SNHL have decreased speech comprehension post-CI [46], which suggests that a RWM perilymph "tap" with metabolic analysis might be useful for predicting speech comprehension after CI. Although further studies are needed to confirm this theory, it is a promising potential tool to determine candidacy for cochlear implantation.

Similar to rat, guinea pig, and mouse models, humans with profound SNHL from multiple etiologies display characteristic metabolites in perilymph. In one human study, the perilymph of patients with profound SNHL was compared to that of those with otosclerosis (CHL). Those with profound SNHL had significantly higher superoxide in perilymph and were positive for the ROS-producing enzyme xanthine [47].

5.2. MicroRNAs as Biomarkers for SNHL

MiRNAs are small non-coding RNAs that can be found in body fluids. They serve as reliable biomarkers and prognostic indicators for multiple other neurodegenerative diseases, including Alzheimer's, amyotrophic lateral sclerosis, and Parkinson's [48–50]. They have also recently been used to differentiate subtypes of SNHL and predict prognosis. In 2018, Shew et al. demonstrated that machine learning algorithms can use miRNA perilymph profiles to delineate between SNHL and CHL and can predict residual hearing after CI with 100% accuracy. In addition, comparison of miRNA profiles between patients with otosclerosis (CHL) and Meniere's disease (SNHL) using microarray has revealed miRNAs differentially expressed in the perilymph of patients with Meniere's disease [51,52]. As shown in recent proteomics studies, miRNA expression may also predict the status of neurotrophin signaling in cochlear implant patients [53].

In summary, we can already derive a wealth of information from a sample of perilymph, including predictors of hearing loss, markers of a pro-inflammatory state, factors predicted to protect the inner ear during surgery, and potential predictors of cochlear implant outcomes. Identifying the mechanisms of hearing loss in real time will also allow optimized pharmacologic intervention. To take advantage of this wealth of data, this information needs to be available prior to initiating a planned treatment such as CI.

6. Applications of Human Perilymph Sampling

Opening the inner ear was historically considered impossible due to the risk of hearing loss; however, recent experience with hearing preservation cochlear implantation and past sampling studies on stapedectomy patients indicates that it is possible to manipulate the inner ear with no or minimal loss of residual hearing in most patients [54]. We propose that perilymph can be sampled as a stand-alone procedure. Several different existing ear surgeries can be used to model the development of a perilymph sampling procedure including cochlear implantation, stapedectomy, and cochleosacculotomy. Initial applications of perilymph sampling will likely be in enhancing CI and evaluating progressive hearing loss. As more targeted therapeutics for hearing loss emerge, further applications will develop [55].

6.1. Cochlear Implantation

A cochlear implant is a prosthetic device inserted into the inner ear of patients with severe SNHL and poor speech perception who have minimal improvement with the use of hearing aids. Criteria for undergoing implantation have been recently expanded from including only patients with profound hearing loss to those patients with significant residual hearing but poor speech understanding. The surgery is performed by drilling a mastoidectomy and then entering the middle ear space through a posterior tympanotomy (the space between the incus, chorda tympani, and facial nerves) [56]. The bony overhang of the round window is then drilled down to visualize the RWM. An incision is made in the RWM, allowing for the sampling of a small amount of perilymph. The electrode can then be advanced through the window.

CI can improve the speech perception ability in 82.0% of adults with post lingual hearing loss and 53.4% of adults with prelingual hearing loss and can markedly improve quality of life in the responders [57]. However, there is a proportion of patients who do not benefit, and most continue to lose hearing that was present before the operation [55]. Unfortunately, clinicians currently have no way to predict which patients will respond to CI. Although duration of hearing loss and pre-implantation speech perception are thought to be correlated to outcomes, studies have shown mixed results in small sample sizes, and there is still no consensus regarding which patient factors predict functional hearing over time [58]. Characteristics such as sex and age also have mixed results regarding correlation to residual hearing, and do not account for the large variability in patient response to CI [55]. In animal models, some groups have shown that trauma during surgery can induce inflammation and affect post-op hearing [59]; however, human studies have shown that hearing continues to decline long after post-operative inflammation has resolved [55]. Taken together, this has led to the hypothesis that etiology of SNHL rather than patient profile or surgical factors may have the most influence on CI outcomes, further demonstrating the need for subclassification of SNHL.

Most of the current perilymph sampling studies have focused on perilymph sampled from cochlear implant patients and information derived from these studies may yield information on optimal pharmacologic intervention to protect hearing during the implantation process. Sampling could also help predict who would be a candidate for supplementation with neurotrophins or who could benefit from drug eluting cochlear implant electrodes [60]. Since patients with significant residual hearing are being successfully implanted, perilymph sampling at the time of implantation can give us initial safety data on the procedure when it is performed at the same time as cochlear implantation. Hannover Medical School has been routinely sampling perilymph on all implant patients and has not seen a decline in their hearing preservation rates [13,61]. However, safety data should not be gleaned solely from CI procedures. Both the perilymph sampling procedure and CI electrode insertion require puncture of the RWM, which causes perilymph egress. Therefore, if these are done simultaneously, it will be difficult to draw conclusions regarding the safety of perilymph sampling specifically.

6.2. Stapedectomy and Cochleosacculotomy

Several other operations access the inner ear fluid spaces. Stapedectomy is commonly performed for patients with otosclerosis, a cause of CHL. Stapedectomy is well tolerated and significantly improves hearing, with some studies showing up to 70% of patients achieving an air–bone gap of 20 dB or better [62,63].

Although opening the stapes footplate accesses the perilymphatic spaces of the inner ear, this approach would probably not be applicable in routine perilymph sampling in patients without a fixed stapes footplate. Additionally, in patients undergoing workup for SNHL, the stapes supra-structure would impede access to the inner ear. Access to the middle ear, which contains the stapes bone, is gained by making an incision in the auditory canal and lifting the tympanic membrane. The bony scutum is then shaved down, allowing for the visualization of multiple middle and inner ear structures, including the round window niche.

Stapedectomy is generally not indicated for SNHL and is therefore not useful for directly profiling patients with SNHL. However, it is commonly performed for CHL, which provides an opportunity for a control group. Although sampling during stapedectomy is a debated topic among some clinicians, multiple groups have reported safety using this methodology, and stapedectomy has yielded valuable information on pathogenesis of CHL [18,22,46,64–75]. In this technique, perilymph is not collected from the stapedotomy opening, but from the surrounding footplate where perilymph has already egressed out of the vestibule. Therefore, it is unlikely that collection of perilymph is significantly altering post-operative outcomes.

The RWM itself is accessed during another open ear surgery called cochleosacculotomy, indicated for patients with refractory MD (SNHL) who have minimal or no residual hearing in the affected ear [76]. In this procedure, the middle ear is opened and the bony overhang of the round window niche is removed. A 4 mm right angle pick is then used to obliterate the inner ear. A similar approach to the round window could be used to develop a non-destructive sampling of inner ear fluid.

6.3. Proposed Method of RWM "Tap"

For sampling perilymph, a standard transcanal approach would be used. After making a cut in the ear canal skin, the tympanic membrane is elevated, revealing the structures of the middle ear (Figure 1A). The round window niche is identified, and the bony overhang removed. Next, the stapes is gently palpated to look for a round window reflex to ensure the correct anatomical plane. The window is then punctured for a sample. Optimally, this should be in the inferior portion of the round window to avoid the basilar membrane. The RWM is at a median angle of 113 degrees to the ear canal; thus, a curved sampling device would be needed. As can be seen in the temporal bone specimen, this approach allows access to the basal turn of the cochlea (Figure 1B) [77]. At the conclusion of sampling, a small tissue patch can be applied. The eardrum is then moved back into position.

6.4. Progress in the Design of Sampling Devices

Successful perilymph sampling depends on developing a device that safely accesses the scala tympani and atraumatically withdraws a small sample. In humans, sterile glass capillary tubes are commonly used for intraoperative sampling via the RWM with preservation of residual hearing [13,29,30,35,52]. When placed in perilymph, the capillary tube forms a meniscus. This creates a pressure gradient, causing the fluid to move into the tube. The amount of fluid drawn up depends on the radius of the tube, density of the liquid, and surface tension. The angle of approach is also an important factor, as this determines the curvature of the meniscus and thus affects the size of the pressure gradient. Benefits of using the glass capillary tube include a simple methodology and low cost. However, volume aspirated into the capillary can be non-uniform due to variable tube diameter and user technique. In addition, puncture of the RWM with the glass capillary tube can cause CSF outflow into the scala tympani and contamination of the sample [78]. A specific capillary tube has not been validated for intraoperative use in humans; however, multiple research groups have used various sterile glass capillary tubes for perilymph extraction without complication [13,29,30,35,52].

Microneedles can also be used for sampling. There are multiple types, most of which have been developed and optimized in animal models. To collect perilymph, the needle is advanced into the RWM and perilymph is drawn up using a syringe. Multiple studies have shown that perforation of the RWM with microneedles does not affect hearing threshold in animals and are generally atraumatic [79–82]. Microneedles have not yet been tested in humans intraoperatively; however Early et al. recently tested a novel microneedle in fresh frozen human temporal bones. They found that the microneedle with syringe could reliably withdraw 5 µL of perilymph from the scala tympani with minimal contamination and little trauma to the RWM [83]. Although microneedles have a more complex design than the glass capillary tubes, they allow for controlled aspiration of perilymph. This may result in more consistent volumes sampled and may decrease the likelihood of CSF contamination. Using the approach to the round window outlined above and a curved sampling device, articulated instruments that allow incremental advancement of a needle through the round window and subsequent microfluidic withdrawal of 10 µL of perilymph could also be designed (Figure 1C–F).

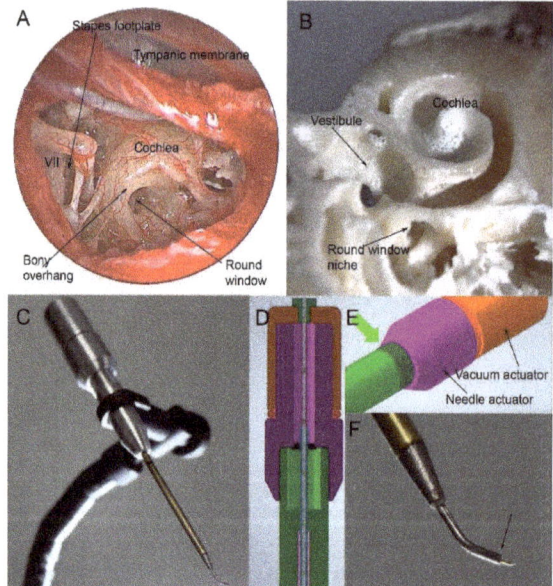

Figure 1. Endoscopic view of the right human middle ear (**A**). After lifting the tympanic membrane, the round window can be seen but is partially obscured by a bony overhang. Only a small area of the stapes footplate is visible next to the facial nerve (VII), making it difficult to access. The anatomy of the cochlea can be seen in a human temporal bone in which the cochlea has been opened (**B**). The round window niche allows access to the basal turn of the cochlea. A prototype sampling device features a 56 mm long shaft that can be passed down the ear canal to reach the round window (**C**). The device has two internal actuators, one advancing a needle and one allowing a plunger to be withdrawn from the needle/internal reservoir (**D**,**E**) through threading built into the device (green arrow, (**E**)). This allows advancement of a needle from the curved tip of the device in submillimeter increments and withdrawal of up to 10 µL of fluid. The tip of the device is shown in (**F**) and measures 0.86 mm at the tip (arrow) from which the needle is deployed.

6.5. Safety and Limitations

Although sampling has been conducted for many years across multiple institutions, there are very few studies directly examining the effects of intraoperative perilymph sampling on post-operative outcomes. Schmitt et al. is the only group to specifically address potential effects on post-CI residual hearing. They compared pre- and post-operative hearing thresholds between patients who underwent CI plus perilymph sampling and randomly selected patients that underwent only CI. No significant differences in residual hearing or speech perception were found between the groups [13].

There is a long history of sampling perilymph in stapedectomy patients. This technique has been used previously for profiling perilymph with no apparent complications but, as noted above, is probably not applicable to routine perilymph sampling for sensorineural hearing loss. Some additional insight can be gained from the surgical procedures in which the inner ear is opened. Stapedectomy is considered a safe procedure having only a minimal incidence of SNHL [84]. However, sampling through the stapes footplate would require manipulation of a mobile stapes. Hearing preservation CI in which the ear is not only opened but an implant placed has shown complete hearing preservation rates of 45%, and partial hearing preservation rates of 100% [85,86]. Analysis of cochlear microphonics during implantation suggests that if hearing loss occurs, it is not related to opening the RWM but occurs fairly late in the implantation process [86]. Therefore, a controlled puncture with a sampling of 5–10 µL is unlikely to cause any hearing loss.

There are also some technical limitations of the sampling procedure. Studies in guinea pigs show that perforation of the RWM induces perilymph outflow driven by CSF pressure, leading to possible CSF contamination of the sample, and that samples greater than 10 µL can be significantly contaminated with CSF [87]. There can also be interparticipant variations in perilymph volume, and samples can contain differing amounts of CSF and blood contamination. However, these limitations can be overcome through proper training, sample quality checks, and further optimization of instrumentation such as the microneedles used for extraction. Individual anatomic differences in the cochlear aqueduct must also be considered in sampling methodology. If the cochlear aqueduct is widely patent, there may be excessive perilymph and CSF outflow when the RWM is punctured during CI prior to electrode placement [88]. Only the fluid that first flows out of the RWM is pure perilymph. Therefore, if there is a large volume outflow, the fluid is likely to be contaminated with CSF that has entered the inner ear via the cochlear aqueduct. The likelihood of a CSF gusher is not entirely predictable but has been associated with malformation of inner ear structures, which may be detected on CT [89]. Finally, to move forward with developing this technique, large animal models such as pigs will be needed to test novel devices [90].

7. Conclusions

New diagnostic techniques are needed to further subclassify SNHL. As proposed here, a round window membrane "tap" can be performed to profile perilymph and determine SNHL subtype and candidacy for adjunctive medical treatment with cochlear implantation. Although perilymph sampling has been performed intraoperatively in humans for decades, it remains controversial due to paucity of literature on post-operative effects on hearing, and further safety studies are needed.

Author Contributions: Conceptualization, M.S.P., A.W. and H.S.; original draft preparation, review, and editing, M.S.P., A.W. and H.S.; funding acquisition, M.S.P. and H.S. All authors have read and agreed to the published version of the manuscript.

Funding: This work was supported in part by the Alpha Omega Alpha Carolyn Kuckien Student Research Fellowship.

Institutional Review Board Statement: Not applicable.

Informed Consent Statement: Not applicable.

Conflicts of Interest: The authors declare no conflict of interest. The funders had no role in the design of the study; in the collection, analyses, or interpretation of data; in the writing of the manuscript, or in the decision to publish the results.

References

1. World Health Organization. Global Costs of Unaddressed Hearing Loss and Cost-Effectiveness of Interventions. *Health Report.* 2017. Available online: https://apps.who.int/iris/handle/10665/254659 (accessed on 11 February 2019).
2. Wong, A.C.; Ryan, A.F. Mechanisms of sensorineural cell damage, death and survival in the cochlea. *Front. Aging Neurosci.* 2015, 7, 58. [CrossRef]
3. Kunelskaya, N.L.; Levina, Y.V.; Garov, E.V.; Dzuina, A.V.; Ogorodnikov, D.S.; Nosulya, E.V.; Luchsheva, Y.V. Presbyacusis. *Vestnik Otorinolaringol.* 2019, 84, 67–71. [CrossRef]
4. Ouda, L.; Profant, O.; Syka, J. Age-related changes in the central auditory system. *Cell Tissue Res.* 2015, 361, 337–358. [CrossRef] [PubMed]
5. Kemp, D.T. Otoacoustic emissions, their origin in cochlear function, and use. *Br. Med. Bull.* 2002, 63, 223–241. [CrossRef]
6. Rask-Andersen, H.; Liu, W.; Erixon, E.; Kinnefors, A.; Pfaller, K.; Schrott-Fischer, A.; Glueckert, R. Human Cochlea: Anatomical Characteristics and their Relevance for Cochlear Implantation. *Anat. Rec. Adv. Integr. Anat. Evol. Biol.* 2012, 295, 1791–1811. [CrossRef] [PubMed]
7. Arriaga, M. Schuknecht's Pathology of the Ear, Third Edition. *Otol. Neurotol.* 2002, 32, 1039. [CrossRef]
8. Prentiss, S.; Sykes, K.; Staecker, H. Partial Deafness Cochlear Implantation at the University of Kansas: Techniques and Outcomes. *J. Am. Acad. Audiol.* 2010, 21, 197–203. [CrossRef]
9. Gantz, B.J.; Turner, C.; Gfeller, K.E.; Lowder, M.W. Preservation of Hearing in Cochlear Implant Surgery: Advantages of Combined Electrical and Acoustical Speech Processing. *Laryngoscope* 2005, 115, 796–802. [CrossRef]
10. Chirtes, A.V.; Mures, T.; Mitrică, M. Normal pressure hydrocephalus–Diagnosis and therapeutic challenges. *Rom. J.* 2020, 123, 354.
11. Waltner, J.G.; Raymond, S. On the chemical composition of the human perilymph and endolymph. *Laryngoscope* 1950, 60, 912–918. [CrossRef]
12. Warnecke, A.; Prenzler, N.K.; Schmitt, H.; Daemen, K.; Keil, J.; Dursin, M.; Lenarz, T.; Falk, C.S. Defining the Inflammatory Microenvironment in the Human Cochlea by Perilymph Analysis: Toward Liquid Biopsy of the Cochlea. *Front. Neurol.* 2019, 10, 665. [CrossRef] [PubMed]
13. Schmitt, H.A.; Pich, A.; Schröder, A.; Scheper, V.; Lilli, G.; Reuter, G.; Lenarz, T. Proteome Analysis of Human Perilymph Using an Intraoperative Sampling Method. *J. Proteome Res.* 2017, 16, 1911–1923. [CrossRef]
14. Palva, T.; Tikanmäki, P. Sodium and Potassium Concentrations in Post-Mortem Human Labyrinthine Fluids. *J. Laryngol. Otol.* 1969, 83, 147–159. [CrossRef] [PubMed]
15. Gamov, V.P.; Vel'Tishchev, I.E. Potassium and sodium content in the perilymph and endolymph of man (a postmortem study). *Zh. Ushn. Nos. Gorl. Bolezn.* 1973, 33, 21–24. [PubMed]
16. Silverstein, H.; Naufal, P.; Belal, A. Causes of elevated perilymph protein concentrations. *Laryngoscope* 1973, 83, 476–487. [CrossRef]
17. Palva, T.; Raunio, V.; Forsén, R. Esterases in Post-Mortem Inner Ear Fluids. *Acta Oto-Laryngol.* 1971, 71, 140–146. [CrossRef]
18. Schindler, K.; Schnieder, E.A.; Wullstein, H.L. Vergleichende Bestimmung Einiger Elektrolyte und Organischer Substanzen in Der Perilymphe Otosklerosekranker Patienten. *Acta Oto-Laryngol.* 1965, 59, 309–319. [CrossRef]
19. Arrer, E.; Oberascher, G.; Gibitz, H.-J. Protein distribution in the human perilymph:A Comparative Study between Perilymph (Post Mortem), CSF and Blood Serum. *Acta Oto-Laryngol.* 1988, 106, 117–123. [CrossRef]
20. Rohde, M.; Sinicina, I.; Horn, A.; Eichner, N.; Meister, G.; Strupp, M.; Himmelein, S. MicroRNA profile of human endo-/perilymph. *J. Neurol.* 2018, 265, 26–28. [CrossRef]
21. Nadol, J.B., Jr.; Burgess, B. A study of postmortem autolysis in the human organ of corti. *J. Comp. Neurol.* 1985, 237, 333–342. [CrossRef]
22. Niedermeyer, H.P.; Zahneisen, G.; Luppa, P.; Busch, R.; Arnold, W. Cortisol Levels in the Human Perilymph after Intravenous Administration of Prednisolone. *Audiol. Neurotol.* 2003, 8, 316–321. [CrossRef] [PubMed]
23. Bird, P.A.; Begg, E.J.; Zhang, M.; Keast, A.T.; Murray, D.P.; Balkany, T.J. Intratympanic Versus Intravenous Delivery of Methylprednisolone to Cochlear Perilymph. *Otol. Neurotol.* 2007, 28, 1124–1130. [CrossRef]
24. Yang, C.J.; Chung, J.W. Pathophysiology of Noise Induced Hearing Loss. *Audiol. Speech Res.* 2016, 12, S14–S16. [CrossRef]
25. Ohlemiller, K.K.; Wright, J.S.; Dugan, L.L. Early Elevation of Cochlear Reactive Oxygen Species following Noise Exposure. *Audiol. Neurotol.* 1999, 4, 229–236. [CrossRef] [PubMed]
26. Pirttilä, K.; Pierre, P.V.; Haglöf, J.; Engskog, M.; Hedeland, M.; Laurell, G.; Arvidsson, T.; Pettersson, C. An LCMS-based untargeted metabolomics protocol for cochlear perilymph: Highlighting metabolic effects of hydrogen gas on the inner ear of noise exposed Guinea pigs. *Metabolomics* 2019, 15, 1–12. [CrossRef] [PubMed]
27. Fetoni, A.R.; Picciotti, P.M.; Paludetti, G.; Troiani, D. Pathogenesis of presbycusis in animal models: A review. *Exp. Gerontol.* 2011, 46, 413–425. [CrossRef] [PubMed]
28. Harman, D. Aging: A Theory Based on Free Radical and Radiation Chemistry. *J. Gerontol.* 1956, 11, 298–300. [CrossRef] [PubMed]
29. Lin, H.-C.; Ren, Y.; Lysaght, A.C.; Kao, S.-Y.; Stankovic, K.M. Proteome of normal human perilymph and perilymph from people with disabling vertigo. *PLoS ONE* 2019, 14, e0218292. [CrossRef] [PubMed]
30. Lysaght, A.C.; Kao, S.-Y.; Paulo, J.A.; Merchant, S.N.; Steen, H.; Stankovic, K.M. Proteome of Human Perilymph. *J. Proteome Res.* 2011, 10, 3845–3851. [CrossRef]

31. Ms, E.E.L.S.; Peppi, M.; Chen, Z.; Ba, K.M.G.; Evans, J.E.; McKenna, M.J.; Mescher, M.J.; Kujawa, S.G.; Sewell, W.F. Proteomics analysis of perilymph and cerebrospinal fluid in mouse. *Laryngoscope* **2009**, *119*, 953–958. [CrossRef]
32. Palmer, J.; Lord, M.S.; Pinyon, J.L.; Wise, A.K.; Lovell, N.H.; Carter, P.; Enke, Y.L.; Housley, G.D.; Green, R.A. Understanding the cochlear implant environment by mapping perilymph proteomes from different species. In Proceedings of the 38th Annual International Conference of the IEEE Engineering in Medicine and Biology Society (EMBC), Orlando, FL, USA, 16–20 August 2016; pp. 5237–5240. [CrossRef]
33. Rasmussen, J.E.; Laurell, G.; Rask-Andersen, H.; Bergquist, J.; Eriksson, P.O. The proteome of perilymph in patients with vestibular schwannoma. A possibility to identify biomarkers for tumor associated hearing loss? *PLoS ONE* **2018**, *13*, e0198442. [CrossRef]
34. Tornabene, S.V.; Sato, K.; Pham, L.; Billings, P.; Keithley, E.M. Immune cell recruitment following acoustic trauma. *Hear. Res.* **2006**, *222*, 115–124. [CrossRef]
35. Lee, K.Y.; Nakagawa, T.; Okano, T.; Hori, R.; Ono, K.; Tabata, Y.; Lee, S.H.; Ito, J. Novel therapy for hearing loss: Delivery of insulin-like growth factor 1 to the cochlea using gelatin hydrogel. *Otol. Neurotol.* **2007**, *28*, 976–981. [CrossRef] [PubMed]
36. Hayashi, Y.; Yamamoto, N.; Nakagawa, T.; Ito, J. Insulin-like growth factor 1 induces the transcription of Gap43 and Ntn1 during hair cell protection in the neonatal murine cochlea. *Neurosci. Lett.* **2014**, *560*, 7–11. [CrossRef]
37. Nakagawa, T.; Kumakawa, K.; Usami, S.-I.; Hato, N.; Tabuchi, K.; Takahashi, M.; Fujiwara, K.; Sasaki, A.; Komune, S.; Sakamoto, T.; et al. A randomized controlled clinical trial of topical insulin-like growth factor-1 therapy for sudden deafness refractory to systemic corticosteroid treatment. *BMC Med.* **2014**, *12*, 1–8. [CrossRef]
38. Rejali, D.; Lee, V.A.; Abrashkin, K.A.; Humayun, N.; Swiderski, D.L.; Raphael, Y. Cochlear implants and ex vivo BDNF gene therapy protect spiral ganglion neurons. *Hear. Res.* **2007**, *228*, 180–187. [CrossRef]
39. Schmidt, N.; Schulze, J.; Warwas, D.P.; Ehlert, N.; Lenarz, T.; Warnecke, A.; Behrens, P. Long-term delivery of brain-derived neurotrophic factor (BDNF) from nanoporous silica nanoparticles improves the survival of spiral ganglion neurons in vitro. *PLoS ONE* **2018**, *13*, e0194778. [CrossRef]
40. Mou, K.; Husberger, C.; Cleary, J.; Davis, R.L. Synergistic effects of BDNF and NT-3 on postnatal spiral ganglion neurons. *J. Comp. Neurol.* **1997**, *386*, 529–539. [CrossRef]
41. De Vries, I.; Schmitt, H.; Lenarz, T.; Prenzler, N.; Alvi, S.; Staecker, H.; Durisin, M.; Warnecke, A. Detection of BDNF-Related Proteins in Human Perilymph in Patients with Hearing Loss. *Front. Neurosci.* **2019**, *13*, 214. [CrossRef]
42. Park, S.-N.; Yeo, S.W.; Park, K.-H. Serum Heat Shock Protein 70 and its Correlation with Clinical Characteristics in Patients with Sudden Sensorineural Hearing Loss. *Laryngoscope* **2006**, *116*, 121–125. [CrossRef]
43. Rauch, S.D.; San Martin, J.E.; Moscicki, R.A.; Bloch, K.J. Serum antibodies against heat shock protein 70 in Ménière's disease. *Am. J. Otol.* **1995**, *16*, 648–652.
44. Schmitt, H.; Roemer, A.; Zeilinger, C.; Salcher, R.; Durisin, M.; Staecker, H.; Lenarz, T.; Warnecke, A. Heat Shock Proteins in Human Perilymph: Implications for Cochlear Implantation. *Otol. Neurotol.* **2018**, *39*, 37–44. [CrossRef]
45. Trinh, T.-T.; Blasco, H.; Emond, P.; Andres, C.; Lefevre, A.; Lescanne, E.; Bakhos, D. Relationship between Metabolomics Profile of Perilymph in Cochlear-Implanted Patients and Duration of Hearing Loss. *Metabolites* **2019**, *9*, 262. [CrossRef]
46. Niparko, J.K. Spoken Language Development in Children Following Cochlear Implantation. *JAMA* **2010**, *303*, 1498–1506. [CrossRef] [PubMed]
47. Ciorba, A.; Gasparini, P.; Chicca, M.; Pinamonti, S.; Martini, A. Reactive oxygen species in human inner ear perilymph. *Acta Oto-Laryngol.* **2010**, *130*, 240–246. [CrossRef]
48. Geekiyanage, H.; Jicha, G.A.; Nelson, P.T.; Chan, C. Blood serum miRNA: Non-invasive biomarkers for Alzheimer's disease. *Exp. Neurol.* **2012**, *235*, 491–496. [CrossRef]
49. Ricci, C.; Marzocchi, C.; Battistini, S. MicroRNAs as Biomarkers in Amyotrophic Lateral Sclerosis. *Cells* **2018**, *7*, 219. [CrossRef]
50. Staff, T.P.O. Correction: Profiles of Extracellular miRNA in Cerebrospinal Fluid and Serum from Patients with Alzheimer's and Parkinson's Diseases Correlate with Disease Status and Features of Pathology. *PLoS ONE* **2014**, *9*, e106174. [CrossRef]
51. Wichova, H.; Shew, M.; Staecker, H. Utility of Perilymph microRNA Sampling for Identification of Active Gene Expression Pathways in Otosclerosis. *Otol. Neurotol.* **2019**, *40*, 710–719. [CrossRef]
52. Shew, M.; Wichova, H.; Bur, A.; Koestler, D.C.; Peter, M.S.; Warnecke, A.; Staecker, H. MicroRNA Profiling as a Methodology to Diagnose Ménière's Disease: Potential Application of Machine Learning. *Otolaryngol. Neck Surg.* **2020**, *164*, 399–406. [CrossRef]
53. Shew, M.; Wichova, H.; Warnecke, A.; Lenarz, T.; Staecker, H. Evaluating Neurotrophin Signaling Using MicroRNA Perilymph Profiling in Cochlear Implant Patients with and Without Residual Hearing. *Otol. Neurotol.* **2021**, *42*, e1125–e1133. [CrossRef]
54. Pillsbury, H.C.; Dillon, M.T.; Buchman, C.A.; Staecker, H.; Prentiss, S.M.; Ruckenstein, M.J.; Bigelow, D.C.; Telischi, F.F.; Martinez, D.M.; Runge, C.; et al. Multicenter US Clinical Trial with an Electric-Acoustic Stimulation (EAS) System in Adults: Final Outcomes. *Otol. Neurotol.* **2018**, *39*, 299–305. [CrossRef]
55. Schilder, A.G.; Su, M.P.; Mandavia, R.; Anderson, C.R.; Landry, E.; Ferdous, T.; Blackshaw, H. Early phase trials of novel hearing therapeutics: Avenues and opportunities. *Hear. Res.* **2019**, *380*, 175–186. [CrossRef]
56. Snels, C.; IntHout, J.; Mylanus, E.; Huinck, W.; Dhooge, I. Hearing Preservation in Cochlear Implant Surgery: A Meta-Analysis. *Otol. Neurotol.* **2019**, *40*, 145–153. [CrossRef]
57. Smulders, Y.E.; Hendriks, T.; Eikelboom, R.; Stegeman, I.; Maria, P.L.S.; Atlas, M.D.; Friedland, P.L. Predicting Sequential Cochlear Implantation Performance: A Systematic Review. *Audiol. Neurotol.* **2017**, *22*, 356–363. [CrossRef]

58. Moteki, H.; Nishio, S.-Y.; Miyagawa, M.; Tsukada, K.; Iwasaki, S.; Usami, S.-I. Long-term results of hearing preservation cochlear implant surgery in patients with residual low frequency hearing. *Acta Oto-Laryngol.* **2016**, *137*, 516–521. [CrossRef]
59. Astolfi, L.; Simoni, E.; Giarbini, N.; Giordano, P.; Pannella, M.; Hatzopoulos, S.; Martini, A. Cochlear implant and inflammation reaction: Safety study of a new steroid-eluting electrode. *Hear. Res.* **2016**, *336*, 44–52. [CrossRef]
60. Pfingst, B.E.; Colesa, D.J.; Swiderski, D.L.; Hughes, A.P.; Strahl, S.B.; Sinan, M.; Raphael, Y. Neurotrophin Gene Therapy in Deafened Ears with Cochlear Implants: Long-term Effects on Nerve Survival and Functional Measures. *J. Assoc. Res. Otolaryngol.* **2017**, *18*, 731–750. [CrossRef]
61. Sargsyan, G.; Kanaan, N.; Lenarz, T.; Lesinski-Schiedat, A. Comparison of speech recognition in cochlear implant patients with and without residual hearing: A review of indications. *Cochlea-Implant. Int.* **2021**, 1–8. [CrossRef]
62. Alzhrani, F.; Mokhatrish, M.M.; Al-Momani, M.O.; AlShehri, H.; Hagr, A.; Garadat, S.N. Effectiveness of stapedotomy in improving hearing sensitivity for 53 otosclerotic patients: Retrospective review. *Ann. Saudi Med.* **2017**, *37*, 49–55. [CrossRef]
63. Persson, P.; And, H.H.; Magnuson, B. Hearing Results in Otosclerosis Surgery after Partial Stapedectomy, Total Stapedectomy and Stapedotomy. *Acta Oto-Laryngol.* **1997**, *117*, 94–99. [CrossRef] [PubMed]
64. Levenson, M.J.; Desloge, R.B.; Parisier, S.C. Beta-2 Transferrin: Limitations of use as a clinical marker for perilymph. *Laryngoscope* **1996**, *106*, 159–161. [CrossRef]
65. Rauch, S.D. Transferrin Microheterogeneity in Human Perilymph. *Laryngoscope* **2000**, *110*, 545–552. [CrossRef] [PubMed]
66. Attanasio, G.; Viccaro, M.; Covelli, E.; De Seta, E.; Minni, A.; Pizzoli, F.; Filipo, R. Cyclo-oxygenase enzyme in the perilymph of human inner ear. *Acta Oto- Laryngol.* **2010**, *131*, 242–246. [CrossRef] [PubMed]
67. Ribári, O.; Sziklai, I. Cathepsin D Activity in Otosclerotic Bone and Perilymph. *Acta Oto-Laryngol.* **1988**, *105*, 549–552. [CrossRef]
68. Causse, J.R.; Uriel, J.; Berges, J.; Shambaugh, G.E.; Bretlau, P.; Causse, J.B. The enzymatic mechanism of the otospon-giotic disease and NaF action on the enzymatic balance. *Am. J. Otol.* **1982**, *3*, 297–314.
69. Fritsch, J.H.; Jolliff, C.R. XC Protein Components of Human Perilymph. *Ann. Otol. Rhinol. Laryngol.* **1966**, *75*, 1070–1076. [CrossRef]
70. Hladk, R.; Brada, Z.; Kočent, A. Versuch Einer Biochemischen Biopsie Der Perilymphe Bei Operierten Kranken. *Acta Oto- Laryngol.* **1960**, *51*, 424–428. [CrossRef]
71. Jacob, M.; Causse, J.; Gaudy, D.; Duru, C.; Causse, J.B.; Puech, A. Antibacterial therapy in surgery of the inner and middle ear. A study of co-trimoxazole penetration into the perilymph (author's transl). *Nouv. Presse Med.* **1982**, *11*, 2205–2209.
72. Rüedi, L.; Sanz, M.C.; Fisch, U. Untersuchung Der Perilymphe Nach Stapedktomie in Otosklerosefàallen. *Acta Oto-Laryngol.* **1965**, *59*, 289–308. [CrossRef]
73. Altmann, F.; Kornfeld, M.; Shea, J.J. I Inner Ear Changes in Otosclerosis: Histopathological Studies. *Ann. Otol. Rhinol. Laryngol.* **1966**, *75*, 5–32. [CrossRef] [PubMed]
74. Chevance, L.-G.; Causse, J.R. 1-Antitrypsin Activity of Perilymph: Occurrence During Progression of Otospongiosis. *Arch. Otolaryngol. Head Neck Surg.* **1976**, *102*, 363–364. [CrossRef]
75. Shew, M.; Warnecke, A.; Lenarz, T.; Schmitt, H.; Gunewardena, S.; Staecker, H. Feasibility of microRNA profiling in human inner ear perilymph. *NeuroReport* **2018**, *29*, 894–901. [CrossRef] [PubMed]
76. Kinney, W.C.; Nalepa, N.; Hughes, G.B.; Kinney, S.E. Cochleosacculotomy for the treatment of meniere's disease in the elderly patient. *Laryngoscope* **1995**, *105*, 934–937. [CrossRef]
77. Fujita, T.; Shin, J.E.; Cunnane, M.; Fujita, K.; Henein, S.; Psaltis, D.; Stankovic, K.M. Surgical anatomy of the human round window region: Implication for cochlear endoscopy through the external auditory canal. *Otol. Neurotol.* **2016**, *37*, 1189–1194. [CrossRef] [PubMed]
78. Plontke, S.K.; Hartsock, J.J.; Gill, R.M.; Salt, A.N. Intracochlear Drug Injections through the Round Window Membrane: Measures to Improve Drug Retention. *Audiol. Neurotol.* **2016**, *21*, 72–79. [CrossRef]
79. Aksit, A.; Arteaga, D.N.; Arriaga, M.; Wang, X.; Watanabe, H.; Kasza, K.; Lalwani, A.K.; Kysar, J.W. In-vitro perforation of the round window membrane via direct 3-D printed microneedles. *Biomed. Microdevices* **2018**, *20*, 1–12. [CrossRef] [PubMed]
80. Chiang, H.; Yu, M.; Aksit, A.; Wang, W.; Stern-Shavit, S.; Kysar, J.W.; Lalwani, A.K. 3D-Printed Microneedles Create Precise Perforations in Human Round Window Membrane in Situ. *Otol. Neurotol.* **2020**, *41*, 277–284. [CrossRef]
81. Watanabe, H.; Cardoso, L.; Lalwani, A.K.; Kysar, J.W. A dual wedge microneedle for sampling of perilymph solution via round window membrane. *Biomed. Microdevices* **2016**, *18*, 1–8. [CrossRef] [PubMed]
82. Szeto, B.; Aksit, A.; Valentini, C.; Yu, M.; Werth, E.G.; Goeta, S.; Tang, C.; Brown, L.M.; Olson, E.S.; Kysar, J.W.; et al. Novel 3D-printed hollow microneedles facilitate safe, reliable, and informative sampling of perilymph from guinea pigs. *Hear. Res.* **2020**, *400*, 108141. [CrossRef]
83. Early, S.; Moon, I.S.; Bommakanti, K.; Hunter, I.; Stankovic, K.M. A novel microneedle device for controlled and reliable liquid biopsy of the human inner ear. *Hear. Res.* **2019**, *381*, 107761. [CrossRef] [PubMed]
84. Lippy, W.H.; Berenholz, L.P. Revision Stapedectomy. *Ear Nose Throat J.* **2009**, *88*, 1260. [CrossRef]
85. Gstoettner, W.; Helbig, S.; Settevendemie, C.; Baumann, U.; Wagenblast, J.; Arnoldner, C.; Gstoettner, W.; Helbig, S.; Settevendemie, C.; Baumann, U.; et al. A new electrode for residual hearing preservation in cochlear implantation: First clinical results. *Acta Oto-Laryngol.* **2009**, *129*, 372–379. [CrossRef]
86. Adunka, O.F.; Mlot, S.; Suberman, T.A.; Campbell, A.P.; Surowitz, J.; Buchman, C.A.; Fitzpatrick, D.C. Intracochlear Recordings of Electrophysiological Parameters Indicating Cochlear Damage. *Otol. Neurotol.* **2010**, *31*, 1233–1241. [CrossRef]

87. Salt, A.N.; Kellner, C.; Hale, S. Contamination of perilymph sampled from the basal cochlear turn with cerebrospinal fluid. *Hear. Res.* **2003**, *182*, 24–33. [CrossRef]
88. Bianchin, G.; Polizzi, V.; Formigoni, P.; Russo, C.; Tribi, L. Cerebrospinal Fluid Leak in Cochlear Implantation: Enlarged Cochlear versus Enlarged Vestibular Aqueduct (Common Cavity Excluded). *Int. J. Otolaryngol.* **2016**, *2016*, 6591684. [CrossRef]
89. Hongjian, L.; Guangke, W.; Song, M.; Xiaoli, D.; Daoxing, Z. The prediction of CSF gusher in cochlear implants with inner ear abnormality. *Acta Oto- Laryngol.* **2012**, *132*, 1271–1274. [CrossRef]
90. Yi, H.J.; Guo, W.; Wu, N.; Li, J.N.; Liu, H.Z.; Ren, L.L.; Liu, P.N.; Yang, S.M. The temporal bone microdissection of miniature pigs as a useful large animal model for otologic research. *Acta Oto-Laryngol.* **2013**, *134*, 26–33. [CrossRef]

MDPI AG
Grosspeteranlage 5
4052 Basel
Switzerland
Tel.: +41 61 683 77 34

Journal of Clinical Medicine Editorial Office
E-mail: jcm@mdpi.com
www.mdpi.com/journal/jcm

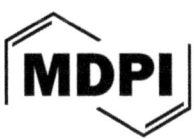

Disclaimer/Publisher's Note: The statements, opinions and data contained in all publications are solely those of the individual author(s) and contributor(s) and not of MDPI and/or the editor(s). MDPI and/or the editor(s) disclaim responsibility for any injury to people or property resulting from any ideas, methods, instructions or products referred to in the content.

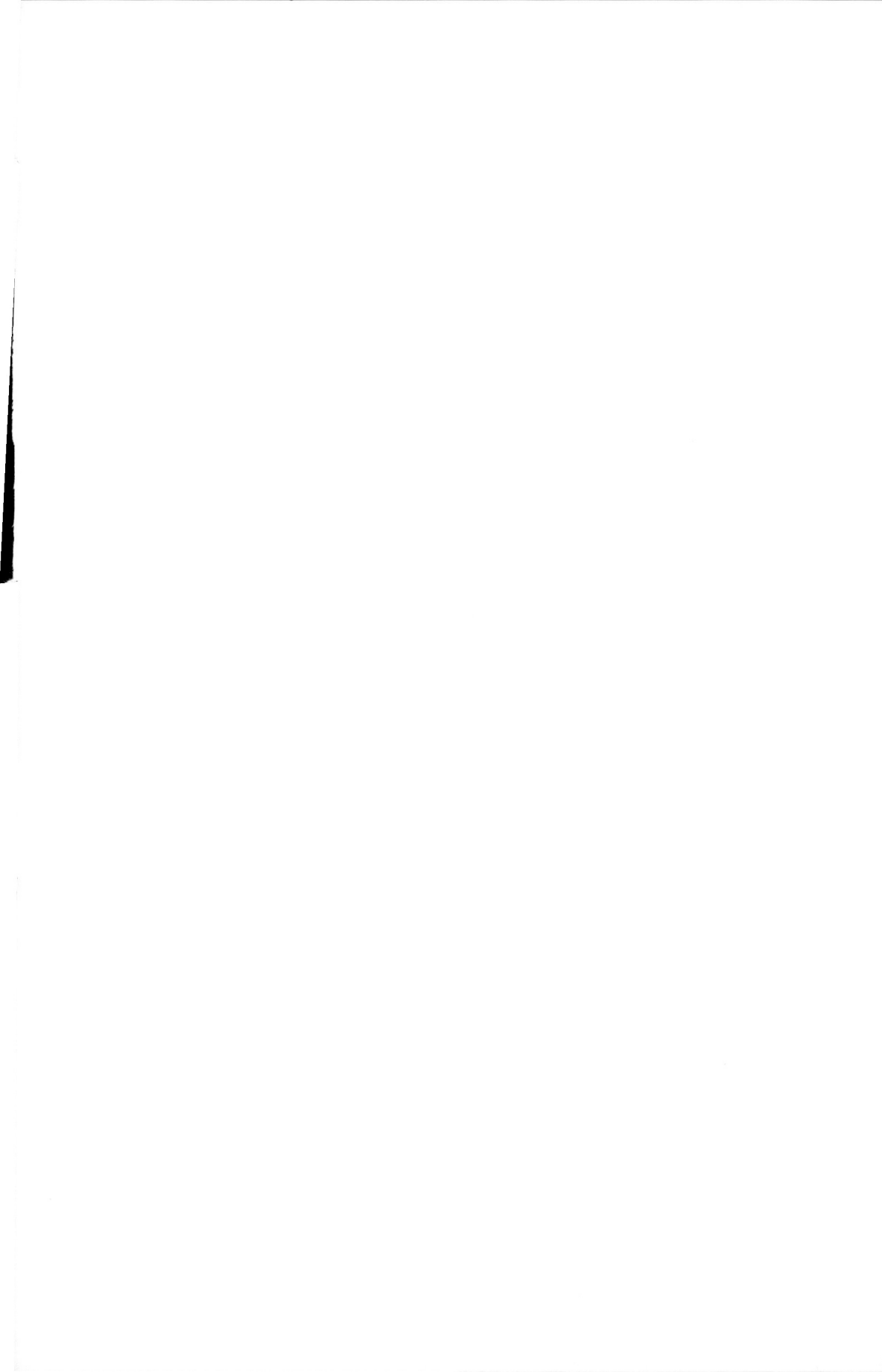

www.ingramcontent.com/pod-product-compliance
Lightning Source LLC
LaVergne TN
LVHW070615100526
838202LV00012B/652